Strabismus Management

Strabismus Management

William V. Good, M.D.

Ben and Louise Tate Professor and Chairman of Ophthalmology,
University of Cincinnati College of Medicine; Director, Abrahamson
Pediatric Eye Institute, Cincinnati Children's Hospital, Cincinnati

Creig S. Hoyt, M.D.

Professor of Ophthalmology and Pediatrics, University of California,
San Francisco, School of Medicine, San Francisco

with 6 contributing authors

Foreword by
Frank A. Billson, A.O., M.B.B.S. (Melb), D.O., F.R.A.C.O., F.R.C.S.
(Ed), F.R.C.S. (Eng), F.R.A.C.S., F.A.C.S.
Professor of Clinical Ophthalmology, University of Sydney;
Professor of Ophthalmology and Eye Health,
Sydney Eye Hospital, Australia

BUTTERWORTH-HEINEMANN
Boston   Oxford   Melbourne   Singapore
Toronto   Munich   New Dehli   Tokyo

Library of Congress Cataloging-in-Publication Data
Good, William V.
    Strabismus management / William V. Good, Creig S. Hoyt ; foreword
by Frank A. Billson.
      p. cm.
    Includes bibliographical references and index.
    ISBN 0-7506-9075-5 (alk. paper)
    1. Strabismus. I. Hoyt, Creig Simmons, 1942–   . II. Title.
    [DNLM: 1. Strabismus—therapy. 2. Strabismus—physiopathology.
WW 415 G646s 1995]
RE771.G66 1995
617.7'62—dc20
DNLM/DLC
for Library of Congress   95-40719
                                   CIP

British Library Cataloguing-in-Publication Data
A catalogue record for this book is available from the British Library.

The publisher offers discounts on bulk orders of this book.
For information, please write:

Manager of Special Sales
Butterworth–Heinemann
313 Washington Street
Newton, MA 02158–1626
10 9 8 7 6 5 4 3 2 1

Printed in the United States of America

To Laurie, Ben, and Sam

Contents

Contributing Authors

Michael C. Brodsky, M.D.
Associate Professor of Ophthalmology and Pediatrics, University of Arkansas for Medical Sciences; Chief of Pediatric Ophthalmology, Department of Ophthalmology, Arkansas Children's Hospital, Little Rock

J. Raymond Buncic, M.D., F.R.C.S.(C)
Associate Professor of Ophthalmology, University of Toronto; Chief, Department of Ophthalmology, Hospital for Sick Children, Toronto

Luis C. F. deSa, M.D.
Attending Physician, Department of Ophthalmology, Hospital das Clinicas, University of São Paulo, Brazil

William V. Good, M.D.
Ben and Louise Tate Professor and Chairman of Ophthalmology, University of Cincinnati College of Medicine; Director, Abrahamson Pediatric Eye Institute, Cincinnati Children's Hospital, Cincinnati

Richard Gregson, M.A., D.Phil., B.M., B.Ch., F.R.C.Ophth
Consultant and Honored Lecturer in Ophthalmology, Queen's Medical Centre and University Hospital, Nottingham, England

Creig S. Hoyt, M.D.
Professor of Ophthalmology and Pediatrics, University of California, San Francisco, School of Medicine, San Francisco

David S. I. Taylor, F.R.C.S., F.R.C.P., F.R.C.Ophth
Senior Lecturer in Vision Science, Institute of Child Health; Consultant
    Ophthalmologist, Department of Ophthalmology,
    Great Ormond Street Hospital, London

Harry E. Willshaw, B.Sc., M.B.ChB., F.R.C.S., F.R.C.Ophth
Honorary Lecturer of Medicine, University of Birmingham;
    Consultant Pediatric Ophthalmologist, Department of Pediatric
    Ophthalmology, Children's Hospital, Birmingham, England

Foreword

Individuals outstanding in their knowledge of strabismus, its practical management, and its basic science substrate who, in addition, have special training in pediatric neurology and neuropsychiatry are rare. To have them as colleagues in the same institution provides a special opportunity for collaboration. William V. Good and Creig S. Hoyt working together have made an important contribution to the understanding and practical management of strabismus.

The strength of this book is that it not only provides the intellectual framework for a clinical approach to strabismus, with individual chapters reflecting distinct clinical entities, but that it also addresses strabismus in the context of neurologic and systemic diseases. The section on strabismus and neurologic disease is one of the highlights of the book. This book has particular relevance for general ophthalmologists and residents in training but will also interest the specialist in strabismus.

The references include a number of original articles written by the authors during their professional association. Dr. Good and Dr. Hoyt, in critically analyzing their clinical and research experiences, have made a significant contribution to pediatric ophthalmology and the tradition of teaching at the University of Cincinnati and the University of California, San Francisco.

Frank A. Billson

Preface

Strabismus Management has been written to provide the reader with easily accessible information on various clinical strabismus problems. In writing the book, we chose to divide strabismus conditions into chapters. Some of this division of information is arbitrary, but we had the goal of providing the reader a format that lends itself to quick and easy-to-find information.

Strabismus Management does not have separate sections on strabismus diagnosis. We have included diagnostic issues in each chapter so that the reader is not obligated to flip through the book to find information about diagnostic problems.

If management issues appear idiosyncratic in places, it is because strabismus management is highly individualized. The interested reader will note that we have avoided much detail concerning quantification of eye muscle surgery for the management of strabismus. The manner in which each individual surgeon performs his or her dissection and muscle placement is quite variable. Each doctor must determine his or her own surgical outcome and make alterations in surgical management accordingly.

Writing this book was a great pleasure. We surely gained as much in its preparation as the reader will gain in studying it. The book is intended for an audience of general ophthalmologists and residents. We would be especially pleased if residents found it useful, since so much of our efforts in Cincinnati and San Francisco are devoted to educating the future generation of ophthalmologists.

William V. Good, M.D.
Creig S. Hoyt, M.D.

Strabismus Management

I

Introduction and Background

1

Epidemiology of Strabismus

PREVALENCE

The prevalence of strabismus has been studied in various populations. Frandsen (1960) studied children in Copenhagen and found that strabismus most often develops within the first 6–7 years of life. Among Copenhagen schoolchildren, 3.1% had amblyopia related to strabismus. Horizontal strabismus was far more common than vertical strabismus. Approximately 7% of children aged 6–7 years had strabismus. Strabismus affected approximately 1% of infants (<12 months).

The prevalence of strabismus and amblyopia was studied in a group of 21,446 men, who were examined at a military induction center in Pennsylvania (Glover and Brewer, 1944). The incidence of amblyopia was 2.39%, but only 0.75% of these men had strabismus. In this study amblyopia was defined as 20/70 or less with correction. "Convergent squint" with amblyopia occurred in 0.6% of the subjects and without amblyopia in 0.76%. Divergent strabismus was less common and occurred in approximately 0.25% of the subjects. All of the individuals examined in this study were young adults.

Helveston (1965) also studied young men in Minnesota and had the opportunity to compare his results with those of a previous study in a similar population, performed 20 years earlier by Downing (1945). In Downing's study the prevalence of amblyopia ex anopsia was 3.2%. This rate had decreased to 1% in Helveston's study.

In a study performed in Finland in 1971, the prevalence of manifest strabismus was 4.6% in a population of 2,100 seven-year-old students. Anisometropic amblyopia occurred in 0.5% of these children. Latent nystagmus occurred in 1.9% of them. Of all the types of strabismus, esotropia was most common, representing 55% of the population. Exotropia occurred in 45%, and there were no cases of hypertropia in this study (Rantanen and Tommila, 1971).

Wyatt and Boyd (1973) found a lower prevalence of esotropia in their study in Canada, compared with studies performed in Denmark (*see also,* Frandsen, 1960). In the Canadian study, the overall prevalence of strabismic amblyopia was similar to previous studies. The authors reviewed the rates of "convergent" versus "divergent" strabismus noted in previous studies. (These terms were used previously to indicate esotropia [convergent] and exotropia [divergent].) In most earlier studies, the ratio of esotropia to exotropia was at least 5:1, and as high as 20:1 (Thompson, 1924), but in the Canadian study this ratio was lower.

Graham (1974) studied the epidemiology of strabismus in Cardiff in the United Kingdom. He found that 7.1% of children had strabismus, similar to the results of Frandsen (1960).

From these studies it can be concluded that in virtually every population, the prevalence of esotropia is higher than that of exotropia in young children. Most cases of strabismus probably occur by the ages of 6 and 7 years. A surprisingly large number of children have strabismus, indicating that the problem is exceptionally important. Because so many children with strabismus also have amblyopia, a preventable form of vision loss can be identified with a simple strabismus examination.

The actual rate of development of strabismus has also been studied by many authors (Worth, 1906; Nordlow, 1953, 1964; Scobee, 1951). Fifteen percent of strabismus cases will occur in the first year of life (Frandsen, 1960). The rate increases in the second and third years of life, so that as many as 50% of strabismus cases will have occurred by 3 years of age.

RISK FACTORS FOR STRABISMUS

A variety of risk factors have been identified in strabismus in children (Table 1.1).

Maternal Cigarette Smoking

Several studies have indicated an association between heavy cigarette smoking early in pregnancy and esotropia (Hakim and Tielsch, 1992; Christianson, 1980). The risk appears to be greatest for low-birth-weight infants and high-birth-weight infants, but not for infants of normal birth weight. There appears to be no relationship between smoking during pregnancy and exotropia.

TABLE 1.1   Risk factors for strabismus

1. Cigarette smoking during pregnancy
2. Neurologic disorders
3. Use of other drugs during pregnancy (opiates, marijuana, barbiturates)
4. Lead poisoning
5. Twins
6. Heredity
7. Ethnicity
8. Refractive errors
9. Low birth weight (prematurity)
10. Anatomic factors (craniofacial anomalies)

Neurologic Disorders

Substance Abuse During Pregnancy

The studies on cigarette smoking point toward the fact that other drugs used during pregnancy also pose a risk for strabismus in offspring. It is possible that exposure to certain chemicals may lead to central nervous system damage. There certainly is an association of strabismus with neurologic disorders, including cerebral palsy and speech disorders (von Noorden, 1985; Blazso and Giesel, 1971; Dunn et al., 1977). Higher rates of strabismus have been shown to occur in children of drug-dependent women (Nelson, 1987), particularly women who use opiates, marijuana, and barbiturates (Butler and Goldstein, 1973).

At least one study has demonstrated an increased risk of strabismus in children who were exposed to cocaine in utero (Dominguez et al., 1991).

Lead Exposure

A relationship between maternal lead exposure and strabismus probably exists (Hakim et al., 1991). Lead exposure in utero is associated with neurologic impairment (Bellinger et al., 1987; Dietrich et al., 1987). As noted previously, events that lead to neurologic impairment in offspring apparently may also be the cause of strabismus.

Heredity

Despite the widespread belief that strabismus frequently occurs among family members, the exact genetic pattern of inheritance remains elusive in most cases. Certainly, some cases may be inherited in a clearly mendelian fashion, particularly autosomal dominant. An autosomal dominant inheritance pattern has been noted for exotropia (Brodsky and Fritz, 1993), for example. One study (DeVries and Houtman, 1979) demonstrated a concordance rate (in identical twins) of approximately 50% for strabismus.

Refractive Errors

A relationship between hyperopia and esotropia has been studied by Aurell and Norrsell (1990). They demonstrated that in children with a family history of strabismus, the presence of high amounts of hyperopia (4.00 D or more) correlated with a significant risk for developing strabismus. The *persistence* of high amounts of hyperopia through the first several years of life was a risk factor. The authors speculated that a lack of emmetropization may have been present in children who develop strabismus.

From a slightly different perspective, Fantl and Perlstein (1961) examined the incidence of refractive characteristics in children with cerebral palsy. Children with cerebral palsy had a higher rate of hyperopia than normal children (or children with physical handicaps other than cerebral palsy). The rate of emmetropization in this group of children was also slow, with many children remaining hyperopic until their teenage years.

High amounts of refractive error can also cause strabismus. We have seen high myopia cause exotropia as well as esotropia. Children with large refractive errors may obtain ocular alignment with spectacles, regardless of the type of refractive problem.

Low Birth Weight

The relationship of low birth weight (or prematurity) to strabismus is a complicated one. Studies have shown that the risk of strabismus is greater in children of low birth weight (Kushner, 1982). However, when neurologic risk factors are excluded (e.g., intraventricular hemorrhage), the risk of strabismus is lower. Nevertheless, the risk is probably greater than it is in full-term babies.

Anatomic Factors

Craniofacial anomalies are notorious for causing strabismus. The usual abnormality is exotropia, presumably related to one of several factors. The angle of the orbits as they are directed into the skull is wider than in children with normal craniofacial arrangements, and this can lead to strabismus. There may be ocular defects as well, leading to asymmetric visual input. An eye that sees poorly is at greater risk for strabismus. Kushner (1985) has proposed that the orientation of extraocular muscles to the globe is altered in children with craniofacial defects. The medial rectus, for example, sometimes inserts from a more superonasal origin. This can cause apparent inferior oblique overaction, because adduction of the eye also causes the eye to elevate.

Ocular Disease

Unilateral or asymmetric eye disease can result in strabismus. In children the strabismus may be esotropic or exotropic (Sidikaro and von Noorden, 1982). However, adults are more likely to show exotropia due to monocular or asymmetric vision loss.

REFERENCES

Aurell E, Norrsell K. A longitudinal study of children with a family history of strabismus: factors determining the incidence of strabismus. Br J Ophthalmol 1990;74:589–594.

Bellinger D, Leviton A, Waternaux C et al. Longitudinal analysis of prenatal and postnatal lead exposure and early cognitive development. N Engl J Med 1987;316:1037–1043.

Blazso S, Giesel V. Correlation between strabismus and central nervous system injuries. J Pediatr Ophthalmol 1971;8:18–22.

Brodsky MC, Fritz KJ. Hereditary congenital exotropia: A report of three cases. Binoc Vis Eye Muscle Surg 1993;8:133–137.

Butler NR, Goldstein H. Smoking in pregnancy and subsequent child development. Br Med J 1973;4:573–575.

Christianson RE. The relationship between maternal smoking and the incidence of congenital anomalies. Am J Epidemiol 1980;112:684–695.

De Vries B, Houtman WA. Squint in monozygotic twins. Doc Ophthalmol 1979;46:305–308.

Dietrich KN, Krafft KM, Bronschein RL et al. Low-level fetal lead exposure effect on neurobehavioral effect in early infancy. Pediatrics 1987;80:721–730.

Dominguez R, Aguirre Vila-Coro A, Slopis JM, Bohan TP. Brain and ocular abnormalities in infants with in utero exposure to cocaine and other street drugs. Am J Dis Child 1991;145:688–695.

Downing AH. Ocular defects in sixty thousand selectees. Arch Ophthalmol 1945;33:137–141.

Dunn HG, McBurney AK, Ingram S, Hunter CM. Maternal cigarette smoking during pregnancy and the child's subsequent development. II: Neurologic and intellectual maturation to the age of 6 1/2 years. Can J Public Health 1977;68:43–50.

Fantl EW, Perlstein MA. Periocular refractive characteristics in cerebral palsy. Am J Dis Child 1961;102:36–41.

Frandsen AD. Occurrence of squint. Acta Ophthalmol 1960(Suppl 62):1–122.

Glover LP, Brewer WR. Ophthalmologic review of more than 20,000 men at Altoona induction center. Am J Ophthalmol 1944;27:346–348.

Graham PA. Epidemiology of strabismus. Br J Ophthalmol 1974;58:224–231.

Hakim RB, Stewart WF, Canner JK, Tielsch JM. Occupational lead exposure and strabismus in offspring: A case control study. Am J Epidemiol 1991;133:351–356.

Hakim RB, Tielsch JM. Maternal cigarette smoking during pregnancy. A risk factor for childhood strabismus. Arch Ophthalmol 1992;110:1459–1462.

Helveston E. The incidence of amblyopia ex anopsia in young adult males in Minnesota in 1962–63. Am J Ophthalmol 1965;60:75–77.

Kushner BJ. Strabismus and amblyopia associated with repressed retinopathy of prematurity. Arch Ophthalmol 1982;100:256–261.

Kushner BJ. The role of ocular torsion on the etiology of A and V patterns. J Pediatr Ophthalmol Strabismus 1985;22:171–179.

Nelson LB, Ehrlich S, Calhoun JH et al. Occurrence of strabismus in infants born to drug-dependent women. Am J Dis Child 1987;141:175–178.

Nordlow W. Age distribution of onset of esotropia. Br J Ophthalmol 1953;37:593–600.

Nordlow W. Squint—The frequency of onset at different ages and the incidence of some associated defects in a Swedish population. Acta Ophthalmol (Copenhagen) 1964;42:1015–1037.

Rantanen A, Tommila V. Prevalence of strabismus in Finland. Acta Ophthalmol 1971;49:506–509.

Scobee RG. Esotropia: incidence, etiology and results of therapy. Am J Ophthalmol 1951;34:817–833.

Sidikaro Y, von Noorden GK. Observations in sensory heterotropia. J Pediatr Ophthalmol Strabismus 1982;19:12–19.

Thompson E. Some considerations regarding aetiology, the incidence and the course of concomitant convergent strabismus, which have a bearing on its treatment. Trans Ophthalmol Soc UK 1924;44:23.

von Noorden GK. Burian–von Noorden's Binocular Vision and Ocular Motility: Theory and Management of Strabismus (3rd ed). St. Louis: Mosby–Year Book, 1985.

Worth C. Squint: Its Causes, Pathology and Treatment. Philadelphia: Blakiston, 1906.

Wyatt HT, Boyd TA. Strabismus and strabismic amblyopia in Northern Canada. Can J Ophthalmol 1973;8:244–251.

2

Refractive Errors in Children

EPIDEMIOLOGY

The management of refractive errors is of the utmost importance in children with strabismus. In subsequent chapters on accommodative esotropia and intermittent exotropia, the reader will note that spectacle correction is often curative. The management of refractive errors in other types of strabismus is equally important. The principle that both eyes should be in the best possible focus should be adhered to. For that reason, many children with strabismus, no matter what type, will end up wearing spectacles.

What refractive error should be corrected? To answer this question, it is helpful to have an understanding of the refractive status of children throughout different stages.

Premature Infants

The exact relationship of myopia to prematurity continues to be debated (Howland, 1993). Quinn and associates (1992) studied the relationship of myopia to birth weight of less than 1,251 g. They concluded that a lower birth weight and increasing severity of retinopathy of prematurity correlated with myopia. Posterior pole complications of retinopathy of prematurity also correlated with higher rates of myopia in the study group and in another study (Majima, 1977). Page and colleagues (1993) reported a direct link between low birth weight and myopia, with the prevalence of myopia more directly associated with actual birth weight. In this study, myopia could develop even up to the age of 2 years. On the other hand, Scharf and co-authors (1975) suggested that myopia could regress once it had developed in premature babies. In our experience, the majority of children with myopia, and also with a history of retinopathy of prematurity, remain myopic throughout their life. The etiology of myopia in premature babies has also been debated and may be multifactorial. The cornea is often steeper in babies born prematurely (Fledelius, 1977), perhaps due to a failure of the cornea to flatten in the immediate newborn period (Fielder et al., 1986). The axial length may increase as a result of prematurity, which could also contribute to myopia (Majima, 1977; Hibino et al., 1978). Finally, a forward shift of the lens-iris diaphragm, or thickening of the lens itself, could cause myopia (Gordon and Donzis, 1986).

Refractive Errors in the First Year of Life

Most full-term babies show hyperopic refractive errors (Atkinson et al., 1984). The amount of hyperopia is somewhat variable and also dynamic, but probably averages 2.00 D (Banks, 1980). Perhaps 5% of babies will show myopia (Atkinson et al., 1984). The incidence of anisometropia and high hyperopia is less than 1% and 5%, respectively (Atkinson et al., 1984).

Astigmatism apparently is also very common in the first year of life (Dobson et al., 1984). Most white children show against-the-rule astigmatism, with amounts of astigmatic error varying from zero to as much as 2.50 D. Interestingly, the orientation of the astigmatic error may depend on ethnicity. Chinese children, for example, often show with-the-rule astigmatism (Thorn et al., 1987).

Rapid changes in refractive status of children under the age of 1 year are known to occur. Jampolsky (personal communication) recommends delaying surgery for essential infantile esotropia until the baby approaches 1 year of age, because the refractive status may be unstable until then. Because preoperative or postoperative optical correction may be important in maintaining ocular alignment, it is desirable to have a stable refractive error before undertaking surgery. In addition, the globe size and muscle relationship changes but stabilizes toward the end of the first year of life.

Refractive Errors in Childhood

The average refractive error in children shows increasing amounts of hyperopia in the first 5–7 years of life. In our experience, the average 6-year-old will show approximately 2.00 D of hyperopia. However, at least one study has demonstrated an average amount of hyperopia of 3.50 D at age 5 years (Slataper, 1950).

Meanwhile, astigmatic errors diminish with time (Atkinson et al., 1980; Gwiazde et al., 1984; Howland and Sayles, 1984). A 5- or 6-year-old with high amounts of astigmatism, unfortunately, is likely to retain this, and therefore might require corrective management.

After 7 years of age, refractive errors gravitate toward a distribution that is comparable to that seen in adults (Brown, 1938). Myopia becomes more prevalent, and the percentage of children and young adults with myopic refractive errors approaches 33% worldwide (Wallman, 1994).

ETIOLOGY

The four components of ocular refraction are corneal curvature, anterior chamber depth, lens thickness, and axial length. In most cases, though, the origin of an individual refractive error is unknown. There are tantalizing bits of epidemiologic and genetic data that would suggest that certain factors may play a role in causing refractive errors in some children. The special situation of myopia and prematurity is discussed above.

The role of heredity should not be underestimated. Twin studies show a genetic influence on the development of myopia (Sorsby and Fraser, 1964; Hu, 1981). Twins reared apart are likely to show comparable refractive errors (Knobloch et al., 1985). Myopia can be inherited as either a dominant or recessive trait (Avetisov, 1990). Dominant myopia usually develops later in childhood, but recessive myopia can be present very early, even at birth (Avetisov, 1990). Similarly, hyperopia can also be inherited as a dominant or recessive trait.

The environment can also have an effect on the refractive status of children. Near vision effort may induce myopia in some cases (Curtain, 1985; Dunphy et al., 1968; Wong et al., 1993). A relationship between intelligence quotient and myopia has been noted (Ashton, 1985; Rosner and Belkin, 1987). This relationship is not graded because there appears to be no linear relationship between intelligence and the amount of myopia (Teasdale et al., 1988). Rather, some myopization process may be triggered by near work, but once myopization is triggered, it occurs inexorably without dependence on further near work.

The argument can be made that, in general, children who spend a lot of time doing near work do so because they are more intelligent. The reverse may also be true, in that children who are myopic may spend more time reading simply for adaptive reasons, since they are unable to see things in the distance very well.

In epidemiologic studies, it has been shown that peoples of cultures in which reading and near work are not a factor have less myopia

(Curtain, 1985). When members of these populations move to industrialized areas (and therefore take up reading), the incidence of myopia becomes comparable to that of the surrounding population (Morgan and Munro, 1973; Morgan et al., 1975; Johnson et al., 1979).

The mechanism for environmentally induced myopization is unknown. Accommodation could raise intraocular pressure, which, in turn, could lead to axial elongation and myopia (Young, 1977). Alternatively, blurring of visual images on the nonfoveal retina could induce localized eye growth (Wallman et al., 1987).

Myopia can be associated with certain systemic disorders. Stickler syndrome may be the best known association, but others include Down's syndrome, hereditary retinal disorders (Avetisov, 1990), and Marfan, Noonan, and Rubinstein-Taybi syndromes (Jones and Smith, 1988).

A relationship between progressive myopia and glaucoma occurs because the sclera is relatively less rigid in the first 3–5 years of life. Increased intraocular pressure allows expansion of the sclera. Increases in axial length then lead to axial myopia. Progressive myopia in African-American adolescents may signify juvenile glaucoma (Lotufo et al., 1989).

Visual form deprivation early in life can produce myopia. Eyelid hemangiomas (Robb, 1977), unilateral eyelid closure (Hoyt et al., 1981), and congenital cataracts (Rasooly and BenEzra, 1988) can all cause axial elongation and unilateral myopia.

Refractive Errors in Children with Strabismus

A relationship between esotropia and hyperopia was noted in 1864 by Donders and confirmed by many others (Lepard, 1975; Duke-Elder and Wybar, 1983; Aurell and Norrsell, 1990; Otsuka and Sato, 1984). Nevertheless, an exact threshold at which esotropia is likely to occur cannot be established, based on refraction alone. Von Noorden and Avilla (1990) showed that the risk for esotropia is less in the presence of a low accommodation convergence to accommodation (AC:A) ratio; therefore, excessive accommodative convergence, high AC:A ratio, and inadequate (motor) fusion amplitudes are all risk factors for esotropia.

Abrahamsson and colleagues (1992) studied refractive errors in esotropic and exotropic children. Hyperopia was more common in esotropia at the time of diagnosis. A few exotropic children were myopic, but most exotropic children were hyperopic, just like esotropic children. The strabismic eye had a greater chance of becoming anisometropic in esotropia, but emmetropization could occur in the fixing eye.

MANAGEMENT

The most important question regarding these various refractive errors involves the decision whether to correct them. In general, low amounts of myopia in the first few years of life are well tolerated and do not cause abnormal visual development. As long as refractive errors are bilaterally equal, the use of spectacles is not necessary.

Rather large astigmatic errors in the first year of life can also be tolerated. Howland (1993) has commented on the potential value of these large astigmatic errors. In his view, they may allow an increased depth of focus and therefore be adaptive. On the other hand, large amounts of hyperopia are probably best dealt with by early spectacle correction. The risk of acquiring accommodative esotropia when hyperopia exceeds 4.00 D is substantial (von Noorden and Avilla, 1990). Hyperopia in excess of 5.00 D is potentially amblyogenic and may lead to bilateral amblyopia (Werner and Scott, 1985; Schoenleber and Crouch, 1987). We would choose to treat high hyperopia with a spectacle correction that deliberately undercorrects the refractive error by 1.00 or 2.00 D. For example, a +8.00-D hyperope might be given a prescription for glasses of +6.00 D. We have found that full refractive correction is sometimes poorly tolerated, because these children are used to accommodating. Exceptions to this practice would include the child with esotropia associated with hyperopia. In this situation we would be inclined to prescribe the full refractive error.

The existence of high amounts of hyperopia (>5.00 D) can lead to bilateral amblyopia (Schoenleber and Crouch, 1987; Werner and Scott, 1985), irrespective of the presence of esotropia. Based on the above studies (von Noorden and Avilla, 1990), it would seem prudent to correct children who have more than 4.00 D of hyperopia and to carefully evaluate, via AC:A ratio and motor fusion examinations, children in the 2.00–4.00 D range. Children with abnormalities may require correction.

Anisometropia is uncommon in the first year of life (Atkinson et al., 1980). Its incidence apparently increases somewhat with increasing age. Anisometropia can lead to anisometropic amblyopia, particularly when the difference between the two eyes exceeds 1.25 D. The eye that is closest to emmetropia usually has better vision. Management of anisometropia should consist of full refractive correction and also attempts to ensure that no anisometropic amblyopia has developed or that amblyopia is being effectively treated.

No treatment is available to prevent myopia or progression of myopia. One nonrandomized study showed a benefit from antiaccommodative intervention (i.e., bifocals) (Oakley and Young, 1975), but carefully controlled studies in this area are unavailable.

REFERENCES

Abrahamsson M, Fabian G, Sjostrand J. Refraction change in children developing convergent or divergent strabismus. Br J Ophthalmol 1992;76:723–727.

Ashton GC. Near work, school achievement and myopia. J Biosoc Sci 1985;17:223–233.

Atkinson J, Braddick O, Durden K et al. Screening for refractive errors in 6–9 month old infants by photorefraction. Br J Ophthalmol 1984;68:105–112.

Atkinson J, Braddick OJ, French J. Infant astigmatism: Its disappearance with age. Vision Res 1980;20:891–893.

Aurell E, Norrsell K. A longitudinal study of children with a family history of strabismus: Factors determining the incidence of strabismus. Br J Ophthalmol 1990;74:589–594.

Avetisov ES, Kashshenko TP, Smol'ianinova IL et al. The clinical characteristics and treatment tactics of vertical strabismus. Oftalmologicheskii Zhurnal 1990:193–197.

Banks M. Infant refraction and accommodation. Int Ophthalmol Clin 1980;20:205–232.

Brown EVL. Net average yearly changes in refraction of atropinized eyes from birth to beyond middle life. Arch Ophthalmol 1938;19:719–734.

Curtain BJ. The myopias: Basic science and clinical management. Philadelphia: Harper & Row, 1985.

Dobson V, Fulton AB, Sebris SL. Cycloplegic refractions of infants and young children: The axis of astigmatism. Invest Ophthalmol Vis Sci 1984;25:83–87.

Duke-Elder S, Wybar K. Ocular Motility and Strabismus. In S Duke-Elder (ed), System of Ophthalmology. London: Henry Kimpton, 1983;VI:577–641.

Dunphy EB, Stoll MR, King SH. Myopia among American male graduate students. Am J Ophthalmol 1968;65:518–521.

Fielder AR, Levene MI, Russell-Eggett IM, Weale RA. Temperature—A factor in ocular development? Dev Med Child Neurol 1986;28:279–284.

Fledelius H. Myopia of Prematurity: Oculometric Considerations Based Upon a Danish Material. In White D, Brown RE (eds), Ultrasound in Medicine: Clinical Aspects (Vol 3A). New York: Plenum, 1977:959–963.

Gordon RA, Donzis PB. Myopia associated with retinopathy of prematurity. Ophthalmology 1986;93:1593–1598.

Gwiazda J, Scheiman M, Mohindra I, Held R. Astigmatism in children: Changes in axis and amount from birth to six years. Invest Ophthalmol Vis Sci 1984;25:88–92.

Hibino Y, Takahashi M, Majima A. Studies on ocular functions of cicatricial retinopathy of prematurity. Measurements of refractive elements. Jpn J Ophthalmol 1978;32:655–662.

Howland HC, Sayles N. Photorefractive measurements of astigmatism in infants and young children. Invest Ophthalmol Vis Sci 1984;25:93–102.

Howland HC. Early Refractive Development. In K Simon (ed), Early Visual Development: Normal and Abnormal. New York: Oxford University Press, 1993;5–26.

Hoyt CS, Stone RD, Fromer C, Billson FA. Monocular axial myopia associated with neonatal eyelid closure in human infants. Am J Ophthalmol 1981;91:197–200.

Hu D. Twin study on myopia. Chinese Med J 1981;94:51–55.

Johnson GJ, Matthews A, Perkins ES. Survey of ophthalmic conditions in a Labrador community. I. Refractive errors. Br J Ophthalmol 1979; 63:440–448.

Jones KL, Smith S. Recognizable patterns of human malformation. Philadelphia: Saunders, 1988;718–719.

Knobloch WH, Leavenworth NM, Bouchard TJ, Eckert ED. Eye findings in twins reared apart. Ophthalmol Paediatr Genet 1985;5:59–66.

Lepard CW. Comparative changes in the error of refraction between fixing and amblyopic eyes during growth and development. Am J Ophthalmol 1975;80:485–490.

Lotufo D, Ritch R, Szmyd L, Burris JE. Juvenile glaucoma, race, and refraction. JAMA 1989;261:249–252.

Majima A. Studies on retinopathy of prematurity. II. Fundus appearance and ocular functions in cicatricial phase of very low birth weight infants. Jpn J Ophthalmol 1977;21:421–435.

Morgan RW, Munro M. Refractive problems in northern natives. Can J Ophthalmol 1973;8:226–228.

Morgan RW, Speakman JS, Grimshaw SE. Inuit myopia as environmentally induced epidemic? Can Med Assoc J 1975;112:575–577.

Oakley KH, Young FA. Bifocal control of myopia. Am J Optometr Physiol Optics 1975;52:758–764.

Otsuka J, Sato Y. Supplementary study of comparison of refractive components of orthophoric hyperopic eyes with those of accommodative esotropic eyes. Acta Soc Ophthalmol Jpn 1984;88:58–64.

Page JM, Schneeweiss S, Whyte HE, Harvey P. Ocular sequelae in premature infants. Pediatrics 1993;92:787–790.

Quinn GE, Dobson V, Repka MX, et al. Development of myopia in infants with birth weights less than 1251 grams. Ophthalmology 1992;99:329–340.

Rasooly R, BenEzra D. Congenital and traumatic cataract: The effect on ocular axial length. Arch Ophthalmol 1988;106:1066–1068.

Robb RM. Refractive errors associated with hemangiomas of the eyelids and orbits in infancy. Am J Ophthalmol 1977;83:52–58.

Rosner M, Belkin M. Intelligence, education and myopia in males. Arch Ophthalmol 1987;105:1508–1511.

Scharf J, Zonis S, Zeltzer M. Refraction in Israeli premature babies. J Pediatr Ophthalmol 1975;12:193–196.

Schoenleber DB, Crouch ER. Bilateral hypermetropic amblyopia. J Ped Ophthalmol Strabismus 1987;24:75–77.

Slataper FJ. Age norms of refraction and vision. Arch Ophthalmol 1950;43:466–481.

Sorsby A, Fraser GR. Statistical note on the components of ocular refraction in twins. J Med Genet 1964;1:47–49.

Teasdale TW, Fuchs J, Goldschmidt E. Degree of myopia in relation to intelligence and educational level. Lancet 1988;2:1351–1354.

Thorn F, Held R, Fang LL. Orthogonal astigmatic axes in Chinese and Caucasian infants. Invest Ophthalmol Vis Sci 1987;28:191–194.

von Noorden GK, Avilla CW. Accommodative convergence in hypermetropia. Am J Ophthalmol 1990;110:287–292.

Wallman J. Nature and nurture of myopia. Nature 1994;371:201–202.

Wallman J, Gottlieb MB, Rajaram V, Fugate-Wentzek LA. Local retinal regions control local eye growth and myopia. Science 1987;237:73–77.

Werner DB, Scott WE. Amblyopia case reports. Bilateral hypermetropic ametropic amblyopia. J Ped Ophthalmol Strabismus 1985;22:203–205.

Wong L, Coggon l, Cruddas M, Hwang CH. Education, reading and familial tendency as role factors for myopia in Hong Kong fishermen. J Epidemiol Comm Health 1993;47:50–53.

Young FA. The nature and control of myopia. J Am Optom Assoc 1977;48:451–457.

3

Amblyopia Management

Strabismic amblyopia is a decrease in visual acuity in the nonfixing eye, which occurs as the result of the strabismic deviation itself. Any patient whose onset of strabismus is prior to 6 years of age is at risk for development of amblyopia. Nevertheless, there is great variability in the actual prevalence rate of amblyopia in association with specific strabismic disorders. For example, amblyopia is uncommon in Duane's syndrome and occurs frequently in accommodative esotropia. If free alternation of fixation continues throughout the course of strabismus management the patient may avoid amblyopia. If a head-tilt, face-turn, or chin position allows the patient to fuse a nonconcomitant strabismus, amblyopia may also be avoided. Every child with strabismus needs to be carefully and periodically reevaluated for any evidence of monocular visual loss in an effort to detect amblyopia at the earliest possible time.

ETIOLOGY AND PATHOPHYSIOLOGY

The underlying cause of amblyopia in the patient with strabismus is presumably the establishment of a preferred fixing eye. The nonfixing eye becomes amblyopic. In general, fixation preference is more likely to occur in the smaller-angle esotropic patient than in the larger-angle esotropic patient, in whom cross fixation may persist as a long-standing adaptation, thus precluding the development of amblyopia (Hoyt et al., 1984; Good et al., 1993). Once fixation preference has been established, however, the nonfixing eye is at risk for development of amblyopia under the age of 6 years.

The simplistic view of amblyopia pathophysiology described above would suggest that amblyopia is caused by an ocular defect. In fact, there is hardly any evidence that a retinal or optic nerve abnormality causes amblyopia (Levi and Carkeet, 1993). Instead, research suggests that cortical defects of form and shape perception are at the heart of the amblyopia defect. Amblyopic eyes have reduced ability to see small objects, particularly with low contrast. These defects are most pronounced at low temporal frequencies (slow flicker) (Schor and Levi, 1980).

DIAGNOSIS

In every child with strabismus, an attempt should be made by the physician to measure visual acuity as early as possible to detect amblyopia. A number of direct and indirect methods are available for determining vision. Strabismic amblyopia is diagnosed when the vision in one eye is two lines or worse compared with the fellow eye. Visual acuity may be reduced to as low as 20/100 but is seldom worse. Visual acuity of 20/200 or less should raise the suspicion of anisometropic amblyopia or other ocular disease.

Amblyopia shows other interesting characteristics. Patients may be able to identify single optotypes, but not similarly-sized letters that are crowded together. Accommodation is also reduced in amblyopic eyes. Amblyopic patients can see equally well in the dark and light with their amblyopic eye, in contrast to healthy individuals or patients with retinal pathology, who lose several lines of vision in the dark (Amman, 1921; von Noorden and Burian, 1959).

Fixation Reflex

In a large percentage of patients with strabismus, the only possible way to evaluate and detect amblyopia is with the use of fixation reflexes (because the child is preverbal). The use of fixation reflexes in the detection and relative quantification of strabismic amblyopia was described by Zipf (1976). In his description of the use of fixation reflexes, the amblyopic eye was detected by evaluating the light reflex and its characteristics in each eye. In the patient with freely alternating strabismus with no amblyopia, each eye under monocular viewing conditions will view a fixation light centrally and steadily without any deviation. Under binocular viewing conditions the patient without amblyopia will continue to fixate on the fixation target with the eye that was being tested under monocular circumstances. In the patient with amblyopia, although the amblyopic eye may view the fixation light under monocular conditions centrally and steadily, under binocular conditions fixation is immediately reestablished with the preferred fixing eye and the amblyopic eye immediately deviates. Thus, under this testing condition the nonfixing eye is said to have central, steady, *unmaintained* fixation. In more dense amblyopia the fixation reflex may even be central and unsteady, so that under monocular viewing conditions the eye does not steadily maintain fixation, and indeed even shows nystagmus (Good et al., 1993b), or it may even be uncentral. In this situation, under monocular viewing conditions, eccentric fixation is detected. In all of these instances any result other than central, steadily maintained fixation is said to be evidence for amblyopia in that eye.

Cross-fixation at the midline indicates no amblyopia (Dickey et al., 1991). When a child cross-fixates to their side of the midline, amblyopia should be suspected. For example, in essential infantile esotropia, amblyopia should be suspected when a baby does not take up visual fixation with the right eye until after the object of regard has passed the midline toward the baby's left.

More recently, Wright and colleagues (1981) described a variation of the fixation light reflex test using a 10-D vertical prism test. Their investigation suggested that in the presence of small angles of strabismus fixation, preference was not always correlated with amblyopia and that some children were being patched when it was not necessary. Therefore, in the patient with a small-angle strabismus (or with no strabismus), the introduction of a 10-D vertical prism further delineates the test to avoid the problem of a patient with a fixation preference but no amblyopia. A normal response to the 10-D vertical prism test would be if the patient always preferred to fixate with the eye without the prism in front of it. If the patient fixates through the prism, this suggests that the other uncovered eye is amblyopic.

Visual Acuity Measurement

Visual acuity measurements are still the gold standard for the evaluation of the patient with amblyopia. Of all the visual acuity measurements, Snellen measurements are preferred. Many other forms of visual acuity measurements will underestimate amblyopia. This is true, in part, because of the crowding phenomenon, where the amblyopic eye performs better when it has a single, isolated target than when it has to read a whole line of letters arranged closely together (Müller, 1951; Flom, 1963; Stuart and Burian, 1962). Also, the psychophysiology of reading letters is not the same as the psychophysiology of detecting figures (e.g., "illiterate" E's or other illiterate symbols). It should also be recalled that the amblyopic eye functions best under mesopic lighting conditions, and therefore the visual acuity of the amblyopic patient may vary depending on the background luminance of the examining room. Visual acuity measurements in a brightly lighted room may be markedly different from those in an ordinary, darkened examining room. In some patients with strabismic amblyopia, the near visual acuity improves before distance visual acuity. For all the above reasons, strabismic patients should have their visual acuity measured at distance and closer up with a full line of Snellen acuity letters, whenever possible.

Forced choice preferential looking techniques and electrophysiologic techniques have been advocated as a way to quantitate amblyopia in the preverbal child. However, data from numerous investigators suggest that the acuity responses of amblyopic eyes to these tests are not always comparable to Snellen acuity measurements (Ellis et al., 1988; Mayer and Fulton, 1985; Birch and Stager, 1985). Both forced choice preferential looking techniques (including Teller cards) and visual-evoked potential techniques may overestimate the visual acuity of the amblyopic eye (i.e., underestimate amblyopia) (Mayer and Fulton, 1985; Birch and Stager, 1985). These tests may be useful in monitoring changes in visual acuity, but caution should be employed in translating directly from grating tests to equivalent Snellen acuity measurement.

DIFFERENTIAL DIAGNOSIS

Not all monocular vision loss in the patient with strabismus is secondary to amblyopia. Only after an extensive examination has been performed can one be certain that coexisting intraocular pathology is not the cause of vision loss. Careful refraction must be performed and any refractive error corrected before it is assumed that the patient's vision loss is secondary to amblyopia. Mild forms of congenital optic nerve pathology as well as small lens opacities can be overlooked and the patient said to be amblyopic, when instead a structural abnormality is responsible for the decrease in visual acuity.

Additional testing may be beneficial when trying to distinguish between amblyopia and other disorders. The amblyopic patient has normal color vision, in contrast to the patient with optic neuropathy. A subtle Marcus Gunn pupil defect has been described in some patients with strabismic amblyopia. In our experience, a clinically detectable Marcus Gunn pupil is rare in strabismic amblyopia.

MANAGEMENT

Critical Period for Amblyopia
From a clinical standpoint, strabismic amblyopia rarely develops after age 6–8 years (Worth, 1903; von Noorden, 1981). However, retrospective

studies concerning the natural history of amblyopia and its treatment have been derived mostly from animal studies (Boothe et al., 1985) as well as from retrospective studies of clinical evaluations of patients (von Noorden, 1981). These data suggest that children are vulnerable to developing strabismic amblyopia at least until the age 5 years (Banks et al., 1975; Hohmann and Creutzfeldt, 1975), with the likelihood of considerable variability between individuals. Sparrow and Flynn (1979) and Scott and Dickey (1988) demonstrated that amblyopia can often be successfully managed with occlusion between the ages of 6 and 9 years.

Because there are multiple psychophysical (visual) functions with different stages of development, it seems likely that amblyopia is not an all-or-none phenomenon; that is, certain aspects of amblyopia may be likely to develop (and therefore susceptible to treatment) at different stages in the first 5–6 years (Levi and Carkeet, 1993). Visual functions that develop early probably are least susceptible to later damage, whereas visual functions that develop later are most susceptible. Levi and Carkeet (1993) have termed this the "Detroit model," jokingly referring to the fact that the "last hired, first fired" principle of psychophysical visual development may apply to susceptibility to amblyopia.

Amblyopia Management Before or After Strabismus Surgery

The management of strabismic amblyopia is usually based on the principle that visual acuity should be equalized before a definitive attempt at realignment of the visual axes is attempted (Friendly, 1985; von Noorden, 1988; Parks and Wheeler, 1992). Not every surgeon would agree with this principle, and there is at least some data that support early surgical alignment, with amblyopia management continuing postoperatively (Lam et al, 1993). In our experience, patching may be more acceptable after surgical alignment in certain uncommon cases due to greater compliance on the part of the family.

Part-Time Patching

Occlusion of the fixing eye is the standard therapy for equalizing visual acuity in amblyopic patients. However, there is great variation in the way in which this patching may be accomplished. Some investigators suggest that total occlusion (patching all but a very short period of time every day for a given period of time) is the most appropriate way to rehabilitate the amblyopic patient. If total occlusion is undertaken, the physician must be aware that the occluded eye may develop amblyopia if treated too long. Close follow-up (e.g., every week in children under 1 year of age) is advised. Others suggest that even short-term occlusion therapy may be effective, even in the patient who has previously failed a total occlusion program (Watson et al., 1985).

Full-Time, Alternate-Day Occlusion

Jampolsky and associates (1994) recommend alternate-day patching (right eye, then left eye) for essential infantile esotropia. This form of patching may delay or prevent the development of pathologic optokinetic nystagmus (OKN) responses. In babies with essential infantile esotropia, an asymmetric OKN response occurs. Smooth pursuit from the temporal to the nasal side is normal, but abnormal with movement from the nasal to the temporal side. Full-time alternate-day occlusion could keep the "binocular slate clean" and help to prevent amblyopia and anomalous retinal correspondence, both of which require some degree of binocular interaction (Jampolsky, 1953, 1978). Full-time, alternate-day occlusion may help to normalize the OKN response, and this, in turn, could lead to better binocular interaction upon realignment of the eyes.

Vision Stimulators

Although attempts have been made to develop specific devices (e.g., CAM [Cambridge] stimulator) to stimulate the amblyopic eye and thus maximize the visual recovery (Banks et al., 1978; Nyman et al., 1983; Lennerstrand and Samuelsson, 1983), the evidence does not suggest that these devices markedly alter the therapeutic results that would have been achieved with occlusion therapy alone. Nevertheless, we usually recommend to the parents of children with strabismic amblyopia that small, detailed visual tasks be performed during some of the patching therapy.

Contact Lens Occlusion

In some patients occlusion therapy is simply not possible. Oftentimes, though, providing the parents with moral support and strong encouragement will result in more success with patching than is initially anticipated. In some circumstances, alternatives to standard patching therapy can be used. In the patient who develops dense amblyopia when patching therapy is not possible, we have, on occasion, used black occluder contact lenses. These lenses have their own distinct problems and carry the risk of corneal infection or damage. Nevertheless, in some patients these lenses offer a viable alternative to standard occlusion therapy.

Penalization

Penalization therapy, in which one uses cycloplegic drops in the fixing eye, thereby intentionally fogging it, may be appropriate in some patients with mild to moderate amblyopia (Repka and Ray, 1993; McKenney and Byers, 1975; Willshaw and Johnson, 1979). Penalization therapy may have a special role in the patient who has strabismus and preexisting nystagmus (in which occlusion of the fixing eye brings out latent nystagmus). In this case penalization therapy may be the preferable form of therapy. Management consists of administration of a drop of atropine into the fixing eye every day or every other day.

Neurotransmitter Therapy

Recent attempts to document whether changes in visual acuity can be achieved in the amblyopic eye using various neurotransmitters hold promise for the future. Preliminary investigations using treatment with levodopa suggest that the neural systems responsible for amblyopia may be partially responsive to these types of compounds (Leguire et al., 1992, 1993; Gottlob and Stangler-Zuschrott, 1990). Currently, there is no compelling information to suggest that any of these forms of therapy should replace occlusion therapy.

Patching therapy needs to be continued in the management of the patient with strabismic amblyopia until visual acuity is equalized. Once visual acuity is equalized the patient may be gradually or relatively quickly withdrawn from patching therapy. In a relatively high percentage of patients (perhaps 40%), slippage of vision in the amblyopic eye occurs once patching therapy is stopped (Dickey and Scott, 1987). Continued careful monitoring of the patient with strabismic amblyopia after patching therapy has been decreased or discontinued is important. If changes in visual acuity in the amblyopic eye occur, patching therapy should be reinstituted to bring the visual acuity back to its previously good level.

REFERENCES

Amman E. Einige beobachtunger be den funktionsprunfungen in der sprechstund: "Zentrales" sehen. – Schen der glaukomatosen – Schen der amblyopen. Klin Monatsbl Augenheilkd 1921;66:564.

Banks MS, Aslin RN, Letson RD. Sensitive period for the development of human binocular vision. Science 1975;190:675–676.

Banks RV, Campbell FW, Hess R, Watson PG. A new treatment for amblyopia. Br Orthopt J 1978;35:1.

Birch EE, Stager DR. Monocular acuity and stereopsis in infantile esotropia. Invest Ophthalmol Vis Sci 1985;26:1624–1630.

Boothe RG, Dobson V, Teller DY. Postnatal development of vision in human and non-human primates. Annu Rev Neurosci 1985;8:495–545.

Dickey CF, Metz HS, Stewart SA, Scott WE. The diagnosis of amblyopia in cross-fixation. J Pediatr Ophthalmol Strabismus 1991;28:171–175.

Dickey CF, Scott WE. Amblyopia—The prevalence in congenital accommodative esotropia. Diagnosis and results of treatment. Proceedings of the Sixth International Orthoptic Conference. Harrogate, England, 1987.

Ellis GS Jr, Hartmann EE, Love A et al. Teller acuity cards versus clinical judgment in the diagnosis of amblyopia with strabismus. Ophthalmology 1988;95:788–791.

Flom MC, Weymouth FW, Kahneman D. Visual resolutions and contour interaction. J Opt Soc Am 1963;53:1026–1032.

Friendly DS. Management of infantile esotropia. Int Ophthalmol Clin 1985;25:37–52.

Good WV, deSa LCF, Lyons CF, Hoyt CS. Monocular visual outcome in untreated, early-onset esotropia. Br J Ophthalmol 1993;77:492–495.

Good WV, Koch TS, Jan JE. Monocular nystagmus caused by unilateral anterior visual-pathway disease. Dev Med Child Neurol 1993;35:1106–1110.

Gottlob I, Stangler-Zuschrott E. Effect of levodopa on contrast sensitivity and scotomas in human amblyopia. Invest Ophthalmol Vis Sci 1990;31:776–780.

Hohmann A, Creutzfeldt OD. Squint and the development of binocularity in humans. Nature 1975;254:613–614.

Hoyt CS, Jastrzebski GB, Marg E. Amblyopia and congenital esotropia. Visually evoked potential measurements. Arch Ophthalmol 1984;102:58–61.

Jampolsky A. The physician and the cross-eyed child. A medical forum. Modern Medicine 1953;21:144–154.

Jampolsky A. Unequal Visual Inputs and Strabismus Management. In Strabismus Symposium. Transactions of New Orleans Academy of Ophthalmology. St. Louis: Mosby, 1978;358–592.

Jampolsky A, Norcia AM, Hamer RD. Preoperative alternate occlusion decreases motion processing abnormalities in infantile esotropia. J Pediatr Ophthalmol Strabismus 1994;31:6–17.

Lam GC, Repka MX, Guyton DL. Timing of amblyopia therapy relative to strabismus surgery. Ophthalmology 1993;100:1751–1756.

Leguire LE, Rogers GL, Bremer DL et al. Levodopa and childhood amblyopia. J Pediatr Ophthalmol Strabismus 1992;29:290–298.

Leguire LE, Walson PD, Rogers GL et al. Longitudinal study of levodopa/carbidopa for childhood amblyopia. J Pediatr Ophthalmol Strabismus 1993;30:354–360.

Lennerstrand G, Samuelsson B. Amblyopia in 4 year old children treated with grating stimulation and full-time occlusion; comparative study. Br J Ophthalmol 1983;67:181–190.

Levi DM, Carkeet A. Amblyopia: A Consequence of Abnormal Visual Development. In K Simons (ed), Early Visual Development: Normal and Abnormal. Oxford, England: Oxford University Press, 1993;391–408.

Mayer DL, Fulton AB. Preferential looking grating acuities of infants at risk of amblyopia. Trans Ophthalmol Soc UK 1985;104:903–911.

McKenney S, Byers M. Aspects and results of penalization treatment. Am Orthopt J 1975;25:85–89.

Müller P. Ueber das sehen der amblyopen. Ophthalmologica 1951;121:143–149.

Nyman KG, Sing G, Ryberg A, Fornander M. Controlled study comparing CAM treatment with occlusion therapy. Br J Ophthalmol 1983;67:178–181.

Parks MM, Wheeler MB. Concomitant Esodeviations. In W Tasman, EA Jaeger (eds), Duane's Clinical Ophthalmology (rev. ed, vol. 1). Philadelphia: Lippincott, 1992;9.

Repka MX, Ray JM. The efficacy of optical and pharmacological penalization. Ophthalmology 1993;100:769–775.

Schor CM, Levi DM. Direction selectivity for perceived motion in strabismic and anisometric amblyopia. Invest Ophthalmol Vis Sci 1980;19:1094–1104.

Scott WE, Dickey CF. Stability of visual acuity in amblyopic patients after visual maturity. Graefes Arch Clin Exp Ophthalmol 1988;226:154–157.

Sparrow JC, Flynn FT. Amblyopia: A long-term follow-up. J Pediatr Ophthalmol Strabismus 1979;14:333–336.

Stuart JA, Burian HM. A study of separation difficulty; its relationship to visual acuity in normal and amblyopic eyes. Am J Ophthalmol 1962;53:471–477.

von Noorden GK. Clinical aspects of stimulus deprivation in amblyopia. Am J Ophthalmol 1981;92:416–421.

von Noorden GK. Bowman lecture. Current concepts of infantile esotropia. Eye 1988;2:343–357.

von Noorden GK, Burian HM. Visual acuity in normal and amblyopic patients under reduced illumination. I. Behavior of visual acuity with and without neutral density filter. Arch Ophthalmol 1959;61:533.

Watson PG, Banks RV, Campbell FW, Hess R. Clinical assessment of new treatment for amblyopia. Trans Ophthalmol Soc UK 1978;98:201–208.

Watson PG, Sanac AS, Pickering MS. A comparison of various methods of treatment of amblyopia. A block study. Trans Ophthalmol Soc UK 1985;104:319–328.

Willshaw HE, Johnson F. Penalization in the treatment of amblyopia. Br Orthopt J 1979;36:57–62.

Worth CA. Squint: Its causes, pathology and treatment. Philadelphia: Blakiston, 1903.

Wright KW, Walonker F, Edelman P. 10-Diopter fixation test for amblyopia. Arch Ophthalmol 1981;99:1242–1246.

Zipf RF. Binocular fixation patterns. Arch Ophthalmol 1976;94:401–405.

II

Esodeviations

4

Infantile Esotropia

Harry E. Willshaw

Infantile esotropia is an ocular deviation that appears for the first time before the age of 6 months. The definition encompasses a number of types of strabismus, which need to be distinguished from one another in order to formulate an appropriate management plan (Table 4.1).

The most common entity in this category was referred to in the past as *congenital esotropia* but is rarely, if ever, truly congenital (Nixon et al., 1985) and is more appropriately designated *essential infantile esotropia* (EIE). It is characterized by a large, stable angle of deviation, a limited potential for single binocular vision, and an association with oblique muscle dysfunction and dissociated vertical deviation. In addition, many affected children show latent or manifest latent nystagmus and asymmetry of the monocular optokinetic response (von Noorden, 1988).

Pursuit eye movements are also abnormal in EIE (Tychsen and Lisberger, 1986). Other esotropias that also need to be included in this group are the nystagmus blockage syndrome (Ciancia syndrome) and esotropia secondary to ocular disease. The following conditions are discussed in subsequent chapters: Duane's syndrome (Chapter 6); Möbius' syndrome (Chapter 7); early-onset accommodative esotropia (Chapter 5), and esotropia associated with neurologic disease (Chapter 25).

ESSENTIAL INFANTILE ESOTROPIA

Theory

The etiology of EIE remains controversial, and it may be that different mechanisms acting early in life lead to the same end point. Early consid-

TABLE 4.1   Differential diagnosis of infantile esotropia

Essential infantile esotropia
Nystagmus blockage syndrome
Early-onset accommodative esotropia
Bilateral abducens palsy
Esotropia secondary to ocular disease
Esotropia secondary to neurologic disease
Duane's retraction syndrome
Möbius' syndrome

eration of the underlying pathology has led to the polarization of two groups of opinion: those who believe there is a basic defect in the sensory fusion mechanism, and those who believe that obstacles existed to the development of motor fusion. Implicit in these theories are contrasting philosophies in management. A defect of sensory fusion suggests some inherent neurophysiologic problem not likely to be amenable to therapy, which argues against early and aggressive treatment.

On the other hand, if obstacles to the development of normal motor fusion exist and were remedied sufficiently early in the course of visual development, the prospects for ultimately achieving single binocular vision would seem to be more encouraging. To some extent these theories are still relevant, albeit in modified form. Von Noorden (1988) has argued that factors such as excessive tonic convergence, uncorrected hypermetropia, anisometropia, high accommodation convergence to accommodation (AC:A) ratio, or anomalies of the brain stem integrator of vergence eye movements might be acting in a sensorially normal child. Thereafter, failure to achieve high-grade (foveal) stereopsis and disturbance of motion processing response are seen as secondary phenomena, and by implication, early elimination of these factors should enable near normal sensorial development.

Several other authors have surmised that an underlying neurologic defect might be responsible for all the phenomena associated with EIE. In support of this argument is the high incidence (up to 40% in some series) of EIE in children with cerebral palsy (Levy, 1976), the occurrence of EIE in children with a skew deviation in the neonatal period (Hoyt, 1980), the frequent association with latent or manifest latent nystagmus, and an asymmetric motion processing response. Indeed, it has been suggested that an optokinetic defect might be the underlying problem rather than a consequence of the strabismus (Kommerell, 1982). A challenging attempt to reconcile many of these apparently conflicting views has appeared (Flynn, 1991), in which the suggestion is put forward that as a consequence of a neurodevelopmental mishap, the scene is set for both motor and sensory distur-bances. Their impact, then, on the developing ocular system will give rise to strabismus, although if they arose in the absence of that initial mishap they would produce no untoward effect.

Diagnosis

Affected children typically have an esodeviation of between 40 and 70 prism diopters, with no more significant hypermetropic refractive error than is normal for their age. In my experience, they are rarely amblyopic, although this is debated (Costenbader, 1961; Good et al., 1993). These children usually have good vision in either eye, as demon-strated by an ability to alternate fixation between eyes. In addition, affected children show a habitual limitation of abduction, preferring to fix objects in their left visual field with their right eye, and vice versa—so-called cross-fixation.

Vertical Strabismus Associated with Esotropia

At first presentation, features of inferior oblique muscle overaction, with updrifting of the adducting eye in contralateral version move-ments, tend not to be apparent. However, they will appear in up to 78% of patients (Hiles, 1980) before the age of 2 years (Figure 4.1).

Similarly, dissociated vertical deviation (DVD) is rarely obvious at first presentation but will eventually become apparent in up to 70% of cases by 18 months to 3 years of age (Parks, 1978). Dissociated verti-cal deviation consists of elevation of an occluded eye and a slow return to fixation when the occlusion is removed (Figure 4.2).

The return to fixation may include a small overshoot into downgaze with a following corrective upward movement. This observed updrifting is accompanied by excyclotorsion of the affected eye, and recovery is accompanied by incyclotorsion; the latter is easier to see clinically. Dissociated vertical deviation is usually bilateral, although sometimes asymmetric, and in severe cases it can become a cosmetic blemish when the updrifting occurs spontaneously, perhaps associated with episodes of illness or inattention.

A problem that occasionally arises is that of distinguishing inferior oblique overaction from the updrifting in adduction, which can be caused by DVD with the patient's nose acting as an occluder. The two entities can and do coexist, so the distinction needs to be made before planning correction. Inferior oblique weakening procedures will have no effect on a DVD and will exaggerate the "A" phenomenon that may accompany DVD (Mein and Johnson, 1981). The distinction is made by asking the patient to look into extreme lateral gaze, thus occluding the abducted eye. The two conditions will then behave quite differently. In inferior oblique overaction, the adducting eye will come down to take up

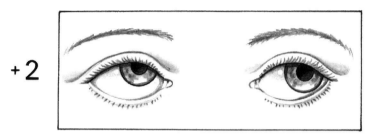

FIGURE 4.1   *Inferior oblique overaction is diagnosed when the involved eye abducts and elevates higher than the fellow eye when moved into the field of action of the inferior oblique muscle (elevation and adduction).*

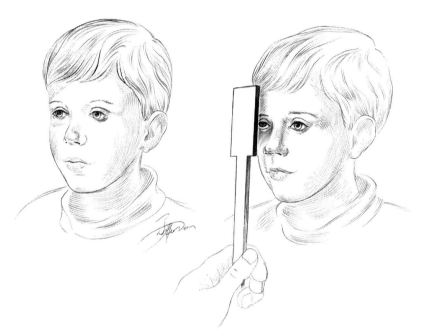

FIGURE 4.2   *Divergent vertical deviation causes the involved eye to drift upward under occlusion or spontaneously. When the cover is removed, the eye may return to normal without a corresponding downward shift of the fellow eye.*

fixation, and that movement will be accompanied by a downward movement of the occluded, abducted eye. Conversely, in DVD, the adducted eye will move down to take up fixation, but the occluded, abducted eye will tend to drift upward. This simple examination should be enough to distinguish the two entities if doubt exists (see also Chap. 15).

Latent Nystagmus
Latent nystagmus is identified by recognizing the appearance of a jerky nystagmus when one eye is occluded or its image markedly degraded

by the use of neutral density filters. The fast phase is always directed toward the fixing eye and the nystagmus is predominantly horizontal, although a torsional component has been described (Hiles, 1980). Eye movement recordings have shown latent nystagmus to have a characteristic decelerating waveform, and this has allowed an oxymoronic diagnosis of manifest latent nystagmus in some children. This simply means that the child has a low-intensity nystagmus with both eyes open and an increasing intensity with one eye occluded, while in each case maintaining the decelerating waveform (Dell'Osso et al., 1979).

The Motion Processing Response in Esotropia

The final phenomenon associated with EIE is asymmetry of the monocular, optokinetic, motion processing response (Norcia et al., 1991; Tychsen et al., 1985). When presenting an optokinetic target to each eye individually, the response to the target moving from the temporal to the nasal field is normal, but the response to targets moving in the opposite direction is grossly disturbed. The presence of this phenomenon in an older patient presenting with esotropia may help establish that the deviation was infantile in origin. It may also be an important observation in trying to understand the basic etiology of the condition, since the pattern described is identical to that seen in the newborn child and disappears at 3–4 months of age, unless EIE develops (Naegele and Held, 1982). It has been suggested that normalization of monocular optokinetic nystagmus is dependent on the development of binocular binocularity (Atkinson, 1979), and persistence of the primitive pattern may indicate a poor prognosis for binocular vision.

Differential Diagnosis

Because of the alternating fixation pattern and the consequent failure to abduct either eye fully in lateral gaze, EIE must be distinguished from those esotropias in which abduction is pathologically limited. It is necessary, therefore, to demonstrate the potential for full abduction (to exclude congenital abducens palsy) and to make sure that there are no synkinetic lid or eye movements occurring with attempted horizontal gaze (to exclude Duane's retraction syndrome). The best way of achieving this is to use vestibular and proprioceptive stimulation, either by rotating the child at arm's length or by performing a "doll's head" maneuver.

Rotating the child at arm's length will stimulate the vestibulo-ocular reflex and tend to drive the eyes in the direction of rotation (Figure 4.3). In younger infants this alone is usually enough to demonstrate that each eye will fully abduct. However, in older children (over 4 months of age), apart from the practical problems of swinging the child at arm's length, the improved vision allows them to fix the examiner's

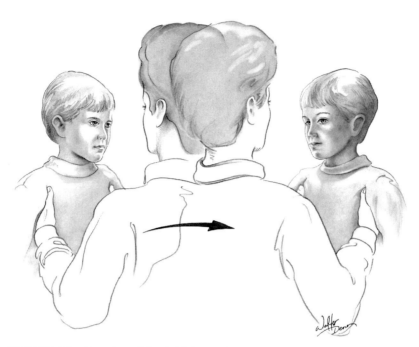

FIGURE 4.3 *Rotation of the child drives the eyes in the direction of rotation. Failure of one eye to move indicates a nuclear, fascicular, or extraocular muscle abnormality.*

face and thus suppress vestibularly driven eye movements. In these older children the doll's head maneuver is more helpful, because both the vestibular/proprioceptive input and the visual drive are in the same direction. Having warned both the child and the parents, the examiner rotate's the child's head briskly, first in one direction and then in the other (Figure 4.4). This maneuver will drive the eyes in a direction opposite that of the head rotation, in the manner of a toy doll. When appropriate, it is equally applicable to vertical eye movements.

One or the other of these techniques should yield full horizontal ocular rotations, but if doubt persists it may be necessary to occlude the child's eye for a period, either briefly in the clinic or for longer periods at home, to assure that the uncovered eye demonstrates its ability to abduct.

Differentiation of EIE from early-onset accommodative esotropia will rest on the identification of a significant hypermetropic refractive error with a high AC:A ratio, and elimination or reduction of the deviation by the wearing of appropriate spectacles. Similarly, careful fundus examination at the first opportunity should identify those children with a sensory cause for their strabismus. However, it may be more difficult in early infancy to identify the child with a subtle neurologic defect. In an unselected series, almost 50% of children presenting with EIE had an associated neurologic problem (Charles and Moore, 1992),

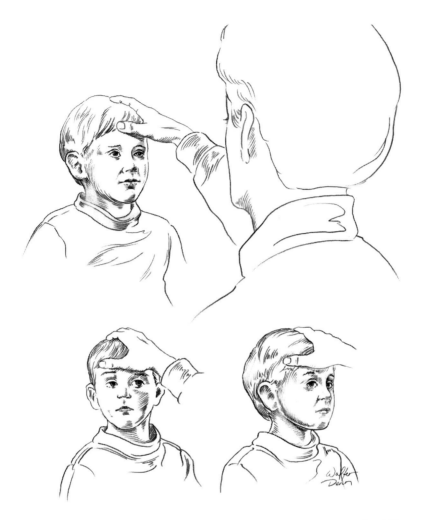

FIGURE 4.4 *In the doll's eye test, only the head is rotated. The eyes should be driven to the side opposite the rotation. Failure of one eye to rotate indicates a nuclear, fascicular, or extraocular muscle abnormality.*

and because these children probably have a poor long-term outlook, both in terms of binocularity and stable ocular alignment, any suspicion of a neurologic handicap should stimulate a detailed evaluation by a pediatric neurologist.

Management
Amblyopia
As with other forms of strabismus, it is of paramount importance to eliminate amblyopia (when it exists), which, in infants, usually means using occlusion until free alternation of fixation is established.

Occlusion may be especially difficult in the child with latent nystagmus, because the process of occlusion further degrades vision in the open eye by virtue of the induced nystagmus. If this proves to be a major barrier to successful amblyopia therapy, then optic and drug penalization can be used (Willshaw and Johnson, 1979). Also, bilateral atropinization, reported to allow occlusion without worsening latent nystagmus, can be used (Calcutt and Crook, 1972). Other barriers to fusion must also be removed, particularly anisometropia and astigmatism. Failure to deal adequately with either of these problems results in a markedly poor long-term outcome (Keenan and Willshaw, 1992).

Refraction

Any substantial refractive error should be corrected. Myopia in EIE is uncommon, but its correction could change the angle of deviation. Similarly, hyperopia in EIE can affect the degree of ocular misalignment. In this regard, there is debate as to how much hyperopia must be present to warrant the effort to correct it. Baker and Parks (1980) showed that accommodative esotropia can occur before age 1 year, with as little as 2.25 D of hyperopia. Other physical findings may suggest at least a partial accommodative component to the esotropia. These would include variable amounts of esotropia and/or an amount of esotropia less than usual—e.g., under 40 prism diopters. It is easier to attempt spectacle correction preoperatively than to rush a child into wearing spectacles postoperatively to control a small (residual) deviation.

Surgical Management

The management of EIE is invariably surgical, and the major debate centers around the timing of surgery. Many authorities believe that early surgery, aiming at alignment within 10 prism diopters of straightness by 2 years of age, offers the best prospect for the development of single binocular vision and achievement of stable, long-term, ocular alignment (Ing, 1983). Furthermore, there is some evidence of improved visuomotor development in children following early correction of their EIE (Rogers et al., 1982), so in the absence of any anesthetic contraindication, delaying surgery beyond 2 years of age does not seem warranted. However, prospective studies have failed to show any significant incidence of stereopsis in children corrected early (Dobson and Sebris, 1989), and the realistic expectation in most children with EIE may be peripheral fusion and microtropia with stable ocular alignment.

Because the angle of deviation is commonly large, two schools of thought have evolved regarding the surgical correction of EIE. Some surgeons (including myself) prefer to perform surgery on only two horizontal rectus muscles during one operation. Proponents of this approach usually use symmetric recession of each medial rectus muscle. The theoretic maximum for recession of a medial rectus muscle is 5.5 mm from the original insertion, or to a point 11 mm from the corneoscleral limbus. Several authors have shown that greater recessions can be performed without compromising convergence in the long term. As a result, recession of 6 mm is commonly performed (Willshaw et al., 1986) and reports of successful 7- and 8-mm recessions are available (Szmyd, 1985). For the surgeon wishing to restrict medial rectus recession to 6 mm, further enhancement of the effect can be achieved by using what Helveston and associates (1978) described as the "en bloc" recession. This technique involves recessing not only the medial rectus muscle but also the nasal conjunctiva and Tenon's capsule. The nonmuscular tissue is recessed to a point just anterior to the original insertion of the medial rectus muscle, and this en bloc recession will consistently increase the effect of medial rectus recession. Depending on the age of the child, a mean correction in excess of 4 prism diopters per millimeter of recession can be achieved (Willshaw, 1986), thus allowing correction of deviations up to 50 prism diopters.

Because of the enormous variation in the correction achieved by the same surgeon in different children, restricting surgery to two muscles in the first operation seems reasonably cautious. However, it must be accepted that this approach will yield a significant number of undercorrections, particularly in the larger deviations, and the surgeon must be prepared to reoperate early when there has been a significant undercorrection. The second operation will usually be a resection of each lateral rectus muscle, although that decision must be based on the nature of the residual esotropia.

An alternative approach is to use graded bilateral medial rectus recessions for deviations up to 40 prism diopters, but for greater deviations, reduce the size of the medial rectus recessions and introduce a resection of one or more lateral recti muscles. Scott and colleagues (1986) have reviewed their results in 107 patients using both of these approaches, and they have found that a smaller number of those children receiving a graded procedure require a second operation. Readers must select the approach that seems most appropriate and most effective, but it is relevant to point out that in the United Kingdom, but perhaps not in the United States, most parents are happy to accept the need for a second procedure if the surgical objectives and the inevitable inaccuracies are made clear at the outset.

Inferior Oblique Overaction
Because EIE is so commonly associated with overaction of the inferior oblique muscles, it may be necessary to deal with this overaction either

at the time of surgery of the horizontal muscle or as a separate surgical procedure. Inferior oblique overaction is commonly encountered (40% of the children in my unit) (Keenan and Willshaw, 1992), and only rarely is it unilateral. However, marked asymmetry of the overaction is not unusual, and before considering a unilateral inferior oblique weakening procedure, a careful examination should be undertaken to exclude overaction in the fellow eye. The risk that inferior oblique overaction will occur in the fellow eye after surgery in the involved eye is 33% (Raab and Costenbader, 1973).

The inferior oblique overaction may represent a substantial cosmetic blemish, but more important, oblique muscle dysfunction can be an important factor in disrupting binocular vision and contributing to the generation of large-angle esotropia. Evidence exists that simultaneous correction of any oblique dysfunction will increase the frequency with which stable binocular single vision is achieved postoperatively (Gobin, 1969). The correction of the inferior oblique overaction, again, is surgical and is best achieved using a graded approach to the surgical procedure. The overaction can be classified as grades 1–4, with the surgical approach selected according to that grading (Figure 4.5). This grading of surgery is debated, and there are many who would perform the same surgery regardless of the amount of inferior oblique overaction.

Grade 1 overactions are dealt with using a recession of between 8 mm and 10 mm. Grade 2 overactions require a myectomy of the inferior oblique muscle. Grade 3 overactions require extirpation of the muscle, achieved by combining a myectomy with division of the neurovascular bundle as it enters the posterior border of the muscle. Finally, grade 4 overactions are dealt with by using a denervation (as above) in conjunction with anteropositioning of the inferior oblique tendon (Parks, personal communication, 1991). If these guidelines are followed, a more predictable correction of inferior oblique dysfunctions of differing severity will be achieved. However, of even greater importance in any inferior oblique muscle surgical procedure is the accurate identification and isolation of the muscle. Inaccurate localization (as caused by a blind sweep of the muscle hook) may well cause disruption of the orbital septum, leading to the admixture of orbital fat, blood, and muscle tissue. This is a potent combination for the creation of scar tissue, and the subsequent fibrous contraction can give rise to an inferior adhesive syndrome (Figure 4.6). This usually appears several months after the original operation, with the operated eye becoming tethered in depression and showing defective elevation (most marked in adduction). It is an extremely difficult problem to deal with and may require the use of protective sheets to prevent further scarring and

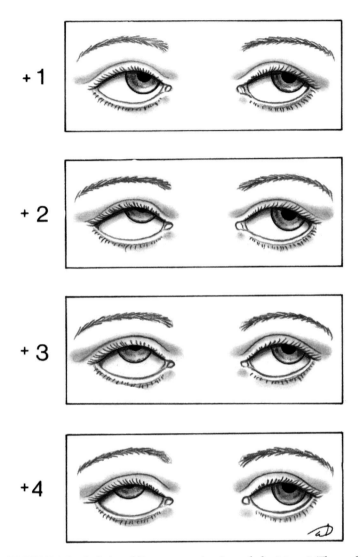

FIGURE 4.5 *Inferior oblique overaction is graded +1 to +4. The evaluation should be objective, even though we are not aware of any exact criteria for grading inferior oblique overaction. Each grade indicates further displacement of the eye from normal in the field of action of the inferior oblique muscle.*

restriction of movement. Undoubtedly the best prophylaxis is avoidance of excessive trauma at the time of the initial operation.

The other element of EIE that may require surgical correction is DVD. The reported incidence of DVD varies from 15% (Keenan and Willshaw, 1992) to 90% (Lang, 1967), but the frequency of surgery is much lower than the overall incidence. In the 1992 series by Keenan and Willshaw only 1 child out of 40 required surgery for DVD. Opinions vary as to the best surgical approach, and this may reflect the

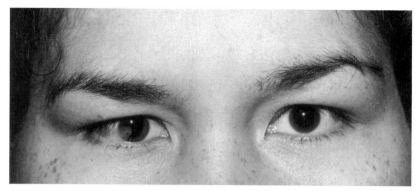

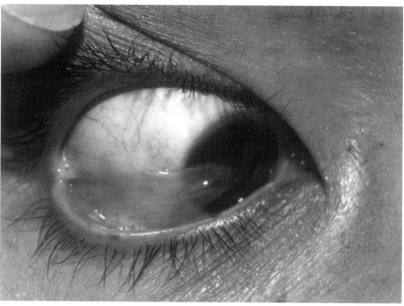

FIGURE 4.6 *Fat adherence syndrome can complicate weakening procedures of the inferior oblique muscle. This patient presented with a right hypotropia (A). Close inspection showed scarring in the inferior cul de sac and a pseudopterygium. (B).*

relatively disappointing outcome reported by most authors (Scott et al., 1982). There is agreement, in principle, that the correct approach is to compromise the function of the superior rectus muscle. Magoon and associates (1982) have advocated the use of unusually large superior rectus muscle recessions of 10–15 mm. Possible dangers of this approach include the development of upper lid retraction or the induction of hypotropia of the operated eye. It is useful, therefore, to place the recessed superior rectus muscle on an adjustable suture (in adults) to allow correction of either of these problems. To avoid such large recessions a combination of superior rectus muscle recession and ipsilateral inferior rectus muscle resection has been used (Knapp, 1976), or, more commonly, small superior rectus muscle recessions have been used in combination with a Faden or posterior fixation suture on the same muscle. The latter approach showed a notably superior outcome in a retrospective review of 42 patients (Lorenz et al., 1992).

It is worth bearing in mind that the child with EIE plus DVD is most unlikely to develop useful binocular vision, and that the surgeon is dealing with an essentially cosmetic defect. Furthermore, the cosmetic defect may increase with age, so surgical correction should only be undertaken when all parties are confident that a cosmetic problem really exists.

Inevitably the surgeon dealing with EIE will be called on, from time to time, to deal with either residual esotropia or consecutive exotropia following surgery. If exotropia occurs in the immediate postoperative period, the possibility of a slipped muscle should be considered. A complete examination of the ocular rotations of each eye will clarify the situation. In the presence of a slipped muscle, early reoperation is indicated (MacEwen et al., 1992). More commonly, however, these problems arise despite normal ocular rotations, and although not ignoring the original operation, it is important to evaluate fully the new deviation and plan management appropriately.

In the case of residual esotropia, once again, amblyopia must be eliminated, if possible. Repeat refraction may reveal a level of hypermetropia that now warrants correction in the context of the new, smaller angle of deviation. After assessing vision and checking the refraction, if the residual esotropia shows no great variation in angle between distance and near fixation, then bilateral lateral rectus muscle resection is a potential second surgical procedure. This is probably best performed within 3–4 months of the initial operation before increasing tone develops in the recessed medial recti muscles, but still allowing time to accurately evaluate the effect of the original surgery. Nonetheless, in my experience bilateral lateral rectus muscle resections performed up to 12 months after the medial rectus muscle recessions can still be effective.

If the esotropia remaining after bilateral medial rectus muscle recessions shows a substantial accommodative component with the near deviation exceeding the distance deviation by 10 prism diopters or more, then further surgery to the medial recti muscles is indicated. The medial recti muscles should be explored to ensure that a full recession has been achieved by the original surgical procedure and that there has been no inadvertent misplacement of the medial recti muscles or, more commonly, migration forward of the insertion. This last event is likely to occur if the original recession has been performed using a "hangback" technique (Repka et al., 1990). If either of these situations exists, then the medial recti muscles should be rerecessed to the desired position on the globe. If, in fact, the recession proves to be adequate, then the choice of another medial rectus muscle weakening procedure is between a posterior fixation suture placed through the muscle and fixed to the sclera at the equator or a partial myotomy. These procedures can be impressively effective, though they are known to be less predictable than the original recession (Zak and Morin, 1983).

If a consecutive exotropia develops following bilateral medial rectus muscle recessions, then a trial with myopic spectacles (to stimulate accommodative convergence) or an attempt to correct the deviation with base in fresnel prisms might be deemed necessary in an attempt to encourage motor fusion. There is evidence that a small overcorrection in the early postoperative period is beneficial in terms of long-term stability of the ocular alignment (Scott et al., 1986). However, if cooperation with optical maneuvers is limited and the exotropia persists beyond 3 months, the surgeon should not hesitate to recommend another surgery. Only rarely is the consecutive exotropia greater for near than for distance, and, therefore, only rarely is simple readvancement of the medial recti muscles adequate to correct the deviation. If the exotropia is equal for near and for distance, it is best dealt with by recessing one lateral rectus muscle and readvancing the ipsilateral medial rectus muscle. If the exotropia is substantially greater for distance fixation, the preferred operation would be recession of both lateral recti muscles.

With the increased use of botulinum toxin chemodenervation in the management of adult strabismus, some reference to that modality should be made in this management section. Despite reports of its use in children in the early 1980s (Magoon, 1984), the procedure has found little favor. In young children the technique of injecting extraocular muscles with botulinum neurotoxin requires general anesthesia. A major advantage of botulinum treatment in adults is that it does not require general anesthesia. In addition, the need for repeated injections and the lack of any permanent effect in children means that surgical management is likely to remain the mainstay for the foreseeable future.

Prognosis

The long-term outcome in EIE will depend on a variety of factors, but most important are the presence or absence of amblyopia, the age at which surgical alignment is achieved, and the absence of associated neurologic or ocular anomalies. The incidence of stereopsis following good surgical alignment is a controversial subject, and arguments have depended on the criteria used for evaluating stereopsis (Ing, 1983; Charles and Moore, 1992). The frequency of long-term, stable ocular alignment, whether maintained by peripheral fusion or not, is, on the other hand, very encouraging. More than 80% of children adequately aligned by 2 years of age will fall into the category of "favourable outcome" (Keenan and Willshaw, 1992), and this is most certainly a worthwhile goal.

It is very important in the prognosis for these children to ensure that the possibility of amblyopia is not overlooked in the postoperative period simply because the ocular alignment is satisfactory. Indeed, it may well be that the greatest risk of amblyopia occurs after good ocular alignment (Good et al., 1993). It has been shown that following surgical correction (and removal of the alternating pattern of fixation), the likelihood of amblyopia increases (Hoyt et al., 1980). In our series, 9 children out of 40 who were not amblyopic at the time of surgery required amblyopia therapy in the postoperative period.

NYSTAGMUS BLOCKAGE SYNDROME (CIANCIA SYNDROME)

Theory

The nystagmus blockage syndrome, recognized by Alberto Ciancia, but first named in 1966 by Adelstein, has a much more clearcut etiology than does EIE. Some children with congenital nystagmus possess a so-called "null zone," a direction of gaze in which the intensity of their nystagmus either diminishes or disappears altogether. If the null zone is in eccentric gaze, affected children develop a compensatory head posture in order to view objects with their eyes directed into their null zone. In this way they achieve their optimum visual acuity. For example, if the null zone is within 20 degrees of the left gaze, then a face turned 20 degrees to the right will allow objects straight ahead to be viewed with the least amount of nystagmus. (Nystagmus degrades the quality of vision by virtue of a reduced time for foveation of objects of regard.) There are children with congenital nystagmus in whom the position of least nystagmus is with the eyes convergent. These children adopt a large-angle esotropia to minimize or eliminate their nystagmus and, where necessary, use a head posture to allow fixation with the dominant eye in its adducted position. These children will also appear to have limitation of abduction. Their large-angle esotropia commonly appears in the first 6 months of life, although it is not usually present at birth.

Diagnosis

From the foregoing description it is obvious that nystagmus blockage syndrome must be distinguished from EIE with manifest latent nystagmus. Ultimately the distinction is possible using eye movement recordings, but few departments have these routinely available, and the distinction usually can be drawn following careful clinical examination.

Unlike manifest latent nystagmus, congenital nystagmus does not increase in intensity with occlusion of one eye, and if its pattern is "jerky" in nature, the direction of the fast phase does not vary with occlusion. In fact, every manifest nystagmus has some latent component, but this is usually not clinically apparent. In nystagmus blockage syndrome, the eyes show manifest nystagmus as soon as they move from the adducted position, without needing occlusion to render the nystagmus manifest. In addition to the above features, von Noorden (1976) has described pupillary constriction at the time of appearance of the esotropia, which would lend further support to the concept of an active process of convergence being used to block the nystagmus.

The frequency with which nystagmus blockage will be the underlying mechanism in children presenting with it in the first 6 months of life is unclear. The original proponents of the nystagmus blockage mechanism invoke it as the explanation for most cases of early-onset esotropia, but this view is, for the most part, unpopular today. Now, a distinction is clearly drawn between latent nystagmus and congenital idiopathic nystagmus. On this basis, relatively few cases (probably less than 5%) are attributed to nystagmus blockage (von Noorden, 1976).

Management

Children with nystagmus blockage syndrome develop amblyopia far more frequently than do children with EIE. When amblyopia has developed, it causes the child to show a face turn, which is used to allow the viewing of objects with the dominant eye in adduction. Observation of this phenomenon should alert the clinician to the probability of amblyopia, and appropriate remedial steps should be taken. As with children with latent nystagmus, tolerance of occlusion regimens is often limited, and recourse to optic and drug penalization (blurring vision with atropine drops) may be necessary.

From a surgical standpoint, the importance of recognizing this apparently uncommon condition is that it responds less predictably to conventional management. Because of the tonic drive to converge and the resultant hypertonicity of the medial recti muscles, simple recessions of the medial recti muscles are rarely sufficient to deal with the esotropia in the long term. More success has accompanied the use of small medial rectus muscle recessions (of about 4 mm) coupled with placement of a Faden suture at the equator of the globe, or at least 10.5 mm behind the original muscle insertion.

Anxiety is sometimes expressed such that, by denying the eyes their convergent position, the nystagmus will no longer be dampened and hence the quality of vision will be reduced. This appears not to be the case, indicating that it is the "neurologic drive" to converge that is instrumental in dampening the nystagmus, rather than a mechanical effect dependent on the position of the eyes. This observation accords well with the observed benefits of Kestenbaum surgery in those children with nystagmus and who employ a face turn to use a null zone in lateral gaze.

Optical means alone are insufficient to deal with nystagmus blockage, but having reduced the angle of deviation, the use of prisms may be helpful in older patients. The nature of the prism combination required may not be entirely predictable from the measured deviation, and a subjective assessment is essential for accurate prescription.

ESOTROPIA SECONDARY TO OCULAR DISEASE

Theory and Management

Contrary to popular view, strabismus in children with ocular disease is equally divided between esotropia and exotropia and is not primarily exotropia. So long as the ocular pathology is sufficient to degrade the vision in one eye below a level of 6/24 to 6/36 (20/80 to 20/120), strabismus is likely to result. Diseases that reduce the vision in both eyes (e.g., cataract, albinism, optic nerve hypoplasia), while also likely to give rise to strabismus (again, commonly esotropia), do not usually present with strabismus but rather with nystagmus and poor vision.

With monocular pathology, the onus is on diagnosis and management of the ocular pathology, rather than on the strabismus. In this context, it is worth noting that in a review of 117 children with retinoblastoma, 18 (15%) presented initially with strabismus (Parks, 1992). However, if the barrier to good vision can be overcome, and this applies especially to cataract and congenital glaucoma, then attention should be directed toward the strabismus. A detailed assessment of the management of monocular cataracts would not be appropriate in this context, and the generally held view is that strabismus surgery in these children is directed primarily at eliminating an unsightly cosmetic deviation. Nonetheless, more aggressive management of monocular cataract has spawned a number of reports of good monocular vision having been achieved and, more recently, of suggestions that some binocular vision might be recovered (Wright et al., 1992). With early surgical correction and attention to amblyopia and the associated anisometropia, children with glaucoma may also be capable of retrieving some binocularity.

Unlike some older patients, in whom removing the underlying pathology will also eliminate the strabismus (Cole et al., 1988), children require strabismus surgery if they are to achieve binocular vision. Despite a more optimistic approach to the management of these conditions, it remains important to retain a realistic perspective. Even in ideal circumstances, the establishment of any evidence of motor fusion remains unusual, and overly aggressive surgical management of the esotropia is likely to yield a significant number of children with consecutive exotropia. At this time it would be reasonable to reserve the aggressive early alignment of the eyes to those children who have their underlying pathology treated within the first 2–3 months of life, who cooperate well with amblyopia therapy, and who, by virtue of their fixation preference or their measured acuity, have had any amblyopia eliminated before the age of 6 months. It will be interesting to observe the long-term impact of our increasingly ambitious management regimens.

A final cautionary note: In children with disease in one eye (unlike most others in the EIE category), it is a wise precaution to restrict surgery to the already compromised eye. The incidence of sight-threatening complications following strabismus surgery is thankfully low. In one report, no cases of endophthalmitis were identified in 12,000 strabismus operations (Weinstein et al., 1979). Nonetheless, scleral perforation with its vision-threatening potential occurs in at least 3% of strabismus procedures (Morris et al., 1990), and even a slight risk to the better eye would seem unreasonable when the prospect is for motor alignment without sensory fusion.

REFERENCES

Abrahamsson M, Fabian G, Sjonstrant J. Refraction changes in children developing convergent or divergent strabismus. Br J Ophthalmol 1992;76:723–727.

Adelstein FE, Cupers C. Zum problem der echten und der scheinbaren Abducenslahmung (Das sogenannte Blockierungssyndrom). Buch Augenarzt 1966;46:272–278.

Atkinson J. Development of Optokinetic Nystagmus in Human Infant and Monkey Infant: An Analogue to Development in Kittens. In RD Freeman (ed), Developmental Neurobiology of Vision. New York: Plenum, 1979:277–287.

Baker JD, Parks MM. Early-onset accommodative esotropia. Am J Ophthalmol 1980;90:11–18.

Calcutt C, Crook W. Treatment of amblyopia in patients with latent nystagmus. Br Orthop J 1972;29:70–72.

Charles SJ, Moore AT. Results of early surgery for infantile esotropia in normal and neurologically impaired infants. Eye 1992;6:603–606.

Cole MD, Hay A, Eagling EM. Cyclic esotropia in a patient with unilateral traumatic aphakia: Case report. Br J Ophthalmol 1988;72:305–308.

Costenbader FD: Infantile esotropia. Trans Am Ophthalmol Soc 1961;59:397–429.

Dell'Osso LF, Schmidt D, Daroff RB. Latent, manifest latent and congenital nystagmus. Arch Ophthalmol 1979;97:1877–1885.

Dobson V, Sebris SL. Longitudinal study of acuity and stereopsis in infants with or at risk for esotropia. Invest Ophthalmol Vis Sci 1989; 30:1146–1158.

Flynn JT. Strabismus: A Neurodevelopmental Approach. New York: Springer-Verlag, 1991.

Gobin MH. Cyclotropia and Squint. Antwerp: Krol & Courtin, 1969.

Good WV, de Sa LCF, Lyons CJ, Hoyt CS. Monocular visual outcome in untreated early onset esotropia. Br J Ophthalmol 1993;77:492–494.

Helveston EM, Ellis FD, Patterson JH et al. Augmented recession of the medial recti. Ophthalmology 1978;85:507–511.

Helveston EM, Ellis FD, Schott J et al. Surgical treatment of congenital esotropia. Am J Ophthalmol 1983;96:218–228.

Hiles DA, Watson BA, Biglan A. Characteristics of infantile esotropia following early bimedial rectus recession. Arch Ophthalmol 1980;98:697–703.

Hoyt CS, Mousel DK, Weber AA. Transient supranuclear disturbance of gaze in healthy neonates. Am J Ophthalmol 1980;89:708–713.

Ing MR. Early surgical alignment for congenital esotropia. Ophthalmology 1983;90:132–135.

Keenan JM, Willshaw HE. Outcome of strabismus surgery in congenital esotropia. Br J Ophthalmol 1992;76:342–345.

Kommerell G. Indications for nystagmus operation. Buch Augenarzt 1982;89:165–172.

Knapp P. Dissociated Vertical Deviations. In P Fells (ed), Second Congress, International Strabismological Association. Marseilles: Diffusion Generale de Librairie, 1976.

Kushner BJ, Fisher MR, Lucchese NJ, Morton CO. Factors influencing response to strabismus surgery. Arch Ophthalmol 1993;111:75–79.

Lang J. Cited in GK von Noorden (ed), Binocular Vision and Ocular Motility. St. Louis: Mosby, 1967;295.

Levy NS, Cassin B, Newman M. Strabismus in children with cerebral palsy. J Pediatr Ophthalmol Strabismus 1976;13:72–74.

Lorenz B, Raab I, Boergen KP. Dissociated vertical deviation: What is the most effective surgical approach? J Pediatr Ophthalmol Strabismus 1992;29:21–29.

MacEwen CJ, Lee JP, Fells P. Aetiology and management of the "detached" rectus muscle [editorial]. Br J Ophthalmol 1992;76:131–136.

Magoon E, Cruciger M, Jampolsky A. Dissociated vertical deviation: An asymmetric condition treated with large bilateral superior rectus recession. J Pediatr Ophthalmol Strabismus 1982;19:152–156.

Magoon EH. Botulinum toxin chemo-denervation for strabismus in infants and children. J Pediatr Ophthalmol Strabismus 1984;21:110–113.

Mein J, Johnson F. Dissociated Vertical Divergence and Its Association with Nystagmus. In J Mein, S Moore (eds), Orthoptics, Research and Practice. Kimpton, England, 1981;14–16.

Morris RJ, Rosen PH, Fells P. Incidence of inadvertent globe perforations during strabismus surgery. Br J Ophthalmol 1990;74:490–493.

Naegele JR, Held R. The postnatal development of monocular optokinetic nystagmus in infants. Vision Res 1982;22:341–346.

Nixon RB, Helveston EM, Miller K et al. Incidence of strabismus in neonates. Am J Ophthalmol 1985;100:798–801.

Norcia AM, Jampolsky A, Hamer RG, Orel BD. Plasticity of human motion processing following strabismus surgery. Invest Ophthalmol Vis Sci 1991;32:1044.

Parks MM. Oblique Muscle Dysfunction, Dissociated Hyperdeviations. In MM Parks (ed), Ocular Motility and Strabismus. Hagerstown, MD: Harper & Row, 1978.

Raab EL, Costenbader FD. Unilateral surgery for inferior oblique overaction. Arch Ophthalmol 1973;90:180–182.

Repka MX, Fishman PJ, Guyton DL. The site of reattachment of the extraocular muscle following hang-back recession. J Pediatr Ophthalmol Strabismus 1990;27:286–290.

Rogers GL, Chazan S, Fellows R et al. Strabismus surgery and its effect upon infant development in congenital esotropia. Ophthalmology 1982;89:479–483.

Scott WE, Sutton VJ, Thalacker JA. Superior rectus recessions for dissociated vertical deviation. Ophthalmology 1982;89:317–322.

Scott WE, Reese PD, Hirsh CR et al. Surgery for large angle congenital esotropia. Two vs. three and four horizontal muscles. Arch Ophthalmol 1986;104:374–377.

Szmyd SM, Nelson LB, Calhoun JH et al. Large bimedial rectus recessions in congenital esotropia. Br J Ophthalmol 1985;69:271–274.

Tychsen L, Lisberger SG. Maldevelopment of visual motion processing in humans who had strabismus with onset in infancy. J Neurosci 1986;6:2495–2508.

Tychsen LR, Hurtig R, Scott WE. Pursuit is impaired but the vestibulo-ocular reflex is normal in infantile esotropia. Arch Ophthalmol 1985;103:536–539.

von Noorden GK, Isaza A, Parks ME. Surgical treatment of congenital esotropia. Trans Am Acad Ophthalmol Otolaryngol 1972;76:1465–1478.

von Noorden GK. The nystagmus compensation (blockage) syndrome. Am J Ophthalmol 1976;82:283–290.

von Noorden GK. Current concepts of infantile esotropia. Eye 1988;2:343–357.

Weinstein GS, Mondino BJ, Weinberg RJ et al. Endophthalmitis in a pediatric population. Ann Ophthalmol 1979;11:935–943.

Willshaw HE, Johnson F. Penalization as the primary treatment of strabismic amblyopia. Br Orthop J 1979;36:67–72.

Willshaw HE. Rectus muscle surgery—How to do it. Trans Ophthalmol Soc UK 1986;105:583–588.

Willshaw HE, Mashhoudi N, Powell S. Augmented medial rectus recession in the management of esotropia. Br J Ophthalmol 1986;70:840–843.

Wright KW, Matsumoto E, Edelman PM. Binocular fusion and stereopsis associated with early surgery for monocular congenital cataracts. Arch Ophthalmol 1992;110:1607–1609.

Zak TA, Morin JD. Surgery of infantile esotropia: A critical evaluation of marginal myotomy of the medial recti as a primary and secondary procedure. J Pediatr Ophthalmol Strabismus 1983;20:52–57.

5

Accommodative Esotropia

Harry E. Willshaw

The majority of patients with acquired esotropia seen in clinical practice will have some disturbance of the normal relationship between accommodation and convergence. Because this relationship is not present at birth but develops within the first 2 years of life (coinciding with the anatomic maturation of the fovea and relating to the ability of the retina to appreciate "blur"), most of these esotropias will appear between the ages of 18 and 36 months. It is important, however, to consider the possibility of an accommodative esotropia when assessing any convergent deviation, even if its onset seems to lie outside this age range. The onset of accommodative esotropia as early as 5 months of age (Baker and Parks, 1980) and as late as 6 years of age (Costenbader, 1958) is well recognized.

THEORY

A synkinetic relationship between accommodation, convergence, and pupillary constriction develops early in life to eliminate blurring of the retinal image of a near object. The link between accommodation and convergence may be measured in a number of ways (von Noorden, 1980) and yields a measure of the number of prism diopters of accommodation—the accommodative convergence to accommodation (AC:A) ratio. The absolute value of the AC:A ratio varies between individuals but normally lies within the range of 3 to 1 to 5 to 1 (Sloan et al., 1960). It is unclear whether this ratio is fixed genetically or develops in response to visual stimulation and can then be modified by further visual experience. Clinical studies have suggested a fairly constant value, at least into the presbyopic age range (Breinin and Chin, 1973).

TABLE 5.1   Types of accommodative esotropia

Esotropia	Distance	Near	Treatment
Fully accommodative	ET	ET	Optical
Convergent XS (high AC:A ratio)	Orthotropic	ET	Optical, miotics, surgery
Convergent XS (normal AC:A ratio)	Orthotropic	ET	Surgery
Accommodative plus high AC:A ratio	ET	ET++	Optical, surgery
Partially accommodative	ET	ET	Accommodative treatment, surgery

ET = esotropia; ET++ = increasing esotropia.

However, studies in which optical devices have been used demonstrate a more adaptive system (Judge and Miles, 1980). When viewing a near object, accommodative convergence is inadequate to direct both foveas onto the target; therefore, accommodative convergence is augmented by fusional convergence (Leigh and Zee, 1991).

From a clinical standpoint it seems appropriate to regard the AC:A ratio as a fixed, innate ratio so that if it is disordered it must be modified rather than relearned. This modification may be by mechanical means (optical or surgical) or by use of pharmacologic agents. Orthoptic exercises to help control the consequences of the disturbed AC:A ratio may also be helpful but do not fundamentally alter its value.

Accommodative esotropias arise either because of a demand for accommodation, which is inappropriate for the fixation distance, or because of an abnormally high AC:A ratio so that excessive convergence results from a unit of accommodation. Some esotropes show elements of both mechanisms. For a child viewing a distant object with +3.00 D of hypermetropia, 3.00 D of accommodation will be exercised to eliminate blurring of the retinal image. In the case of a normal AC:A ratio, this will generate an esophoria of up to 15 prism diopters, which must then be controlled by the use of fusional divergence.

Once the normal fusional vergence mechanisms are no longer able to deal with the phoria generated by the disturbances of accommodation, a manifest deviation develops. Other factors may then come into play, modifying the clinical characteristics of the deviation. This results in different accommodative esotropias as presented to the clinician; each requires a different approach to management (Table 5.1).

It goes without saying that not all children with hypermetropia will develop an accommodative esotropia. However, as the level of hypermetropia increases, so does the likelihood of strabismus and amblyopia (Ingram and Walker, 1986). Why one child with a +3.00 D refractive error should develop esotropia and not another remains obscure. Genetic influences may play a part, in view of the known familial tendency in esotropia (Mash et al., 1975; Parks, 1974). A basic neurodevelopmental problem predisposing the child to strabismus may also be important (Flynn, 1991). Because accommodation has such a pivotal role in this group of conditions, the emphasis of management should be on accurate identification and the manipulation of that accommodation.

DIAGNOSIS

A careful cycloplegic refraction is the critical step in diagnosis. Cycloplegia is obtained using one of the parasympatholytic agents that competitively inhibits the action of acetylcholine. Adequate cycloplegia is usually obtained within 30–40 minutes of the instillation of 2 drops of cyclopentolate 1% (or 0.5% in children under 6 months of age, because of potential systemic effects). This allows both refraction and fundoscopy to be performed at the first visit to the clinic and has the dual benefits of convenience to the family and early institution of appropriate therapy. In some children, particularly those with darkly pigmented eyes, cyclopentolate may fail to provide adequate cycloplegia, and recourse to atropine sulfate instilled at home will be necessary.

Our preferred regimen is atropine 1% (0.5% in younger children) in ointment form (which leads to less absorption from the tear film) instilled 3 times per day for 3 days prior to the next clinic visit. Considerable debate has been centered on the amount of hypermetropia revealed by different cycloplegic agents. Generally speaking, with lower levels of hypermetropia the difference between atropine and the shorter-acting agents is inconsequential, but may assume greater importance with refractive errors above +3.00 D (Rosenbaum et al., 1981). If a considerable, but incomplete, reduction in the angle of strabismus is achieved by prescription of the hypermetropia revealed by cyclopentolate, it may be that the extra hypermetropia disclosed by atropine would allow full control.

If home cycloplegia is to be used, the family must be cautioned about the features of systemic toxicity from atropine, which include tachycardia, flushing, agitation, and dryness of mucous membranes. As with any medication, the parents also should be warned to discontinue the ointment in the event of local allergic reactions or toxicity.

Meticulous correction of both spherical and astigmatic errors is essential in children. The actual technique of retinoscopy will vary according to personal preference and experience, but making sure that the child is in a subdued mood, which often accompanies feeding of infants, and with a variety of interesting toys available, is always helpful. Forceful restriction of the child is rarely useful, because even with maximum restraint the eyes may be deviated, and the resulting "off axis" refraction can be very misleading (Moore, 1990). Rarely, if ever, is general anesthesia necessary, but if the uncooperative child is to receive an anesthetic agent for some other reason, then the opportunity should be taken to obtain an accurate refraction. The best approach is to accept failure before the child develops an insurmountable aversion to the examination and to retry later when cooperation may be more easily obtained. Needless to say, all refractions should be accompanied by a careful fundus examination.

The suspicion of esotropia with a high AC:A ratio depends on the identification of a near deviation that exceeds the distance deviation by more than 15 prism diopters (Parks, 1958). The AC:A ratio should then be measured formally, as a baseline to monitor future management and to exclude the rare entity of a convergence excess esotropia *without* a high AC:A ratio (von Noorden and Avilla, 1986).

The V phenomenon (see Chapter 10) and hypoaccommodative convergence excess also must be considered in the differential diagnosis of esotropia with a high AC:A ratio. A prism cover test for near in the primary position and in downgaze should reveal the presence of the V phenomenon, and there will usually be an associated hypertropia if the pattern is a manifestation of superior oblique weakness. Hypo-accommodative convergence excess is a rare entity that was first described by Costenbader (1958). The pattern of increased convergence for near seems, in this instance, to be associated with a remote near point of accommodation. It is assumed that in the face of a hypoaccommodative state, the extra "drive" necessary to achieve a focused image at near engenders unnecessarily large amounts of convergence.

Partially accommodative esotropias are those in which the deviation can be reduced but not eliminated by provision of the correct hypermetropic prescription. It is assumed that many of these children are initially fully accommodative, but with the breakdown of motor fusion, secondary changes occur, including increased tonus in the medial recti muscles. These changes then alter the fundamental nature of the deviation, preventing it from being fully corrected by optical means (Parks, 1974). The very existence of this group of children further emphasizes the need for early introduction of a full refractive correction in accommodative esotropia.

MANAGEMENT OF FULLY ACCOMMODATIVE ESOTROPIA

Optical Management

The management of fully accommodative esotropia consists of optical correction, and any hypermetropic refractive error of +2.00 D or more should be prescribed. In the first instance, this is achieved by the use of spectacles, and it is important to prescribe the full hypermetropic correction to eliminate any need for accommodation when viewing distant targets. Ophthalmologists working with children need to be aware of their working distance when refracting (commonly closer than for adults), and the appropriate deduction should be made for this working distance. However, there is no merit in making another deduction to allow for latent hypermetropia, because the objective must be to eliminate all accommodative effort in the distance. With this in mind, it is worth ensuring that clinic staff record the retinoscopy as well as the prescription provided. This allows a check to be made on the level of prescription provided and alerts the supervising physician to the likely presence of residual hypermetropia.

This counsel of full prescription may need to be modified in children over the age of 6 years, when a maximal prescription will occasionally reduce distance vision and be poorly tolerated. In younger children, it should be adhered to until good binocular single vision has been established. Thereafter, if the child is uncomfortable, the level of prescription may be cautiously reduced, while ensuring that ocular alignment and normal binocular cooperation are maintained. In some children who have achieved good-quality binocular single vision, alignment is maintained despite the gradual reduction in the level of hypermetropic correction. This phenomenon can be encouraged by the use of appropriate orthoptic exercises to eliminate suppression, to teach the child to recognize diplopia, and to encourage the development of divergence fusion. These exercises may allow the abandonment of spectacles, though this is rare, and more commonly, some form of optical correction will need to be maintained.

In older children, if resistance to use of spectacles is encountered, transfer to contact lens correction may prove to be an acceptable alternative. Control of the esotropia is usually well maintained with contact lenses, but children should be watched carefully during this transition, because a few of them will lose control of their convergent tendency. These children were obtaining a base-out prism effect from their hypermetropic spectacle lenses (especially if they were appropriately decentered) and should be presumed to require that prismatic effect to maintain full control. They will need to be returned to long-term use of spectacles.

Surgical Management

In recent years, considerable discussion has centered on the role of surgery in fully accommodative esotropia. Some authorities recommend surgery with a view to allowing spectacles to be discarded at an early age (Eustace, personal communication, 1990). This is not a popular view in the United Kingdom or the United States because the consequence of such surgery is seen to be late consecutive exotropia when hypermetropic spectacle use becomes optically necessary. These adults have poorly developed convergence fusion and are unable to deal with their increasing divergence. Not only is the divergence unsightly, but it may well be accompanied by intractable diplopia. Surgery can also be viewed as unnecessary, since good ocular alignment can be obtained without it. With surgery, many children still require spectacles for good vision or good alignment, or both.

MANAGEMENT OF ESOTROPIA WITH HIGH AC:A RATIO

It is possible to modify esotropia with a high AC:A ratio in a number of ways, and the clinician should be prepared to try each of them in an effort to reestablish full binocular functions.

Optical Management

By using bifocal spectacles, it is possible to eliminate the need for accommodation (and hence the drive to converge) when viewing a near object. Most commonly, a reading addition of +2.50 or +3.00 D will be necessary to eliminate the excessive convergence, but the appropriate addition for each child can be evaluated in the clinic. The upper segment of the bifocal may contain no prescription lens if the eyes are straight for distance fixation or, alternatively, could carry the child's hypermetropic correction. The reading segment of the bifocal should be of the "high-executive" type, with the upper border of the reading segment at the level of the lower third of the pupil (Figure 5.1). Only in this way is it possible to ensure that the reading segment is consistently used during near fixation.

The aim of bifocal therapy is to establish binocular single vision and then to reduce the strength of the reading segment by small (0.50 D) increments while still maintaining the binocular single vision. To reduce expense and ensure proper placement of the bifocal segment, fresnel adhesive spheres may be used as an alternative to frequent spectacle prescriptions. The use of fresnel prisms in the lower segment has also been advocated, but the size of prism required will usually degrade vision to such an extent that high-grade stereopsis is impossible.

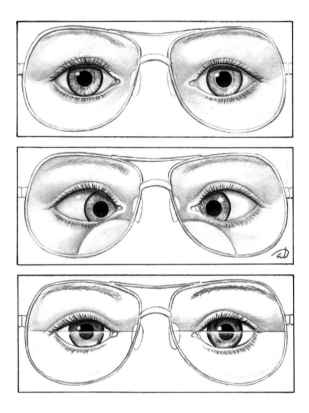

FIGURE 5.1 *Bifocals for children will fail unless the bifocal line transects the pupil, as occurs in "executive-style" bifocals.*

Pharmacologic Management

It is possible, by using anticholinesterase drops, to induce accommodation and thus eliminate the blurring of near objects, which acts as a stimulus to central accommodation. This, in turn, will remove the convergence that accompanies the accommodative effort. The preferred agent for achieving local accommodation is phospholine iodide, and an effective regimen is given in Table 5.2. The reduction in strength and frequency of application depends on the effectiveness of the regimen and the maintenance of binocularity as the dose is reduced. In the United Kingdom, phospholine iodide has been withdrawn and therefore the direct-acting parasympathomimetic, pilocarpine, is used as an alternative.

If phospholine iodide is used in this context, it must be borne in mind that the metabolism of any systemically absorbed drug involves pseudocholinesterase, so that children on long-term therapy may have significant depletion of their red blood cell levels of this enzyme. Such

TABLE 5.2   A pharmacologic regimen for the management of high AC:A ratio convergence-excess esotropia*

Phospholine iodide	*Pilocarpine*
0.12% twice daily	4% four times per day
0.06% twice daily	2% four times per day
0.06% daily	2% twice daily

*Reduction should be continued if binocular single vision is retained. Convert to surgical management if quality of stereopsis deteriorates. Each agent should be given for 2 months.

a depletion becomes important if the child receives succinylcholine as a relaxant during the course of general anesthesia. The failure to metabolize succinylcholine will lead to a delayed recovery of spontaneous respiration (scoline apnea), and the anesthetist needs to be forewarned of this hazard (Kinyon, 1969). The parents should also be warned about local ocular problems, including discomfort and, occasionally, iris cysts.

The aim of either optical or pharmacologic therapy is to establish binocular single vision and to maintain it as therapy is withdrawn slowly. The long-term use of pilocarpine or phospholine iodide is not acceptable, but ophthalmologists' views of long-term bifocal use vary. Concern has been expressed (Mein and Tremble, 1991) about the long-term effect of bifocals on accommodative ability. Because of this, I regard failing stereopsis as the bifocal segment is weakened to be an indication for surgical intervention to reduce the AC:A ratio.

Surgical Management

Because of failure to tolerate or failure to comply with nonsurgical correction, surgical intervention in high AC:A ratio esotropia may become necessary. The surgery should be concentrated on the medial recti muscles since they are the main determinant of ocular alignment during near fixation.

Recession of each medial rectus muscle is the most commonly performed surgical procedure, the amount of recession being dictated by the size of the deviation for *near*. However, with large recessions of 5 mm or more, there is a small danger of inducing a divergence for distance fixation. For that reason, if the near deviation exceeds the distance deviation by more than 25 prism diopters, it may be better to perform a small bilateral medial rectus muscle recession and combine that with a posterior fixation or Faden suture (Helveston, 1986). A Faden suture inhibits the function of the muscle as the eye rotates into the field of action of that muscle and is thus helpful in reducing deviations in one position of gaze (i.e., for near fixation) without altering the primary position distance alignment.

MANAGEMENT OF PARTIALLY ACCOMMODATIVE ESOTROPIA

In a 1992 study of acquired childhood esotropia, 17 of 118 patients fell into the category of partially accommodative, on the basis that their angle of deviation was reduced by at least 10 prism diopters but not eliminated by the use of a hypermetropic spectacle prescription (Keenan and Willshaw, 1992). In dealing with such children, the first priority is to ensure that the hypermetropic refractive error is fully corrected. Occasionally, a slightly increased prescription will effect full control of the deviation. If this fails, then the diagnosis is confirmed, and the aim of treatment must be to eliminate both barriers to sensory and motor fusion—that is, amblyopia and esotropia.

The mean age at presentation of partially accommodative esotropia is 36 months (Keenan and Willshaw, 1992), which is well within the sensitive period for the treatment of strabismic amblyopia (Hubel and Wiesel, 1970). Careful attention to amblyopia therapy should yield a good visual response, and this, in turn, increases the likelihood of a "favorable outcome" following surgery (in terms of both binocular functions and stable ocular alignment). The choice of surgical procedure to correct the esotropia will be guided by personal preference and experience. Commonly, either a unilateral medial rectus muscle recession with resection of the ipsilateral lateral rectus muscle or bilateral medial rectus recessions will be used. As mentioned in connection with esotropia and ocular disease, if dense amblyopia persists despite rigorous attempts to relieve it, then it is wise to concentrate surgery on the amblyopic eye.

The amount of surgery performed will depend on the size of the deviation and the surgical objective. Where amblyopia has been eliminated and the surgeon believes the prospects for binocular single vision are good, then the goal of surgery should be full correction of the deviation or even a small (less than 10 prism diopters) intentional overcorrection (Danker et al., 1978). If the prospects for binocular single vision are perceived as being poor, most surgeons would aim for a small undercorrection leaving 10.00 D of residual esotropia, which is cosmetically acceptable and offers some protection against late consecutive divergence.

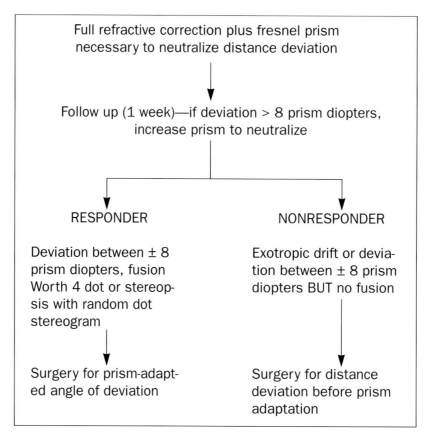

FIGURE 5.2   *Prism adaptation test.*

Evidence from a multicenter, prospective study has demonstrated that determination of the size of deviation to be corrected is best achieved using the prism adaptation test (Prism Adaptation Study Research Group, 1990). This exemplary study demonstrated that not only will a preoperative prism adaptation test regularly reveal a larger angle of deviation than a prism cover test in the clinic, but also that surgery performed to deal with this larger prism-adapted angle yields a much higher incidence of accurate alignment and postoperative binocular single vision. On the basis of this information, any child with equal vision undergoing surgery for an acquired esotropia and old enough to cooperate with the test would appear likely to benefit from a preoperative period of prism adaptation (Figure 5.2).

Keenan and Willshaw (1992) have shown that the best chance of "favorable outcome" is ocular alignment within 15 P.D. of orthotropia 3–6 months after surgery. Failure to achieve this goal should indicate that another surgery is necessary within 6 months of the initial procedure. The second procedure will be dictated to some extent by the first, so that residual esotropia following a bimedial recession will require a bilateral lateral rectus muscle resection, whereas if the initial procedure were a unilateral recession and resection, further recession and resection on the fellow eye is usually indicated. Once again, it is necessary to proceed cautiously where binocular single vision is not the anticipated long-term outcome. A high incidence of late consecutive exotropia may be the cost of overaggressive management.

PROGNOSIS

This group of disorders, if treated sufficiently early in the generation of the esotropia, carries a generally good prognosis. It has been emphasized throughout this chapter that the disorders occur in children most at risk of developing amblyopia, and at all stages in the management this risk has to be borne in mind (Parks, 1986).

Those children with fully accommodative esotropia should retain good-quality stereopsis with refractive correction and are at risk of deteriorating binocularity only when compliance is poor and the strabismus is allowed to deteriorate into a partially accommodative deviation.

In children with high AC:A esotropia, the outlook is again good. Of 24 children followed for a median duration of 46 months (and in no case less than 2 years) following surgical treatment for a high AC:A ratio esotropia, all had a "favorable" outcome. Those children who were initially straight in the distance had a greater chance of developing good-quality stereopsis than those who, at first presentation, were convergent for distance but showed an increase in that convergence for near.

Children with partially accommodative esotropia have the poorest prognosis, and even so, 70% of the children in this series showed either motor fusion alone or stereopsis.

The relatively good prognosis associated with assiduous attention to amblyopia therapy, coupled with elimination of the esotropia, should be used to encourage children and parents to cooperate with what can be a prolonged management course.

REFERENCES

Baker JD, Parks MM. Early onset accommodative esotropia. Am J Ophthalmol 1980;90:11–18.

Breinin GM, Chin NB. Accommodation, convergence and aging. Doc Ophthalmol 1973;34:109–121.

Costenbader FD. Clinical Course and Management of Esotropia. In JH Allen (ed), Strabismus Ophthalmic Symposium 11. St. Louis: Mosby, 1958.

Danker SR, Mash AJ, Jampolsky A. Intentional surgical overcorrection of acquired esotropia. Arch Ophthalmol 1978;96:1848–1852.

Flynn JT. Strabismus: A Neurodevelopmental Approach. New York: Springer-Verlag, 1991.

Helveston EM. Accommodative Esotropia. In JS Crawford (ed), Pediatric Ophthalmology and Strabismus. Transactions of the New Orleans Academy of Ophthalmology. New York: Raven, 1986;111–118.

Hubel DH, Wiesel TN. The period of susceptibility to the physiological effects of unilateral eye closure in kittens. J Physiol (Lond) 1970;206:419–436.

Ingram RM, Walker C, Wilson JM et al. Prediction of amblyopia and squint by means of refraction at age 1 year. Br J Ophthalmol 1986;70:12–15.

Judge SJ, Miles FA. Gain Changes in Accommodative Vergence Induced by Alteration of the Effective Interocular Separation. In AF Fuchs, W Becker (eds), Progress in Oculomotor Research. New York: Elsevier, 1980;587–594.

Keenan JM, Willshaw HE. The outcome of strabismus surgery in childhood esotropia. Eye 1993;7:341–345.

Kinyon GE. Anticholinesterase eye drops—need for caution [letter]. N Engl J Med 1969;280:53.

Leigh JP, Zee DS. Vergence Eye Movements. In The Neurology of Eye Movements. Philadelphia: FA Davis, 1991;262–290.

Mash AJ, Hegmann JP, Spivey BE. Genetic analysis of vergence measurements in populations with varying incidences of strabismus. Am J Ophthalmol 1975;79:978–984.

Mein J, Tremble R. Esotropia. In J Mein, R Tremble (eds), Diagnosis and Management of Ocular Motility Disorders (2nd ed). Cambridge, MA: Blackwell, 1991;217.

Moore AT. Refraction of Infants and Young Children. In D Taylor (ed), Pediatric Ophthalmology. Cambridge, MA: Blackwell, 1990;67–68.

Parks MM. Abnormal accommodative convergence in squint. Arch Ophthalmol 1958;59:364–380.

Parks MM. Management of acquired esotropia. Br J Ophthalmol 1974;58:240–247.

Parks MM. Monocular and Binocular Vision: Expectations in Treatment of Strabismus. In JS Crawford (ed), Pediatric Ophthalmology and Strabismus. Transactions of the New Orleans Academy of Ophthalmology. New York: Raven, 1986;431–448.

Prism Adaptation Study Research Group. Efficacy of prism adaptation in the surgical management of acquired esotropia. Arch Ophthalmol 1990;108:1248–1256.

Rosenbaum AL, Bateman JB, Bremer DL. Cycloplegic refraction in esotropic children. Cyclopentolate versus atropine. Ophthalmology 1981;88:1031–1034.

Sloan LL, Sears ML, Jablonski MD. Convergence accommodation relationships. Arch Ophthalmol 1960;63:283–288.

von Noorden GK. Binocular Vision and Ocular Motility: Theory and Management of Strabismus (2nd ed). St. Louis: Mosby, 1980;91–95, 395–396.

von Noorden GK, Avilla CW. Non-accommodative convergence excess. Am J Ophthalmol 1986;101:70–73.

6

Duane's Retraction Syndrome

David S. I. Taylor and Richard Gregson

ETIOLOGY

Duane's syndrome is an abnormality of eye movements in which one eye usually has markedly limited abduction and variably reduced adduction. The syndrome has been estimated to account for up to 1% of patients with strabismus (Kirkham, 1970a; White and Lee, 1991). In patients with Duane's syndrome, when adduction is attempted, there is marked narrowing of the palpebral fissure on the affected side as well as widening of the palpebral fissure upon regaining the primary position or upon attempted abduction. Affected patients usually retain good vision in each eye with binocular single vision, but also with suppression of the affected eye on lateral gaze. Most patients are remarkably asymptomatic, and their odd eye movements are often noticed only by others. Amblyopia is unusual despite the often marked limitation of voluntary eye movements. Diplopia is also rare. Patients with Duane's syndrome appear to be able to suppress vision in one eye in specific directions of gaze and to have excellent binocular single vision in other directions.

The syndrome is named after Alexander Duane (1858–1926), who published a comprehensive review of the literature of this condition (Duane, 1905), giving credit to earlier authors (Stilling, 1887; Turk, 1898). Some authors prefer to call the condition Stilling-Turk-Duane syndrome. It is a congenital condition. Duane's syndrome is often bilateral (Alexander, 1963; Rowe et al., 1991) but very asymmetric, so its bilaterality may be overlooked (Figure 6.1).

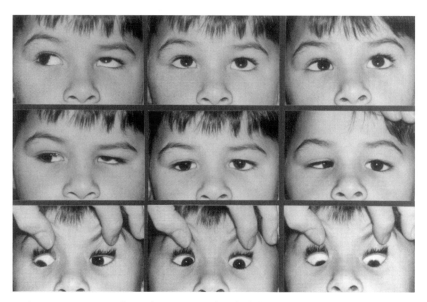

FIGURE 6.1   *Duane's syndrome may often be bilateral. Note its presence in both eyes in this patient.*

Duane concluded that a tight, fibrotic lateral rectus muscle could produce the features of the syndrome, except for the vertical movements, which he concluded were due to inferior oblique tightening because of the retraction of the globe into the orbit. At surgery, the lateral rectus muscle is indeed found to be tight, but when it became possible to measure the electrical activity in the lateral rectus muscle of awake adults, it was found that there was paradoxical firing of the muscle when adduction was attempted, as if the lateral rectus muscle were innervated like a medial rectus (Huber, 1974). Histologic study of postmortem cases shows that twigs from the third nerve innervate the lateral rectus muscle, while the sixth nerve and its nucleus are absent (Hotchkiss et al., 1980; Miller et al., 1982).

Several workers used electromyography (EMG) to investigate the extraocular muscles in awake adult patients with Duane's syndrome (Blodi et al., 1964; Breinin, 1957; Holzman et al., 1990). These EMG recordings revealed the paradoxical activity of the extraocular muscle of the affected eye, the lateral rectus muscle contracting during abduction, and adduction of the eye. The syndrome is now thought to be a congenital misinnervation of the lateral rectus muscle by branches of the third nerve (Hotchkiss et al., 1980), with the lateral rectus muscle contracting on attempted adduction (Hoyt and Nachtigaller, 1965). Co-contraction of both the lateral and medial recti muscles upon adduction is thought to produce the retraction of the globe that is so characteristic of Duane's syndrome. In 1974,

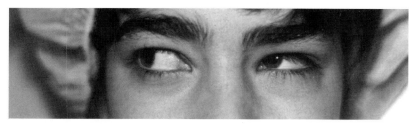

A

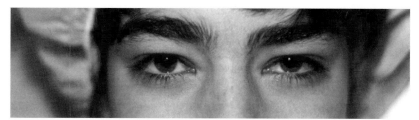

B

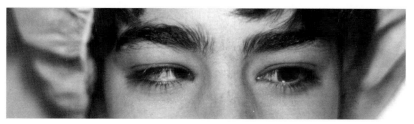

C

FIGURE 6.2 *A. This woman shows the most common variation of Duane's syndrome. Left eye adduction causes enophthalmos, and abduction is deficient. She was concerned by enophthalmos. B, C. Simultaneous left medial and lateral rectus muscle recession (6 and 8 mm) eliminated most of the enophthalmos without affecting eye movements.*

Huber divided the syndrome into three categories based on electromyographic findings:

1. Type 1: markedly deficient abduction but almost normal adduction and marked narrowing of the palpebral fissure on adduction (Figure 6.2).
2. Type 2: normal abduction but adduction is deficient, with an exotropia of the affected eye. Narrowing of the palpebral fissure occurs upon attempted adduction (Figure 6.3).
3. Type 3: limitation of adduction and abduction. Narrowing of the palpebral fissure also occurs upon attempted adduction.

It appears, from the EMG recordings, that this division into three subcategories is not based on a difference in etiology, nor necessarily of management, but merely in the degree to which the lateral rectus muscle attempts to behave like a medial rectus muscle, and the degree to

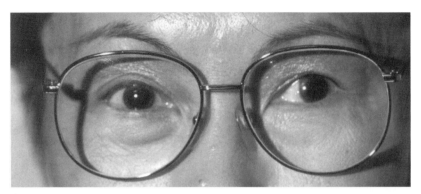

A

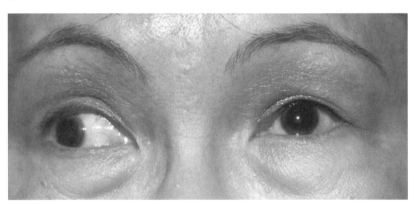

B

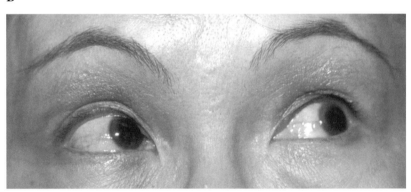

C

FIGURE 6.3   *A. A patient with an exotropia type of Duane's syndrome. Note the left exotropia in gaze straight ahead. B. Her eye adducts poorly and adduction causes enophthalmos. C. Left gaze is nearly normal. She was asymptomatic.*

which the lateral rectus muscle is also fibrotic or otherwise mechanically abnormal due to its misinnervation. If the lateral rectus muscle is fibrotic and contracts only a little, then it is classified as type 1. If the lateral rectus muscle is able to contract and is only partially misinnervated, contracting on both abduction and adduction, it is type 2. If the lateral rectus muscle is able to contract but does so only on adduction, it is type 3. Huber's subclassification is rather difficult to remember so is not often used. Most ophthalmologists, rather than attempting to categorize Duane's syndrome, describe instead the patient's ocular motility defects and will talk of "typical" (Huber's type 1) or "atypical" (all the others) Duane's syndromes.

It is not known why the lateral rectus muscle is misinnervated. Although usually sporadic, Duane's syndrome can be familial—that is, inherited in an autosomal-dominant way (Kirkham, 1970a; Sevel and Kassar, 1974). Most patients with the syndrome, however, have no family history and no other abnormality of their central nervous system (Pfaffenbach et al., 1972), and in them the syndrome probably represents the sequelae of a single insult to the developing brain in utero. Thirty to fifty percent of patients with Duane's syndrome have other congenital anomalies, however subtle. Abnormalities in brain stem auditory-evoked potentials (Jay and Hoyt, 1980) or the association of congenital "crocodile tears" (Ramsey and Taylor, 1980) have been taken as evidence for the anatomic site of the abnormality being in the brain stem. The related abnormalities appear to be of structures that develop between the fourth and eighth weeks of gestation (Huber, 1974; Hughes et al., 1991; Sevel and Kassar, 1974; Pfaffenbach et al., 1972). Sometimes the insult to the embryo may be known; for instance, Duane's syndrome is common in patients with thalidomide embryopathy (Miller and Stromland, 1991) and has been described in association with fetal alcohol syndrome (Holzman et al., 1990).

DIAGNOSIS

The six cardinal features of Duane's syndrome are:

1. Retraction of the globe on adduction
2. Variably reduced adduction
3. Completely or greatly reduced abduction
4. Sometimes, a sharply oblique up or down movement of the affected eye on adduction (Figure 6.4)
5. Partial closure of the eyelids on adduction
6. Paresis or reduction of convergence of the affected eye

Pfaffenbach and colleagues (1972) and Isenberg and Blechman (1983) examined a large number of patients with Duane's syndrome and recorded their other developmental abnormalities, including:

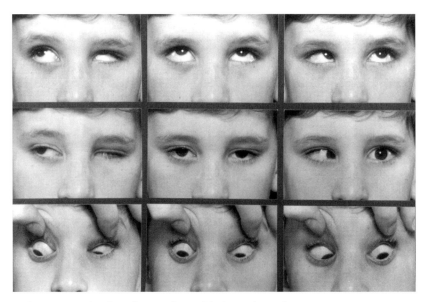

FIGURE 6.4   *Upshoot in a patient with Duane's syndrome.*

Ocular Abnormalities
Nystagmus
Epibulbar dermoids
Anisocoria
Ptosis
Microphthalmos
Prominent epicanthal folds
Persistent hyaloid artery
Ectropion of the lower lid
Myelinated nerve fibers

Auditory Abnormalities
Sensorineural deafness
Preauricular skin tags
Malformed pinnae
Hypoplastic external ear canal
Anomalous ossicles

Central Nervous System Abnormalities
Epilepsy
Hypotonia
Congenital facial palsy
Cerebellar dysgenesis

Skeletal Abnormalities
Abnormalities of the vertebral column
Rib anomalies
Radioulnar synostosis

Genitourinary Abnormalities
Renal agenesis
Bifid ureters
Atrophic testicles
Bladder exstrophy

Skin Abnormalities
Lipomas
Hemangiomas
Café-au-lait spots

Although this list is long, the incidence of each one of these abnormalities in patients with Duane's syndrome is low. The only common association is sensorineural deafness, which occurs in 16% of patients (Parks, 1975); the next most common are minor ocular anomalies of various kinds, which occur in about 8% of patients (Pfaffenbach et al., 1972).

One syndrome of which Duane's syndrome is a part is Wildervank's syndrome (Elsas, 1991; Hughes et al., 1991; Fraser and MacGillivray, 1968), in which the eye movement abnormalities accompany the Klippel-Fiel anomaly, deafness, and mirror movements of the fingers. Wildervank's syndrome is probably inherited in an X-linked dominant way. Duane's syndrome may also be associated with Goldenhar's syndrome (Miller et al., 1989). An association with ipsilateral jaw-winking synkinesis has also been described (Isenberg and Blechman, 1983; Willshaw and Al-Ashkar, 1983).

DIFFERENTIAL DIAGNOSIS
In practicality, sixth nerve palsy figures into the differential diagnosis. Sixth nerve palsy usually is characterized by deviation in primary gaze greater than 30 prism diopters and by a V pattern (due to the greater strength of the unopposed medial rectus muscle in downgaze). There should be no restriction of adduction or enophthalmos on adduction in sixth nerve palsy. Patients with Duane's syndrome may be able to abduct the involved eye in extreme upgaze or downgaze, a finding not seen in sixth nerve palsy.

Duane's syndrome can be simulated by other acquired disease, though rarely (Freeman, 1987; Kivlin and Lundergan, 1985; Timms et al., 1989). These are not what Duane described and differ in etiology, so should be referred to as "Duane-like" or "pseudo-Duane" (Timms et al., 1989). A medial orbit wall blowout fracture, entrapping the medial rectus muscle, could limit abduction, for example. The diagnosis would usually be obvious on other grounds (constant enophthalmos, history of trauma).

MANAGEMENT

It is important to make the diagnosis of Duane's syndrome as soon as possible and to explain the situation to the patient and parents. Eye movement examinations are part of any routine general or neurologic examination, and any physician who is called on to treat the patient in the future may be unnecessarily alarmed by the abnormal ocular motility, unless the patient is able to explain the situation. The best way to establish the diagnosis of Duane's syndrome is by a careful clinical examination of the eye movements and testing of cranial nerve function. In patients with a large-angle esotropia, Duane's syndrome may be masked by the strabismus and become obvious only after successful strabismus surgery (Elsas, 1991). Further studies, such as computed tomography or magnetic resonance imaging (MRI), are unhelpful and are not indicated merely to establish the diagnosis. A full ocular examination is mandatory but usually fails to reveal any other abnormality. Electromyography of the extraocular muscles would be characteristic and therefore diagnostic, but there is no clinical need for this invasive procedure outside of specific research.

Sensorineural deafness occurs in 16% of patients with Duane's syndrome (Parks, 1975; Ro et al., 1990), and the patient may need to be referred for audiometric assessment.

INDICATIONS FOR SURGERY

The majority of patients with Duane's syndrome do not have much in the way of symptoms and do not require surgical intervention. It is enough to reassure them and their parents that the condition is not normally progressive and to emphasize that it is not possible to give them normal eye movements. A refractive error is common (Kirkham, 1970b) and, if present, is more likely to result in amblyopia than is Duane's syndrome itself. The role of anisometropia in causing amblyopia has been discussed by Tredici and von Noorden (1985). It is important to determine the degree of stereopsis present. These patients usually have normal stereoacuity in the primary position or when they are adopting their head posture.

The principal indication for surgery is to improve a cosmetically unacceptable head posture. Usually the head is turned to the side of the eye having the restricted abduction, and improving the abduction of this eye allows the patient to adopt a more normal head posture (Fells and McCarry, 1987; Kraft, 1988; Lyle and Wybar, 1967). Occasionally, the vertical upshoots or downshoots that accompany attempts at horizontal eye movement can be a cosmetic problem, and these, too, can be helped with surgery (Kraft, 1988; von Noorden, 1992).

Surgical guidelines for Duane's syndrome are twofold. First, resection should not be contemplated—the eye muscles are already tight in patients with Duane's syndrome, so only recessions should be used. Second, surgery should not be contemplated for a patient over the age of 8 years without careful consideration (Fells and McCarry, 1987). The reason for this is that the patient develops a complex system of suppression in various directions of gaze by age 8 years, and surgery may disrupt this suppression and cause diplopia. It is better, then, to operate on these patients while their visual system remains plastic, if they require surgery at all.

Temporal Transposition of Vertical Muscles

In an attempt to improve abduction and thereby reduce the head posture, temporal transfer of vertical recti muscles has been performed (Fells and McCarry, 1987; Gobin, 1974), but most authors specifically advise against this procedure, because, in general, it does not increase abduction very much and it may further reduce adduction (Lyle and Wybar, 1967; Parks, 1975) and worsen enopthalmos.

Medial Rectus Recession

Recession of the ipsilateral medial rectus muscle will enable the affected eye to lie more in the primary position but will not help much in improving the poor abduction, because the lateral rectus muscle only contracts on attempted adduction (instead of attempted abduction).

Simultaneous recession of the contralateral medial rectus muscle (i.e., bilateral medial rectus recessions) often effects reduced head posture. Recessing the contralateral medial rectus muscle in incomplete cases of Duane's syndrome results in an increase in the drive to the ipsilateral lateral rectus muscle, by Hering's law, and so can produce better abduction. Another reason for performing medial rectus recessions bilaterally is that Duane's syndrome itself is often bilateral (Rowe et al., 1991), albeit asymmetric. Careful examination usually reveals that the "normal" eye has slightly restricted abduction. During surgery, the medial rectus muscle is found to be tight.

Management of Upshoots and Downshoots

The upshoots and downshoots of the affected eye in Duane's syndrome can be problematic. They can be very obvious, because white sclera shows in the palpebral fissure when the patient attempts to gaze away from the affected eye. Many ophthalmologists believe that the cause is a tight lateral rectus that slides over the globe when the eye adducts (von Noorden, 1992). This may cause an upshoot or downshoot, depending on which way the lateral rectus muscle goes. The evidence for this theory is that the vertical movements tend to occur in patients with a large degree of retraction of the globe, and that the movements tend to be less obvious at birth, rather, developing through childhood. Progressive fibrosis of the poorly contracting lateral rectus muscle would explain these features, and by extension, recession of the lateral rectus muscle helps both the retraction and the upshoots and downshoots (von Noorden, 1992). Restriction of the movement of the lateral rectus muscle by a Faden suture may also be helpful (Burke et al., 1990), although this approach is not often recommended because the Faden suture for a lateral rectus muscle has to be placed in sclera almost overlying the macular region of the underlying retina. The macula may be damaged if the suture is too deep. Another procedure that has been described is the splitting of the lateral rectus muscle into a Y-shaped insertion (Rogers and Bremer, 1984).

The vertical movements may also be caused by misinnervation of the vertical recti muscles. Huber (1974) found in his EMG studies that the vertical recti muscles contracted on attempted adduction. MRI of the orbit in one patient with Duane's syndrome failed to show the lateral rectus muscle sliding over the globe (Bloom et al., 1991). However, the MRI images are probably not sensitive enough to detect tiny movements of a tight lateral rectus muscle, which may be enough to generate a large perturbation in the position of the globe. If there is a progressively increasing vertical deviation of the eye as it is adducted, then it is likely that there is misinnervation of one or the other vertical recti muscles, whereas if the eye begins to adduct normally and then suddenly shoots up or down, then the cause is more likely to be a leash effect of the lateral rectus muscle (Kraft, 1988; Ohtsuki et al., 1992).

It may be possible to distinguish these two kinds of vertical movement clinically, but, if not, then paralyzing the lateral rectus muscle temporarily by injection of botulinum toxin A (White and Lee, 1991) or xylocaine (Kivlin and Lundergan, 1985; Magoon et al., 1982) into the body of the lateral rectus muscle may help. If, once the lateral rectus muscle is paralyzed, the vertical deviations are effectively abolished on adduction, then there must be a leash effect and a recession of the lateral rectus muscle should help abolish the vertical deviations. If, on the other hand, paralysis of the lateral rectus muscle has no effect on the vertical movements of the eye on adduction, then recession of the lateral rectus muscle will not be beneficial and a vertical rectus recession might be considered instead (Kivlin and Lundergan, 1985).

If surgery is to be performed on the vertical recti muscles, after surgery to both horizontal recti muscles, only one vertical rectus muscle should be recessed, because of the risk of anterior segment ischemia. Surgery to the vertical recti muscles should also be delayed for several months after surgery to the horizontal recti muscles. A 3-mm recession of the superior rectus muscle will reduce the upshoot with no effect on the resting position of the eye in the primary position. If further weakening of upgaze is required, a superior rectus Faden suture should be considered. For downshoot, recession of the inferior rectus muscle is helpful, but more than 3 mm of recession of the inferior rectus muscle is not advisable, because this tends to recess the lower lid as well.

Summary

In summary, eye muscle surgery in Duane's syndrome is best restricted to recessions. Recession of the medial rectus muscle tends to help diminish head turn; recession of the lateral rectus helps reduce retraction on adduction and also usually reduces the upshoots or downshoots that may exist. In extreme cases of upshoot or downshoot, recession or fadenization of one vertical rectus muscle can improve cosmesis.

COMPLICATIONS OF SURGERY

If surgery is well planned and carried out early, the outcome is usually very good, with only a small number of patients requiring further surgery. Aside from complications common to all types of strabismus surgery, one complication of surgery for Duane's syndrome is that of overcorrection, with its peculiar characteristics. Adduction of the affected eye (Duane's syndrome) is reduced more than expected for the amount of surgery performed, and exotropia occurs. Paradoxically, abduction remains limited, and the patient shows esotropia. We refer to these phenomena as the "splits," although we do not claim to have coined this expression.

The explanation for the "splits" lies in a change in the innervational tone to extraocular muscles, brought on by surgery. A weakened medial rectus muscle in the involved eye makes it necessary for greater innervation for adduction. Because the lateral rectus muscle is co-innervated, it receives comparably greater innervation. Adduction may actually trigger abduction, resulting in exotropia.

Prevention is the best treatment. The "splits" are likely to occur with unconventionally large recessions (>7 mm) and in the setting where some degree of exotropia already exists in adduction (preoperatively) or where there is marked enophthalmos on adduction, implying marked co-innervation of the lateral rectus muscle.

The "splits" will not spontaneously resolve after surgery. If exotropia is present in primary gaze, partial or complete readvancement of the recessed medial rectus muscle is a reasonable course of action.

REFERENCES

Alexander CM. Bilateral Duane's retraction syndrome. Am J Ophthalmol 1963;60:907–910.

Blodi FC, van Allen MW, Yarborough JC. Duane's syndrome: A brain stem lesion. Arch Ophthalmol 1964;72:171–177.

Bloom JB, Graviss R, Mardelli P. A magnetic resonance imaging study of the upshoot-downshoot phenomenon of Duane's retraction syndrome. Am J Ophthalmol 1991;111:548–554.

Breinin GM. Electromyography—a tool in ocular and neurologic diagnosis: II. Muscle palsies. Arch Ophthalmol 1957;57:165–175.

Burke JP, Orton HP, Strachan IM. Up- and downshoots in Duane's retraction syndrome treated by lateral rectus Faden operation. Br J Ophthalmol 1990;47:41–43.

Duane A. Congenital deficiency of abduction, associated with impairment of adduction, retraction movements, contraction of the palpebral fissure and oblique movements of the eye. Arch Ophthalmol 1905;34:1233–1259.

Elsas F. Occult Duane's syndrome: Co-contraction revealed following strabismus surgery. J Pediatr Ophthalmol Strabismus 1991;28:328–335.

Fells PF, McCarry B. Surgical Options in Duane's Retraction Syndrome. In M Lenk-Schafer, C Calcutt, M Doyle (eds), Transactions of the Sixth International Orthoptics Congress 1987;438–441.

Fraser WI, MacGillivray RC. Cervico-oculo-acoustic dysplasia (the syndrome of Wildervanck). J Ment Defic Res 1968;12:322–329.

Freeman CF. Acquired Duane's retraction syndrome. Br Orthop J 1987;44:70–76.

Gobin M. Surgical management of Duane's syndrome. Br J Ophthalmol 1974;58:301–306.

Holzman A, Chrousos G, Kozma G, Traboulsi E. Duane's retraction syndrome in the fetal alcohol syndrome. Am J Ophthalmol 1990;110:564–565.

Hotchkiss MG, Miller NR, Clark AW, Green WR. Bilateral Duane retraction syndrome: A clinical pathologic case report. Arch Ophthalmol 1980;98:870–874.

Hoyt WF, Nachtigaller I. Anomalies of ocular motor nerves: Neuroanatomical correlation of paradoxical innervation in Duane's syndrome and related congenital ocular motor diseases. Am J Ophthalmol 1965;60:443–448.

Huber A. Electrophysiology of the retraction syndromes. Br J Ophthalmol 1974;58:293–300.

Hughes PJ, Davies PT, Roche SW et al. Wildervanck or cervico-oculo-acoustic syndrome and MRI findings. J Neurol Neurosurg Psychiatry 1991;54:503–504.

Isenberg S, Urist MJ. Clinical observations in 101 consecutive patients with Duane's syndrome. Am J Ophthalmol 1977;84:419–424.

Isenberg S, Blechman B. Marcus Gunn jaw winking and Duane retraction syndrome. J Pediatr Ophthalmol Strabismus 1983;2:235–237.

Jay W, Hoyt CS. Abnormal brainstem auditory evoked responses in Stilling-Turk-Duane syndrome. Am J Ophthalmol 1980;89:814–818.

Kirkham TH. Inheritance of Duane's syndrome. Br J Ophthalmol 1970(a);54:323.

Kirkham TH. Anisometropia in Duane's syndrome. Am J Ophthalmol 1970(b);69:774–777.

Kivlin JD, Lundergan MK. Acquired retraction syndrome associated with orbital metastasis. J Pediatr Ophthalmol Strabismus 1985;22:109–112.

Kraft SP. A surgical approach for Duane syndrome. J Pediatr Ophthalmol Strabismus 1988;25:119–130.

Lyle TK, Wybar KC. In Practical Orthoptics in the Treatment of Squint (5th ed). London: HK Lewis, 1967;575.

Magoon E, Cruciger M, Scott AB et al. Diagnostic injection of xylocaine into extra-ocular muscles. Ophthalmology 1982;89:489–491.

Miller GR, Glaser JS. The retraction syndrome and trauma. Arch Ophthalmol 1966;76:662–663.

Miller NR, Kiel SM, Green WR, Clark AW. Unilateral Duane's retraction syndrome (type 1). Arch Ophthalmol 1982;100:1468–1472.

Miller MT, Ray V, Owens P, Chen F. Möbius' and Möbius-like syndrome. J Pediatr Ophthalmol Strabismus 1989;26:176–188.

Miller MT, Stromland K. Ocular motility in thalidomide embryopathy. J Pediatr Ophthalmol Strabismus 1991;28:47–54.

Ohtsuki H, Hasebe S, Tadozoro Y et al. Synoptometer analysis of vertical shoot in Duane's retraction syndrome. Ophthalmologica 1992;204:82–87.

Papst W, Esslen E. Zur aetiologie der angeborenen abduzenslahmung. Klin Monatsbl Augenheilkd 1960;137:306–327.

Parks MM. Ocular Motility and Strabismus. Hagerstown, MD: Harper & Row, 1975;167.

Pfaffenbach DD, Cross HE, Kearns TP. Congenital anomalies in Duane's syndrome. Arch Ophthalmol 1972;88:635–639.

Ramsey J, Taylor D. Congenital crocodile tears: A key to the aetiology of Duane's syndrome. Br J Ophthalmol 1980;64:518–522.

Ro A, Chernoff G, MacRae D et al. Auditory function in Duane's syndrome. Am J Ophthalmol 1990;109:75–78.

Rogers GL, Bremer DL. Surgical treatment of the upshoot and downshoot in Duane's retraction syndrome. Ophthalmology 1984;91:1380–1383.

Rowe FJ, Wong ML, MacEwen CJ. Duane's retraction syndrome—bilateral until proved otherwise. Br Orthop J 1991;48:36–48.

Sevel D, Kassar BS. Bilateral Duane's syndrome: Occurrence in three generations. Arch Ophthalmol 1974;91:492–494.

Stilling J. Undersuchungen uber die entstehung der kurzsichtigkeit. Wiesbaden: JF Bergman, 1887;13.

Timms C, Russell-Eggitt IM, Taylor D. Simulated (pseudo) Duane's syndrome secondary to orbital myositis. Binoc Vis Quarterly 1989;4:109–112.

Tredici CD, von Noorden GK. Are anisometropia and amblyopia common in Duane's syndrome? J Pediatr Ophthalmol Strabismus 1985;22:23–25.

Turk S. Bemerkungen zu einem falle von retractions bewegung des auges. Zentralb Prakt Augenheilkd 1899;23:14–18.

von Noorden G, Murray E. Up- and downshoot in Duane's retraction syndrome. J Pediatr Ophthalmol Strabismus 1986;23:212–215.

von Noorden G. Recession of both horizontal recti muscles in Duane's retraction syndrome with elevation and depression of the adducted eye. Am J Ophthalmol 1992;114:311–313.

Willshaw HE, Al-Ashkar F. The branchial arch syndromes. Trans Ophthalmol Soc UK 1983;103:331–337.

White JES, Lee JP. Botulinum toxin A in the management of patients with Duane's retraction syndrome. In Transactions of the International Orthoptics Congress 1991;341–345.

White JW, Brown HW. Occurrence of vertical anomalies associated with convergent and divergent anomalies. Arch Ophthalmol 1939;21:999–1009.

7

Möbius' Syndrome

David S. I. Taylor and Richard Gregson

ETIOLOGY

Möbius' syndrome is an unusual condition involving paresis of the cranial nerves along with associated abnormalities, especially of the limbs. The condition is bilateral and congenital. The paresis affects the sixth, seventh, and, often, bulbar cranial nerves (Reed and Grant, 1957).

Ophthalmologists often are asked to confirm the diagnosis in a baby and must ensure that they follow the patient through childhood because of the significance of eye problems.

Möbius' syndrome has generally been regarded as a congenital defect acquired in intrauterine life following an insult occurring between the fourth and fifth weeks of development. In some cases, however, there is clear evidence of a dominant inheritance of the condition (Baraitser, 1977; Dotti et al., 1989; Garcia Erro et al., 1989; MacDermot et al., 1991; Ziter et al., 1977; Slee et al., 1991; Wishnick et al., 1983). Generally, if there are associated limb abnormalities, the case is more likely to be sporadic (Amaya et al., 1990), although dominant inheritance of the combined syndrome has also been reported (Bavinck and Weaver, 1986; Garcia Erro et al., 1989).

The etiology is not clear, but it has been suggested that interruption of the vascular supply is implicated, the deficiency being either genetically determined or due to local accidents in development (Bavinck and Weaver, 1986; Govaert et al., 1989; Legum et al., 1981; Journel et al., 1989). The result is thought to be ischemia, edema, and hypoxia of developing embryonic tissues or the cranial nerves supplied by the affected vessel. In some cases, mineralized deposits form along a

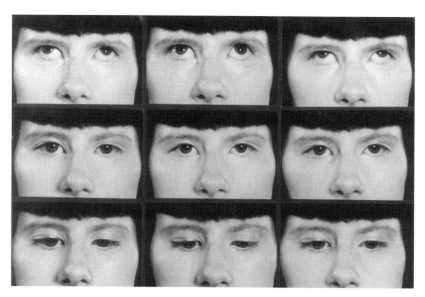

FIGURE 7.1 *Möbius' syndrome. Note that this child has preserved vertical eye movements but bilateral horizontal gaze palsies.*

vascular distribution, and this finding also supports a vascular etiology (D'Cruz et al., 1993). This vascular etiology has been supported by some autopsy findings (Bavinck and Weaver, 1986; Dotti et al., 1989), confirming the idea of a final common pathway for both the sporadic and inherited cases.

DIAGNOSIS

The clinical features present at birth consist of a "flat" facial expression with restricted horizontal extraocular movements and ptosis (Figure 7.1). There is often poor eyelid closure (Figure 7.2).

Although most patients show clear-cut signs of bilateral sixth nerve palsy, nearly half may show a horizontal gaze palsy (Amaya et al., 1990), and many have the appearance of Duane's syndrome (Miller et al., 1989). Vertical movements of the eyes are usually normal. Strabismus may or may not be present (Reed and Grant, 1957), usually an esotropia. Usually these signs are fairly symmetric, but strongly asymmetric cases have been described (Legum et al., 1981; Miller et al., 1989).

Other cranial nerve palsies, particularly bulbar, are usually present (Sudarshan and Goldie, 1985). The affected baby often has feeding difficulties because of the ninth and twelfth nerve palsies. The tongue is usually hypoplastic (Figure 7.3).

Structural abnormalities of the face are common, including micrognathia, dysplastic ears, and defective branchial musculature.

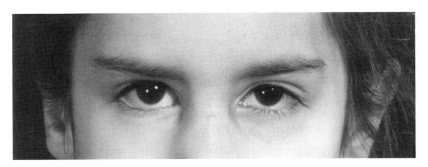

A

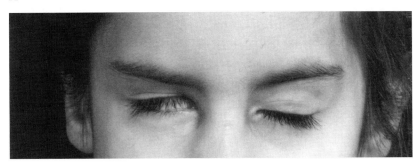

B

FIGURE 7.2 *This child with Möbius' syndrome (A) cannot completely close her eyes (B), due to seventh nerve palsies, which are worse on the right side than on the left.*

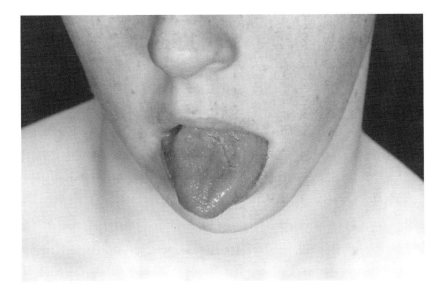

FIGURE 7.3 *The tongue may be hypoplastic in Möbius' syndrome when the twelfth cranial nerve is affected.*

Mild mental retardation has been reported in up to 50% of diagnosed cases (Bavinck and Weaver, 1986; Lipson et al., 1989). The natural history of the condition consists of relatively normal visual development but markedly delayed speech development. If there is a marked strabismus (usually esotropia), amblyopia is common.

The association between restricted horizontal movements of the eyes and facial nerve palsy had been noted in the late 1800s, but Möbius (1888), who classified the different types of ophthalmoplegia, created the separate diagnostic entity that later bore his name. Since then a large number of other congenital abnormalities has been associated with Möbius' syndrome (Legum et al., 1981), especially limb defects (Rogers, 1977; Steigner et al., 1975). Poland's anomaly (syndactyly, shortened phalanges, and ipsilateral absence of all or part of the pectoralis major and the breast) is probably the most common of these (Miller et al., 1989; Sugarman and Stark, 1973; Rojas-Martinez et al., 1991; Mitter and Chudley, 1983). Club foot and tracheal and laryngeal abnormalities have also been reported (Voirin et al., 1991).

MANAGEMENT

The ophthalmic management of Möbius' syndrome first involves assisting the pediatrician in making a correct diagnosis. The unique constellation of physical features limits the differential diagnosis, but congenital myotonic dystrophy, congenital esotropia, congenital sixth nerve palsy, congenital horizontal gaze palsy, and Duane's syndrome all can be confused with this condition. Later, management of the child involves several medical disciplines, as discussed below.

Psychological Management

Careful counseling of the parents is especially important after making the diagnosis of Möbius' syndrome (Amaya et al., 1990). Not only must the appropriate genetic counseling be given, but it must be explained carefully to the parents that the affected child lacks much of the facial expression that a normal infant would show. Their rather blank faces can be interpreted to be a lack of affection, and parents need counseling to overcome this. Appropriate developmental advice and psychologic help need to be provided, and there are parent support groups that will help with this. The development of the patient may be complicated by any other associated congenital abnormalities present.

Language Management

Speech therapy must be commenced early and continued for many years. The presence of the bulbar palsy means that most patients with

Möbius' syndrome do not develop normal speech, although their speech does continue to improve throughout their childhood.

Ophthalmologic Management

The ophthalmologist's specific role is to maximize the affected child's visual potential. Accurate refraction is important, and appropriate amblyopia therapy must be implemented if there is evidence of amblyopia.

Most patients with Möbius' syndrome are incapable of fusional eye movements and are therefore at great risk of strabismic amblyopia. Many patients with Möbius' syndrome have lagophthalmos and must be followed carefully for evidence of corneal exposure. Some of these individuals have reduced corneal sensation as well, and this combination of fifth, sixth, and seventh nerve palsies can produce very severe corneal problems. Corneal protection can be enhanced by asking the parents to instill ointment into the child's eyes at night, or even to tape the child's lids shut during sleep if the condition is very severe. Lid surgery to increase the eye closure is rarely required, but entropion caused by non-functioning orbicularis occasionally necessitates entropion surgery.

SURGERY

Due to the poor eye movements associated with Möbius' syndrome, there is little prospect of obtaining single binocular vision through strabismus surgery. Surgery of the rectus muscles should be contemplated only for cosmetic purposes, and, where indicated, it may be surprisingly successful (Amaya et al., 1990).

At surgery the medial rectus muscles are usually extraordinarily tight, due to the fact that their action has been unopposed throughout the child's life. Rarely, extraocular muscles may be absent (Traboulsi and Maumenee, 1986). Large recessions are required to correct the esotropia. Bilateral, 8- to 9-mm medial rectus recessions will not usually overcorrect the strabismus. Lateral rotations will still be poor, but the cosmetic effect is usually satisfying.

REFERENCES

Amaya LG, Walker J, Taylor D. Möbius' syndrome: A study and report of 18 cases. Binoc Vis Quarterly 1990;5:119–132.

Baraitser M. Genetics of the Möbius' syndrome. J Med Genet 1977;14:415–417.

Bavinck JNB, Weaver DD. Subclavian artery supply disruption sequence: Hypothesis of a vascular etiology for Poland, Klippel-Feil, and Möbius anomalies. Am J Med Genet 1986;23:903–918.

D'Cruz OF, Swisher CN, Jaradeh S et al. Möbius' syndrome: Evidence for a vascular etiology. J Child Neurol 1993;8:260–265.

Dotti MT, Federico A, Palmeri S, Guazzi GC. Congenital oculo-facial paralysis (Möbius' syndrome): Evidence of dominant inheritance in two families. Acta Neurol (Napoli) 1989;11:434–438.

Garcia Erro M, Correale J, Arberas C et al. Familial congenital facial diplegia: Electrophysiologic and genetic studies. Pediatr Neurol 1989;5:262–264.

Govaert P, Vanhaesebrouck P, De Praeter C et al. Möbius' sequence and pre-natal brainstem ischemia. Pediatrics 1989;84:570–573.

Journel H, Roussey M, Le Marec B. MCA/MR syndrome with oligodactyly and Möbius' anomaly in first cousins: New syndrome or familial facial-limb disruption sequence? Am J Med Genet 1989;34:506–510.

Legum C, Godel V, Nemet P. Heterogeneity and pleiotropism in the Möbius' syndrome. Clin Genet 1981;20:254–259.

Lipson T, Webster W, Weaver DD. The Möbius' syndrome: Aetiology, inci-dence of mental retardation, and genetics. J Med Genet 1990;27:533–534 (letter).

Lipson AH, Webster WS, Brown-Woodman PD, Osborn RA. Möbius' syn-drome: Animal model-human correlations and evidence for a brainstem vascular etiology. Teratology 1989;40:339–350.

MacDermot KD, Winter RM, Taylor D, Baraitser M. Oculofacial bulbar palsy in mother and son: Review of 26 reports of familial transmission within the "Möbius spectrum of defects." J Med Genet1991;28:18–26.

Miller MT, Ray V, Owens P, Chen F. Moebius' and Moebius-like syndromes (TTV-OFM, OMLH). J Pediatr Ophthalmol Strabismus 1989;26:176–188.

Mitter NS, Chudley AE. Facial weakness and oligosyndactyly: Independent variable features of familial type of the Möbius' syndrome. Clin Genet 1983;24:350–354.

Moebius PJ. Uber angeborene doppelseitige abducens-facialis-lahmung. Munchen Med Wodhenschr 1888;35:91–94.

Reed H, Grant W. Möbius' syndrome. Br J Ophthalmol 1957;41:731.

Rogers GL. Möbius' syndrome and limb abnormalities. J Pediatr Ophthalmol Strabismus 1977;14:134–138.

Rojas-Martinez A, Garcia-Cruz D, Garcia AR et al. Poland-Möbius syndrome in a boy and Poland syndrome in his mother. Clin Genet 1991;40:225–228.

Slee JJ, Smart RD, Viljoen DL. Deletion of chromosome 13 in Möbius' syn-drome. J Med Genet 1991;28:413–414.

Steigner M, Stewart RE, Setoguchi Y. Combined limb deficiencies and cranial nerve dysfunction: Report of six cases. Birth Defects: Original Article Series 1975;11:133–141.

Sudarshan A, Goldie WD. The spectrum of congenital facial diplegia (Möbius' syndrome). Pediatr Neurol 1985;1:180–184.

Sugarman GI, Stark HH. Möbius' anomaly with Poland's anomaly. J Med Genet 1973;10:192–195.

Traboulsi EI, Maumenee IH. Extraocular muscle aplasia in Möbius' syn-drome. J Pediatr Ophthalmol Strabismus 1986;23:120–122.

Voirin J, Laloum D, Bonte JB et al. Möbius' syndrome associated with pharyngeal and laryngeal paralysis in a premature infant. Arch Fr Pediatr 1991;48:35–38.

Wishnick MM, Nelson LB, Huppert L et al. Möbius' syndrome and limb abnormalities with dominant inheritance. Ophthalmic Paediatr Genet 1983;2:77–81.

Ziter FA, Wiser WC, Robinson A. Three-generation pedigree of a Möbius' syndrome variant with chromosome translocation. Arch Neurol 1977;34:437–442.

III

Exodeviations

8

Exodeviations in the
First Year of Life

ETIOLOGY

This chapter focuses on exotropia in the first year of life, because in babies, constant exotropia may indicate craniofacial or neurologic disease. Given the difficulty of assessing development in very young babies, the surgeon will need to carefully evaluate the attainment of developmental milestones at follow-up visits and make appropriate referrals when necessary.

Upon examination of ocular alignment in neonates, it is evident that up to 60% have a transient constant exodeviation (Archer et al., 1989; Nixon et al., 1985). The incidence of esotropia is very low in neonates, with *intermittent* exotropia accounting for 13% of babies examined and orthotropia accounting for nearly 23%. Although studies on strabismus in babies can be criticized on the basis of not controlling for infant states, these studies still are extremely helpful in demonstrating that many babies have an exodeviation at least some of the time. On the other hand, the presence of esodeviations in infants is extremely uncommon and should suggest the possibility of Duane's syndrome, Möbius' syndrome, or congenital sixth nerve palsy.

Most babies who have exotropia show more than 25 prism diopters of deviation with variability during the examination (Figure 8.1). The majority of children with congenital exotropia show resolution of the strabismus by the age of 6 months. Once a child reaches 6 months of age, the likelihood that the exotropia will diminish sponta-

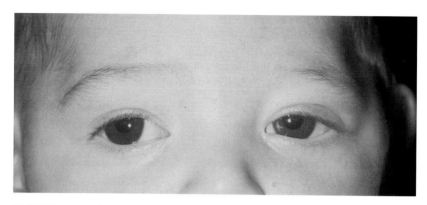

FIGURE 8.1   *This 4-month-old baby suffered herpes simplex encephalitis. A constant head turn to her left is accompanied by a constant exotropia. Confrontational visual field testing indicated a left homonymous hemianopia.*

neously is small, and strabismus management is indicated (Archer and Helveston, 1994).

A link between exotropia and craniofacial anomalies has been well established (Zaki and Kenney, 1957; Nelson et al., 1981; Carruthers, 1988), and therefore, the child with persistent exotropia should be evaluated carefully by the pediatrician for the possibility of an orbital or skull defect. These defects are discussed in Chapter 11. A second reason is that the potential etiology for exotropia is an underlying neurologic disease. For example, exotropia has been reported with homonymous hemianopia (Herzau et al., 1988), and it has been our impression that a variable exotropia frequently accompanies homonymous hemianopia in children of *all* ages (Good et al., 1994). Therefore, the child who presents with exotropia should be evaluated with a confrontational visual field examination for the possibility of a visual field defect (Good et al., 1994).

Other physical findings that suggest homonymous hemianopia in children include a head turn for visual fixation and a specific search strategy for objects of visual interest in the nonseeing visual field. This search strategy involves looking past an object and then centering it with visual fixation with a rapid saccadic eye movement back to the object (Meienberg et al., 1981; Good et al., 1994).

Exotropia in babies may indicate other types of neurologic disease in children, particularly static encephalopathy (cerebral palsy). Once again, the presence of constant exotropia past the age of 6 months is an indication for a very careful pediatric or pediatric neurology examination to exclude the possibility of underlying neurologic abnormalities.

TABLE 8.1 Causes of congenital exotropia

Pseudoexotropia (retinopathy of prematurity)
Vision loss
Oculomotor nerve palsy
Craniofacial anomaly
Neurologic disease (nonlocalizing)
Duane's syndrome
Pure congenital exotropia

Occasionally, exotropia is the result of so-called sensory strabismus. Children respond to asymmetric vision loss or unilateral vision loss by developing either exotropia or esotropia (Sidikaro and von Noorden, 1982). In adults, exotropia will usually develop when unilateral visual loss occurs. A careful, thorough eye examination is always important in cases of childhood strabismus to exclude potentially serious or treatable conditions (e.g., cataract, retinoblastoma).

The possibility of a congenital third nerve palsy should be entertained. Most children with a palsy will show deficiency of elevation, depression, and adduction of the eye. Ptosis may or may not be present. Occasionally, pupil sparing occurs and can cause misinterpretation of an oculomotor nerve palsy (Good et al., 1991).

There is debate as to whether neurologic abnormalities occur in conjunction with congenital third nerve palsies (Balkan and Hoyt, 1984; Hamed, 1991; Miller, 1977). Certainly, enough children have been reported to have other neurologic problems to warrant careful neurologic investigation and possible neuroradiologic evaluation of the child who presents with an exotropia caused by oculomotor nerve palsy.

Exotropia can occur in Duane's syndrome. If, on attempted adduction, the eye abducts almost immediately, it will diverge and cause exotropia. Abduction will still be deficient and result in esotropia when gazing toward the involved eye.

We have emphasized the potential for constant exotropia being caused by some underlying abnormality. Nevertheless, some babies simply show exotropia with no other neurologic or craniofacial defect (Rubin et al., 1988) (Table 8.1).

DIFFERENTIAL DIAGNOSIS

The diagnosis of exotropia is sometimes complicated by the fact that some children show a large-angle kappa, which simulates exotropia (Figure 8.2). If cover testing is possible, the angle kappa nature of an apparent exotropia should be obvious. The penultimate example of

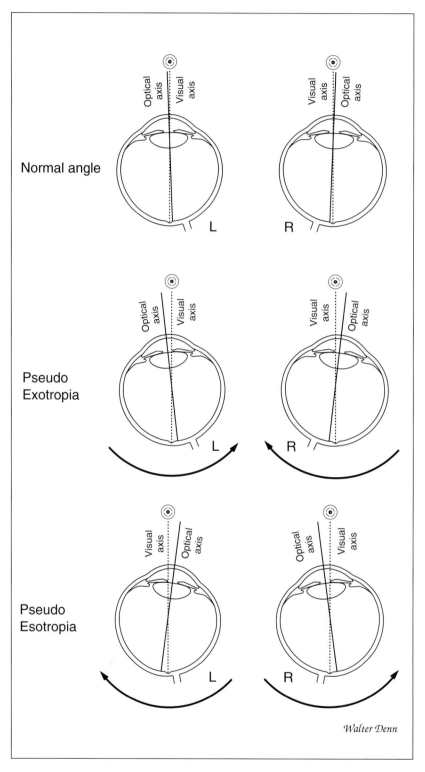

FIGURE 8.2   *A positive-angle kappa simulates exotropia. The visual axis is nasal to and differs substantially from the mid-pupil line direction. In negative-angle kappa, simulating esotropia, the visual axis is temporal to the mid-pupil line.*

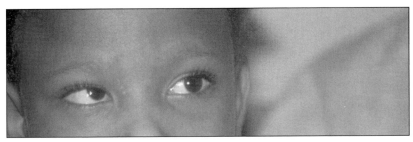

A

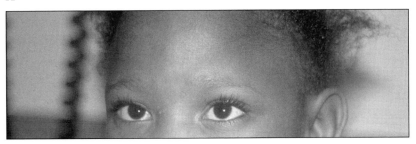

B

FIGURE 8.3   *This 4-year-old girl had bilateral temporally dragged maculae from retinopathy of prematurity. She fixates with a head turn and a positive-angle kappa is present. She has a pseudo-orthotropia (masking an actual esotropia). A. Right eye fixation. B. Left eye fixation.*

positive-angle kappa occurs in children with retinopathy of prematurity and temporal dragging of the macula. The eyes appear divergent, but cover testing indicates no shifting of the eye (Foster et al., 1975). Strabismus can be superimposed on a large-angle kappa (Foster et al., 1975). For example, we have examined a child with bilateral dragging of the macula and good alignment by light reflex testing when not fixating (Figure 8.3). However, she turned her head to fixate due to Ciancia-type esotropia, and then demonstrated the large-angle kappa.

MANAGEMENT

The management of congenital exotropia is similar to the management of congenital esotropia. Exotropia that is noted in the first several months of life should be watched without any particular treatment. Alternating fixation, which implies no amblyopia, is the rule. When exotropia persists beyond 5–6 months of age, intervention may be required.

Congenital exotropia may be accompanied by divergent vertical deviation, oblique muscle overaction, and amblyopia. In our experience, amblyopia is uncommon in congenital exotropia, but congenital exotropia is also very uncommon, so it is difficult to know the real incidence of amblyopia in congenital exotropia. Amblyopia, when present, should be managed in a manner similar to its management in infantile esotropia.

The surgical management of exotropia follows the same course as that for exotropia in older children and adults. First, any signs of amblyopia should be managed. Then, the angle of deviation should be noted and measured as carefully as possible. Once stable measurements are obtained, the exotropia can be treated by strabismus repair, following the guidelines indicated in Chapter 9.

REFERENCES

Archer SM, Helveston EM. Strabismus and Eye Movement Disorders. In Eisenberg SJ (ed), The Eye in Infancy. St. Louis: Mosby, 1994;254–259.

Archer SM, Sondhi N, Helveston EM. Strabismus in infancy. Ophthalmology 1989;96:133–137.

Balkan R, Hoyt CS. Associated neurologic abnormalities in congenital third nerve palsies. Am J Ophthalmol 1984;97:315–319.

Carruthers JD. Strabismus in craniofacial dysostosis. Graefes Arch Clin Exp Ophthalmol 1988;226:230–234.

Foster RS, Metz HS, Jampolsky A. Strabismus and pseudostrabismus. Am J Ophthalmol 1975;79:985–989.

Good WV, Barkovich AJ, Nickel BL, Hoyt CS. Bilateral congenital oculomotor nerve palsy in a child with brain anomalies. Am J Ophthalmol 1991;111:555–558.

Good WV, Jan JE, Barkovich AJ et al. Cortical visual impairment in children. Surv Ophthalmol 1994;38:351–364.

Hamed LM. Associated neurologic and ophthalmic findings in congenital oculomotor nerve palsy. Ophthalmology 1991;98:708–714.

Herzau V, Bleher I, Joos-Kratsch E. Infantile exotropia with homonymous hemianopia: A rare contraindication for strabismus surgery. Graefes Arch Clin Exp Ophthalmol 1988;226:148–149.

Meienberg O, Zangemeister WH, Rosenberg M et al. Saccadic eye movement strategies in patients with homonymous hemianopia. Ann Neurol 1981;9:537–544.

Miller NR. Solitary oculomotor nerve palsy in childhood. Am J Ophthalmol 1977;83:106–111.

Nelson LB, Ingoglia S, Breinin GM. Sensorimotor disturbances in craniostenosis. J Pediatr Ophthalmol Strabismus 1981;18:32–41.

Nixon RB, Helveston EM, Miller K et al. Incidence of strabismus in neonates. Am J Ophthalmol 1985;100:798–801.

Rubin SE, Nelson LB, Wagner RS et al. Infantile exotropia in healthy children. Ophthalmic Surg 1988;19:792–794.

Sidikaro Y, von Noorden GK. Observations in sensory heterotropia. J Ped Ophthalmol Strabismus 1982;19:12–19.

Zaki HAA, Keeney AH. The bony orbital walls in horizontal strabismus. Arch Ophthalmol 1957;57:418–424.

9

Exotropia

The exodeviations can be categorized as exophoria, intermittent exotropia, and constant exotropia. Exophoria denotes a tendency for the visual axes to diverge. This tendency is held in check by fusion, or the use of the eyes together. Intermittent exotropia involves a condition in which the eyes may be diverged at some times but aligned at other times. Constant exotropia describes a condition in which there is continuous divergence of the visual axes.

Exotropia can also be categorized as excess divergence (greater deviation in the distance than at near) or insufficient convergence (greater deviation at near than at distance). Excess divergence deviation is characteristic of intermittent exotropia.

EPIDEMIOLOGY

When the exotropias are grouped together they account for approximately 25% of cases of strabismus in young children (Friedman et al., 1980). Exotropia probably appears within the first few years of life (Cooper and Medow, 1993). In most cases, if left untreated, exotropia progresses throughout the lifespan of the individual. Von Noorden (1990) showed that 75% of cases of exotropia will progress, and that only 9% of cases will not change. The remaining 16% may show improvement over time. Exotropia may begin with exophoria and, with the addition of bitemporal suppression, develop into intermittent and then constant exotropia (Jampolsky, 1954, 1962). The only study that we know of that contradicts the idea that exotropia is progressive was performed by Hiles and associates in 1968. In this study of 48 patients, only 2 actually progressed. The condition of the rest of the patients improved or stayed constant.

Women develop exotropia more commonly than men (Cass, 1937). Most children who have exotropia show refractive errors that are similar to those in age-matched children who do not have strabismus (Bair, 1952; Schlossman and Boruchoff, 1955), despite the perception that refractive errors have a role in causing exotropia.

An interesting relationship between exotropia and exposure to sunlight has been postulated (Eustace et al., 1973; Romano, 1990; MacFarlane, 1960). Intermittent exotropia is more common in latitudes where there are higher levels of sunlight. Sunlight certainly appears to have an effect on intermittent exotropia, because bright illumination often forces patients to close one eye. Indeed, in Australia, constant monocular eyelid closure caused by sunlight has been considered an important indication for surgery (Eustace et al., 1973).

Costenbader (1950) provided data regarding the age of onset of intermittent exotropia. Nearly 50% of intermittent exotropes in his study could be diagnosed at or around the time of birth, and 95% of cases appeared before age 5 years. However, in an important study regarding normal ocular alignment in infants, Sondhi and colleagues (1988) demonstrated that a large number of babies showed intermittent exotropia, yet, when followed past the age of 6 months, they developed ocular alignment. In our experience, the incidence of intermittent exotropia increases at the age of 5 or 6 years, with many children presenting around the time they start school. The exact age of onset is difficult to determine, though.

CRANIOFACIAL ANATOMY

Some cases of exotropia are caused by craniofacial defects. Children who have craniosynostosis are far more likely to show exotropia. But even in cases where no frank craniofacial defect exists, the possibility that exotropia develops from an increased divergent angle of the orbits should be considered (Bielchowsky, 1934). Bielchowsky noted the tendency for a blind or amblyopic eye to become exotropic and ascribed this purely to mechanical factors—e.g., the angle of the orbits in relation to the skull and visual axes.

ABNORMALITIES OF CONVERGENCE AND DIVERGENCE

The possibility that a high accommodation convergence to accommodation (AC:A) ratio could have a role in intermittent exotropia (and excess divergence exotropia) has been discussed at length by Cooper and Medow (1993). These authors present data from von Noorden

(1969), Cooper and co-authors (1982), and Kushner (1988), demonstrating that the AC:A ratio is either normal or just slightly higher than normal in patients who have intermittent exotropia.

It is conceivable, however, that excess lateral rectus muscle activity or diminished medial rectus muscle activity (relaxed convergence) could play a role in some cases of intermittent exotropia. It is clear that the lateral rectus muscle fires during the onset of exotropia (Blodi and Van Allan, 1962), but it is not known whether this excess innervation is the cause or the effect.

ETIOLOGY

Hereditary Defect
A family history of intermittent exotropia can often be found if family members are studied carefully (Burian and Spivey, 1965; Jampolsky, 1962; Parks, 1962). An autosomal-dominant pattern of constant exotropia has been suggested by Brodsky and Fritz (1993), although multifactorial genetic variables cannot be excluded even in their cases.

Hemiretinal Suppression
The possibility of a progression from exophoria to bilateral, bitemporal, hemiretinal suppression to intermittent exotropia has been postulated by Jampolsky (1962, 1954) and Knapp (1953). This theory holds that the ability to suppress temporal vision allows the eye to diverge and may make it difficult to maintain constant ocular alignment. The amount of suppression during divergence may be variable.

Chameleon Theory
Cooper (1977) has proposed the so-called chameleon theory for intermittent exotropia. This theory harkens back to an evolutionary theory of the development of binocularity in vertebrate animals. It is optimal for the eyes to be divergent, thereby giving the animal better panoramic vision when it needs to protect itself. On the other hand, better convergence and bifoveation allow for a better depth perception and may improve tasks that require depth perception. Chameleons have eyes mounted in turret-like protuberances, which can scan independently, then converge to binocularly target an insect in feeding range.

The chameleon theory applies to humans with intermittent exotropia as follows: When relaxed, the eyes are allowed to diverge, but when there are a lot of visual clues and the intermittent exotrope needs to use the eyes together, he or she can augment stereopsis by converging the eyes. Cooper and Medow (1993) explain good stereopsis testing and bifoveation with near work in intermittent exotropes on the basis of better visual cues and greater alertness to near vision tasks.

DIAGNOSIS

Squinting

Many children with intermittent exotropia will close one eye (squint) in bright or direct illumination. There is no completely satisfactory explanation for this finding (Wiggins and von Noorden, 1990). One theory holds that monocular eye closure allows the avoidance of diplopia. Wiggins and von Noorden (1990) discovered that monocular eye closure actually occurs in response to bright light, per se, and occurs before any ocular deviation develops. This finding would suggest that eye closure does not serve the function of allowing an individual to avoid diplopia. Wang and Chryssanthau (1988) found monocular closure much more commonly in patients with normal retinal correspondence, as opposed to anomalous retinal correspondence. They concluded that eye closure may actually be used to avoid diplopia, contrary to the conclusion of Wiggins and von Noorden.

History

Concerning the patient's history of intermittent exotropia it is worth noting that Jampolsky (personal communication) has indicated that a history of intermittent exotropia provided by the patient's parents is usually valid. This is in distinction to histories of esotropia, where the actual examination often indicates a pseudoesotropia.

Strabismus Measurements

Strabismus measurements in intermittent exotropia and exotropia are important and may have some features that require special attention. The first of these is lateral incomitance. Lateral incomitance indicates a limitation in abduction of one eye, thereby reducing the amount of exotropia in lateral gaze, both to the left and to the right. Carlson and Jampolsky (1979) hypothesized that a tight medial rectus muscle could have a role in the etiology and recommended lateral and medial rectus muscle recession as a way of overcoming lateral incomitance. Lateral gaze incomitance has been reported in up to 24% of patients with intermittent exotropia (Moore et al., 1977). Kushner (1988) indicated that perhaps only 5% of exotropes show lateral incomitance. Repka and Arnoldi (1991) indicated that there may be serious flaws in measuring horizontal deviation in lateral gaze, due to the method of placement of the prism in front of the eyes. Measurements may indicate a pseudolateral incomitance when, in fact, the amount of deviation is approximately the same in all horizontal fields of gaze.

The importance of lateral incomitance is this: If it is present, then lateral rectus muscle recessions, which neutralize the deviation in primary gaze, may overcorrect the deviation in left and right gaze. Therefore, the presence of a large amount of lateral incomitance might be an indication for slightly reducing the amount of strabismus surgery that would otherwise be performed.

A second issue in measurements of exotropia has to do with the presence of simultaneous vertical strabismus. Perhaps 50% of patients with intermittent exotropia will show some vertical deviation with distance visual fixation (Dunlap and Gaffney, 1963; Moore et al., 1977). This vertical deviation could be due to superior rectus muscle overaction in the abducted (exotropic), nonfixing eye (Jampolsky, 1986). The vertical deviation may require management if it persists after neutralization (with prisms) of the horizontal deviation.

A and V patterns occur commonly in exotropes. Their diagnosis and management are discussed in Chapter 10. Care should be taken to record strabismus measurements in upgaze and downgaze, as well as in primary gaze.

No one would argue that distance measurements for exotropia should be made and noted using an alternating cover test. However, the best method for making near measurements is debatable (Parks and Mitchell, 1993; Burian and Spivey, 1965). Children will use accommodative convergence to control their exodeviation. They should be asked to fixate on a real symbol (object) at near rather than on a light. This controls accommodative convergence, because the patient must keep the symbol/object in good focus in order to report what it is. Burian and Spivey recommended near measurements through a 3.00+ D lens to control for a high AC:A ratio. Most authorities believe that this maneuver is unnecessary and does not affect management (Parks and Mitchell, 1993).

Finally, it should be noted that the very nature of intermittent exotropia—its intermittency—may pose problems for measurement. Children and adults who are nervous may contain their deviation and show a smaller amount of exotropia than exists under relaxed conditions. It is probably advisable to perform strabismus measurements on more than one occasion and to consider occluding one eye for an hour to allow the true horizontal deviation to emerge.

MANAGEMENT OF INTERMITTENT EXOTROPIA

Amblyopia

Amblyopia is uncommon in intermittent exotropia (Schlossman and Boruchoff, 1955). When it occurs it probably does so in the setting of anisometropia (Moore et al., 1977). Amblyopia management should be undertaken when necessary as a means of restoring vision in the amblyopic eye. The role of amblyopic management in correcting exodeviation is discussed in the next section.

Occlusion

Several investigators have studied the effect of occlusion therapy for the management of unilateral exotropia (Freeman and Isenberg, 1989; Iacobucci and Henderson, 1967; Flynn et al., 1975). Some patients will become orthophoric after part-time occlusion, when exotropia is predominantly unilateral and presumably accompanied by amblyopia (Freeman and Isenberg, 1989). Other patients will show a reduction in the angle of exotropia, possibly indicating an improvement in the ability to control the amount of exotropia (Freeman and Isenberg, 1989). It would certainly seem prudent to manage amblyopia with appropriate occlusion therapy and to monitor the effect on the exotropia in any given patient. Occasionally, exotropia may improve substantially.

Induction of Accommodative Convergence

Deliberately overminusing the prescription for children and young adults who have intermittent exotropia or symptomatic exophoria can be used as a primary means of treating intermittent exotropia as well as managing postoperative undercorrections (Caltrider and Jampolsky, 1983; Iacobucci et al., 1986). The success rate in using minus lenses in the primary management of exotropia may approach 50%. Similarly, when overminus therapy is used for postoperative undercorrections, the success rate also may be approximately 50%.

Prism Therapy

A role for a base-in prism to correct for intermittent exotropia or symptomatic exophoria exists for deviations of approximately 20 prism diopters and less (Pratt-Johnson and Tillson, 1979). These authors noted the difficulty in getting children to wear glasses with prisms, however. When children do wear the glasses, the success rate is probably greater than 50%.

Fusional Convergence Training

There is a role for orthoptics training in the management of exophoria (with symptoms) and probably also for intermittent exotropia. The goal of orthoptics training is to increase *fusional* convergence. Therefore, accommodative convergence should be controlled with proper correction and proper targets—i.e., targets that do not allow the patient to use accommodative convergence.

Treatment should be directed toward symptoms, which usually are asthenopic in nature. The mere presence of exophoria (without symptoms) is not an indication for treatment. Distance deviation should be treated with the patient visually fixating in the distance; near deviations should be managed with near fixation (Parks and Mitchell, 1993).

Orthoptic treatment can involve progressive base-out prisms to induce convergence. Or, stereocards and a variety of other machines are available to stimulate fusional convergence.

Surgery
Timing of Surgery
Surgery for intermittent exotropia in children under 5 years of age is associated with the risk of an overcorrection and possible induction of microtropia and even loss of stereopsis. Richards and Parks (1983) noted overcorrections in 12% of children under the age of 3 years. We would agree with von Noorden (1990) that it may be best to operate on children who have intermittent exotropia after the age of 4 years. Therefore, none of the surgical management options discussed below are particularly valuable in young children.

Types of Surgery
A variety of surgical options are available to manage exodeviations. Some are specific for an underlying defect, but often the choice of treatment is dictated by the surgeon's experience (Table 9.1).

BILATERAL–LATERAL RECTUS MUSCLE RECESSIONS.   Most strabismus surgeons would prefer to treat exotropia with bilateral–lateral rectus muscle recessions (Romano and Wilson, 1990). Even though the near deviation is usually far less than the distance deviation, this form of treatment is effective in correcting distance and near deviations in intermittent exotropia. The amount of surgery performed for the deviation varies from surgeon to surgeon and undoubtedly is dependent on a particular surgeon's surgical technique.

MEDIAL RECTUS MUSCLE RESECTIONS.   Bilateral medial rectus muscle resection can be offered to patients who have convergence paralysis or convergence insufficiency type of exotropia (Kushner, 1988; von Noorden, 1976; Hermann, 1981). The results of this type of treatment may be variable. Patients often experience diplopia due to postoperative esotropia (von Noorden, 1976). This problem can be managed with base-out prisms until it subsides. Most patients report improve-

TABLE 9.1   Surgical treatment of exotropia

Problem	Procedure
Convergence paralysis or insufficiency	Medial rectus muscle resection, both eyes
Concomitant exotropia	Lateral rectus muscle recession, both eyes, or lateral rectus muscle recession with medial rectus muscle resection
Exotropia with lateral inconcomitance	Lateral rectus muscle recession, both eyes, but less recession than indicated by primary gaze measurement
Exotropia greater at near than at distance	Lateral rectus muscle recession, both eyes, (or recess/resect) but more surgery
Sensory exotropia	Recess/resect procedure on amblyopic eye
Large-angle exotropia	Recess/resect bilaterally with or without weakening oblique muscles

ment with surgical treatment, but some patients have a relapse of their convergence insufficiency after long follow-up, in our experience.

RECESS/RESECT PROCEDURES FOR CONSTANT AND SIMULATED EXOTROPIA.   For constant exotropia and simulated intermittent exotropia, the use of a recess/resect procedure may offer some advantage over lateral rectus muscle recession (von Noorden, 1969). Not everyone agrees with this position, though (Kushner, 1988). It is certainly true that a recess/resect procedure may actually produce some lateral inconcomitance as a side effect, as pointed out by Kushner, particularly if a unilateral procedure is performed for more than 30 prism diopters (Parks and Mitchell, 1993), but whether one procedure has an advantage over another may depend on the surgeon's experience.

In cases of constant unilateral exotropia caused by an underlying amblyopia or other sensory defect, a recess/resect procedure on the eye with low vision is obviously desirable, since the "good" eye is not exposed to surgical risk.

Very large angles of exotropia cannot be corrected with a unilateral recess/resect procedure. Horizontal four-muscle surgery for more than 30 prism diopters, and even oblique muscle weakening for deviations in excess of 60 prism diopters, may be required to manage exotropia (Raab, 1979).

Complications of Surgery

UNDERCORRECTION AND OVERCORRECTION.   Surgical results in the management of exotropia are arguably less predictable than in the management of other types of strabismus. Undercorrections occur at a rate of 27%, according to Parks and Mitchell (1993), and persistent overcorrections occur in 5% of patients. Success rates, as reported in the literature, vary from surgeon to surgeon and are dependent on the definition of success. Hardesty and associates (1978) reported a treatment failure rate of only 14%, but approximately 50% of patients with intermittent exotropia required a second operation. On the other hand, Flax and Selenow (1985) reviewed a variety of surgical papers on the subject of the management of exotropia and found that, in total, approximately 78% of patients were successfully aligned from a cosmetic perspective, but less than 50% actually had good binocular vision after surgery.

Small undercorrections (<20 prism diopters) can be managed by orthoptics and prisms. Reoperation may be required if the deviation is large. Overcorrections are desirable in the initial postoperative period, as long as they are under 20 prism diopters. In fact, overcorrection probably carries the best long-term prognosis for alignment (Raab and Parks, 1969; Hardesty et al., 1978; Scott et al., 1981). With a large (>20 prism diopters) overcorrection, realignment may not occur, and further surgery will likely be necessary.

Parks and Mitchell (1993) described a characteristic postoperative course for exotropia. Ideally, the patient is slightly overcorrected at first, but the overcorrection improves by the tenth day; a good (or poor) surgical outcome can be predicted based on the examination 6 weeks after surgery. Good alignment indicates a good prognosis.

REFERENCES

Bair DR. Symposium: Intermittent exotropia; diagnosis and incidence. Am Orthopt J 1952;2:12–17.

Bielchowsky A. Divergence excess. Arch Ophthalmol 1934;12:157–166.

Blodi FC, Van Allen M. Electromyography in intermittent exotropia; recordings before, during, and after corrective operation. Doc Ophthalmologica 1962;16:21–34.

Brodsky MC, Fritz KJ. Hereditary congenital exotropia: A report of three cases. Binoc Vis Eye Muscle Surg Q 1993;8:133–136.

Burian HM, Spivey BE. The surgical management of exodeviations. Am J Ophthalmol 1965;59:603–620.

Caltrider N, Jampolsky A. Overcorrecting minus lens therapy for treatment of intermittent exotropia. Ophthalmology 1983;90:1160–1165.

Carlson MR, Jampolsky A. Lateral incomitancy in intermittent exotropia. Cause and surgical therapy. Arch Ophthalmol 1979;97:1922–1925.

Cass EE. Divergent strabismus. Br J Ophthalmol 1937;21:538–559.

Cooper J. Intermittent exotropia of the divergence excess type. J Am Optometric Assn 1977;48:1261–1273.

Cooper J, Ciuffreda KJ, Kruger PB. Stimulus and response AC/A ratios in intermittent exotropia of the divergence-excess type. Br J Ophthalmol 1982;66:398–404.

Cooper J, Medow N. Intermittent exotropia, basic and divergence excess type. Binoc Vis Eye Muscle Surg Q 1993;8(Suppl 3):185–216.

Costenbader FD. The Physiology and Management of Divergent Strabismus. In Allen JH (ed), Strabismus Ophthalmic Symposium I. St. Louis: Mosby, 1950;349–376.

Dunlap EA, Gaffney RB. Surgical management of intermittent exotropia. Am Orthopt J 1963;13:20–33.

Eustace P, Wesson ME, Drury DJ. The effect of illumination on intermittent divergence squint of the divergence excess type. Trans Ophthalmol Soc UK 1973;93:559–570.

Flax N, Selenow A. Results of surgical treatment of intermittent divergent strabismus. Am J Optom Physiol Optics 1985;62:100–104.

Flynn JT, McKenney S, Rosenhouse M. Eine behandlungsfor des intermittier-entden divergenzschielens. Klin Monastbl Augenheilkd 1975;167:185–190.

Freeman RS, Isenberg SJ. The use of part-time occlusion for early onset uni-lateral exotropia. J Pediatr Ophthalmol Strabismus 1989;26:94–96.

Friedman Z, Neumann E, Hyams SW, Peleg B. Ophthalmic screening of 38,000 children, age 1 to 2-1/2 years, in child welfare clinics. J Pediatr Ophthalmol Strabismus 1980;17:261–267.

Hardesty HH, Boynton JR, Keenan JP. Treatment of intermittent exotropia. Arch Ophthalmol 1978;96:268–274.

Hermann JS. Surgical therapy of convergence insufficiency. J Pediatr Ophthalmol Strabismus 1981;18:28–31.

Hiles DA, Davies GT, Costenbader FD. Long term observations on unoperated intermittent exotropia. Arch Ophthalmol 1968;80:436–442.

Iacobucci IL, Henderson JW. Occlusion in the pre-operative treatment of exodeviations. Am Orthopt J 1967;15:42–47.

Iacobucci IL, Martonyi EJ, Giles CL. Results of overminus lens therapy on post-operative exodeviations. J Pediatr Ophthalmol Strabismus 1986;23:287–291.

Jampolsky A. Differential diagnostic characteristics of intermittent exotropia and true exophoria. Am Orthopt J 1954;4:48–55.

Jampolsky A. Management of Exodeviation. Transactions of the New Orleans Academy of Ophthalmology. New York: Raven, 1962;140–156.

Jampolsky A. Management of Vertical Strabismus. Transactions of the New Orleans Academy of Ophthalmology. New York: Raven, 1986;141–171.

Knapp P. Intermittent exotropia: Evaluation and therapy. Am Orthopt J 1953;3:27–33.

Kushner BJ. Exotropic deviations: A functional classification and approach to treatment. Am Orthopt J 1988;38:81–93.

MacFarlane A. Trans Orthop Assn Australia 1960;17:7.

Moore S, Stockbridge L, Knapp P. A panoramic view of exotropias. Am Orthopt J 1977;27:70–79.

Parks MM. Comitant Exodeviation in Children and Strabismus. In Symposium of the New Orleans Academy of Ophthalmology. St. Louis: CV Mosby, 1962;45–55.

Parks MM, Mitchell PR. Concomitant Exodeviations. In TD Duane (ed), Clinical Ophthalmology. Vol. 1. Philadelphia: Lippincott, 1993.

Pratt-Johnson JA, Tillson G. Prismotherapy in intermittent exotropia: A preliminary report. Can J Ophthalmol 1979;14:243–245.

Raab EL. Unilateral four-muscle surgery for large-angle exotropia. Ophthalmology 1979;86:1141–1150.

Raab EL, Parks MM. Recession of the lateral recti: Early and late postoperative alignments. Arch Ophthalmol 1969;82:203–208.

Repka MX, Arnoldi KA. Lateral incomitance in exotropia: Fact or artifact? J Pediatr Ophthalmol Strabismus 1991;28:125–128.

Richard JM, Parks MM. Intermittent exotropia—Surgical results in different age groups. Ophthalmology 1983;90:1172–1177.

Romano PE. The relationship between light and exotropia. Binoc Vis Eye Muscle Surg Q 1990;5:11–12.

Romano PE, Wilson MF. Survey of Current Management of Exotropia in the USA and Canada. In EC Campos (ed), Strabismus and Ocular Motility Disorders. New York: MacMillan, 1990;391–396.

Schlossman A, Boruchoff SA. Correlation between physiologic aspects of exotropia. Am J Ophthalmol 1955;40:53–64.

Scott WE, Keech R, Mash AJ. The postoperative results and stability of exodeviations. Arch Ophthalmol 1981;99:1814–1818.

Sondhi N, Archer SM, Helveston EM. Development of normal ocular alignment. J Pediatr Ophthalmol Strabismus 1988;25:210–211.

von Noorden GK. Divergence excess and simulated divergence excess: Diagnosis and surgical management. Doc Ophthalmologica 1969;26:719–728.

von Noorden GK. Resection of both medial rectus muscles in organic convergence insufficiency. Am J Ophthalmol 1976;81:223–226.

von Noorden GK. Exo Deviation. In Binocular Vision and Ocular Motility: Theory and Management of Strabismus (4th ed). St. Louis: Mosby, 1990.

von Noorden GK. Some Aspects of Exotropia. In Binocular Vision and Ocular Motility: Theory and Management of Strabismus (4th ed). St. Louis: Mosby, 1990;326.

Wang FM, Chryssanthau G. Monocular eye closure in intermittent exotropia. Arch Ophthalmol 1988;106:941–942.

Wiggins RE, von Noorden GK. Monocular eye closure in sunlight. J Pediatr Ophthalmol Strabismus 1990;27:16–22.

10

Management of A and V Patterns

Duane (1897) was probably the first person to describe changes in the amount of horizontal deviation in upgaze compared to downgaze. The A and V concepts really were not revitalized until Urrets-Zavalia (1948) and Urist (1958) reported a large series of patients with pattern deviations.

DIAGNOSIS

A and V patterns occur commonly in strabismus. The recognition and management of these problems are very important and frequently determine the success or failure of strabismus surgery. *Pattern* refers to the presence of horizontal misalignment, which is greater or lesser in upgaze compared to downgaze. Strabismus patterns are typically categorized as A, V, X, or Y, so named because these letters symbolize the pattern the eyes make when they move up to down.

The most accurate method of measuring patterns is with eyes rotated straight up, approximately 35 degrees, and straight down, approximately 45 degrees (von Noorden, 1965). Adler (1936) believed that flexing the neck could alter the horizontal (mis)alignment of the eyes. Magee (1960) studied this possibility and concurred, but the amount of alteration is seldom very large. Therefore, the more practical method of patient fixation on a target in the distance and flexion or extension of the neck to rotate the eyes up or down works in most cases.

The use of a near target could induce accommodative changes. In patients with abnormal accommodative convergence to accommodation (AC:A) ratios, errors in measurements could occur, particularly if the patient were reluctant to accommodate in upgaze but not downgaze (von Noorden, 1965). A **V** pattern might be erroneously diagnosed in this fashion. An **A** pattern could be missed if the patient accommodated in downgaze and overcame an exodeviation (von Noorden, 1965).

A **V** pattern is defined as a horizontal deviation of the eyes in which there is either an increase in esodeviation or a decrease in exodeviation in downgaze. In nearly every case of strabismus, at least some amount of difference (upgaze versus downgaze) in horizontal alignment is present when careful measurements are made. In fact, some small amount of **V** phoria may occur in the absence of strabismus (Jampolsky, 1965). A **V** pattern should be diagnosed when the difference between upgaze and downgaze measures 15 prism diopters or more (Knapp, 1959). It is at this level of difference that surgical planning, to take into account the **V** pattern, should be formulated.

An **A** pattern occurs when the amount of exotropia is greater in downgaze, or, in the case of esodeviations, the amount of esodeviation is greater in upgaze. The threshold at which horizontal strabismus should be determined as being an **A** pattern should occur when the difference between upgaze and downgaze is 10 prism diopters (Knapp, 1959).

In certain situations, all four oblique muscles overact, leading to a so-called **X** pattern. In this situation the eyes are more divergent both in upgaze and in downgaze. In primary gaze the amount of horizontal misalignment is actually less. A **Y** pattern occurs when the amount of divergence in the eyes is greater in upgaze, but the misalignment of the eyes is the same in primary gaze as it is in downgaze.

EPIDEMIOLOGY

Urist (1958) showed that 79% of patients with horizontal strabismus also have vertical strabismus, where patterns of strabismus could be determined; 54% of these patients showed esotropia with bilateral elevations in adduction (usually a **V** esotropia); 18% had esotropia with bilateral depression on adduction (**A** esotropia); 20% had exotropia with bilateral elevation in adduction (**V** exotropia); and 8% had exotropia with bilateral depression in adduction (**A** exotropia).

A-pattern esotropia is more likely to occur in African-American children. **A** patterns in white children may indicate neurologic disease—for example, hydrocephalus (Rabinowicz, 1974) or Arnold-Chiari malformation (France, 1975, 1976; Maloney et al., 1977).

Originally the **A** pattern was thought to be due to lateral rectus muscle weakness, but now it appears that most cases are caused by superior oblique overaction (Biglan, 1990).

ETIOLOGY

The etiology of **A** and **V** patterns varies from patient to patient. In many cases, a close examination and inspection of the patient's ocular motility and facial and orbital configuration will clarify the exact etiology.

Abnormalities of the insertion of the extraocular muscles and their orientation to the globe can account for some **A** and **V** patterns.

Kushner (1991) and Cheng and associates (1993) noted that the orientation of the rectus muscles to the globe is often more oblique than normal in children with craniofacial defects. The orientation of the medial rectus muscle is more superior. The superior rectus muscle inserts more laterally, the lateral rectus muscle inserts more inferiorly, and the inferior rectus muscle inserts more medially than usual. The result is a change in the vector forces of the extraocular muscles. Efforts at adduction result in adduction plus elevation, simulating inferior oblique overaction. A **V** pattern can result. Cheng and colleagues (1993) performed neuroimaging studies of patients with craniofacial defects and discovered an excyclotortion of the entire globe and muscle column. Their report confirms the work of Kushner (1991) and Urrets-Zavalia (1955, 1981) and demonstrates the importance of inspecting the cranium in patients with **A** and **V** patterns.

The medial recti muscles have their strongest effect in downgaze, and the lateral muscles have their strongest effect in upgaze (Urist, 1958). Sixth nerve palsies, therefore, produce a slight **V** pattern due to the fact that the medial rectus muscle acts relatively unopposed and will have its strongest effect in downgaze. This finding may be useful in distinguishing sixth nerve palsies from other esodeviations—for example, decompensated esophorias.

The fact that vertical rectus muscles are also adductors can be exploited in the management of **A** and **V** patterns (Miller, 1960; Fink, 1959). Transplantation of a vertical rectus muscle will alter the adducting effect of that muscle. For example, movement of an inferior rectus muscle temporally weakens its adducting effect and will help correct a **V**-pattern esotropia. The reason is that, *in downgaze,* the effect of the muscle is converted to an abductor (after transposition) as well as depressor, resulting in downward and outward eye deviation (Miller, 1960). Transplantation of a vertical rectus muscle toward the nasal side will increase the adducting effect of the muscle. A **V**-pattern exotropia could be improved by moving the superior rectus muscle nasally. Miller (1960) reported a correction of 28 prism diopters using this technique, but the procedure has become unpopular because of inconsistencies in its effectiveness.

The oblique muscles may be responsible for A and V patterns (Costenbader, 1965; Jampolsky, 1965). These muscles have an abducting effect in their field of action and therefore can create a pattern. For example, inferior oblique overaction is commonly associated with infantile esotropia. This creates a V pattern and can be corrected by weakening the inferior oblique as well as the medial rectus muscle. A-pattern esotropias caused by superior oblique overaction could be treated with superior oblique weakening procedures. Similarly, A-pattern exotropia with superior oblique overaction could be managed in this fashion.

Superior and inferior oblique overaction frequently accompanies exotropia. Jampolsky (1978) proposed that the constantly abducted eye slackens the inferior and superior oblique muscles. Over time, slackened muscles tighten, and tight oblique muscles overact. Constant abduction could also lead to tightening of the lateral rectus muscle. Attempts at adduction and elevation or depression could cause the eye to shoot up or down, respectively, creating a pseudo-oblique overaction (Jampolsky, 1978; Scott, 1978). Capo and associates (1988) suggested that mechanical limits set by the abducting eye could allow the adducting eye to further elevate or depress, emulating oblique overaction.

Jampolsky's theory that oblique overactions cause patterns is well tested, but oblique overaction may appear to be present without causing the pattern. This is the situation in certain cases where a Y pattern exists. Abduction of an eye on attempted adduction and elevation can occur, presumably as a result of coinnervation of the lateral rectus muscle, i.e., Duane's syndrome variant (Kushner, 1991). A large shift toward exotropia in upgaze (emulating inferior oblique overaction) should lead the surgeon to suspect Duane's syndrome (Jampolsky, personal communication).

The oblique muscle overaction theory accounts for many, but not all, pattern deviations. The individual patient needs to be evaluated on the basis of the clinical ocular motility examination. Simply weakening an oblique muscle may not have much of an effect if the oblique muscle is not overacting. Conversely, successfully weakening the overacting oblique muscle will occasionally fail to eliminate an A or V pattern. Reflecting this problem is the fact that overacting oblique muscles are occasionally associated with the opposite pattern (e.g., inferior oblique overaction with an A pattern) (Khawan and Traboulsi, 1988; Rosenberg et al., 1983).

Scott (1968) studied patients with **A**- and **V**-pattern exotropia using electromyography. He demonstrated that **A** and **V** patterns were not caused by abnormal innervation to horizontal muscles (e.g., in upgaze and/or downgaze). The only other abductors are oblique muscles, so by default, they can be incriminated as causing **A** and **V** patterns. Scott noted, though, that his study did not mean that all the **A** and **V** cases should be managed by oblique muscle weakening.

Patterns that are caused by oblique muscle overaction are due to the abducting effect of the muscle, in its field of action. An oblique muscle that simply overelevates or overdepresses does not contribute to an **A** or **V** pattern.

MANAGEMENT

General Principles

The surgeon has a variety of options to treat patterns. Generally, the surgical choice should be based on the underlying problem. For example, **A** and **V** patterns not associated with oblique muscle overaction should be managed with vertical transposition of the horizontal recti muscles. On the other hand, **A** and **V** patterns associated with oblique muscle overaction should be managed with oblique muscle weakening surgery.

Patterns with No Oblique Muscle Overaction

Elevating or depressing the horizontal rectus muscle tendons can be helpful in the management of **A** and **V** patterns, particularly when there is no accompanying oblique muscle overaction (Knapp, 1959; Costenbader, 1958) (Figure 10.1). The tendons should be moved in the direction of desired weakening or away from the direction that requires the greatest strengthening. For example, elevating the medial rectus muscle tendons at the same time they are recessed will help eliminate an **A**-pattern esotropia. The goal here is to weaken the muscles most in upgaze, where the esotropia is worst. Depressing both medial recti muscles will help eliminate a **V**-pattern esotropia.

Tendons are typically elevated one-half to two-thirds the width of the tendon, but the amount and effect of displacement vary from surgeon to surgeon. The minimum amount of displacement to create an effect is about 4 mm, but displacements of more than 9 mm are technically difficult and add nothing more to the procedure (Dunlap, 1965).

The lateral recti muscles can also be moved to help diminish **A** and **V** patterns. If the lateral recti muscles are transposed in the direction of desired weakening, they will effectively eliminate a considerable

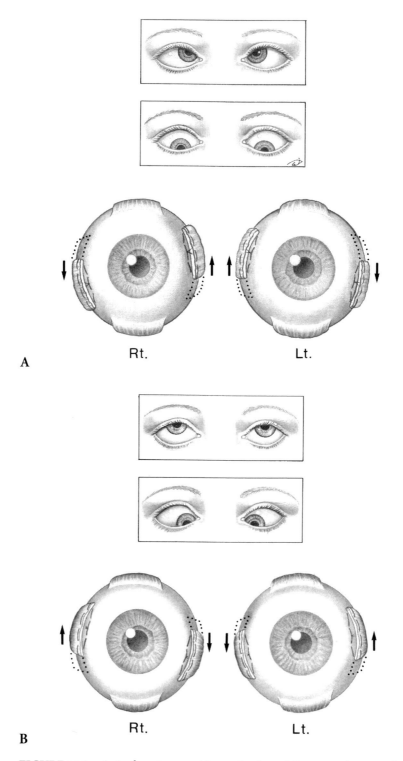

FIGURE 10.1   *A. In **A**-pattern strabismus (and no oblique muscle overaction), medial recti muscles can be moved up, or lateral recti muscles down, to collapse the pattern. B. In **V** patterns, medial recti muscles can be moved down, or lateral recti muscles up, to collapse the pattern.*

TABLE 10.1   Effect of surgical procedures
on **A**- or **V**-pattern esotropia

Goal	Procedure
V patterns collapse 20–25 PD	Transpose medial recti muscles down
V pattern with IO overaction 15–25 PD	Weaken both inferior oblique muscles
Collapse 30 PD **V** pattern	Transpose medial recti muscles down and weaken inferior oblique muscles
Monocular surgery 15 PD of **V** pattern	Transpose medial rectus muscle down and lateral rectus muscle up
Bilateral superior oblique palsy	Tuck both superior oblique muscles
A patterns collapse 15–20 PD	Transpose medial rectus muscle up
SO overaction, **A** patterns collapse 30–45 PD	Superior oblique tenotomies
Collapse >40 PD of **A** pattern	Superior oblique tenotomies and transpose medial recti muscles up
Monocular surgery for **A** pattern	Move medial rectus muscle up and lateral rectus muscle down

IO = inferior oblique; PD = prism diopters; SO = superior oblique.

amount of pattern. Elevating the lateral rectus muscle tendon will reduce a **V**-pattern exotropia. The muscles are weakened by moving them up, thus collapsing the increased exotropia in upgaze. Depressing the lateral rectus muscle tendon will reduce an **A** pattern.

Combinations of medial rectus and lateral rectus muscle transposition can also be performed. For example, a **V**-pattern esotropia can be dealt with through a medial rectus recession and inferior transposition, accompanied by a lateral rectus resection and superior transposition (Goldstein, 1967). This procedure may be ideal for patients who have amblyopia, in whom monocular surgery is advisable. Almost no torsion occurs, and 15 prism diopters of correction of **A** or **V** pattern can, on average, be expected (Metz and Schwartz, 1977) (Table 10.1). Monocular transposition should probably be avoided in cases where oblique overaction is present (Goldstein, 1967).

Displacing the recti muscles without recession or resection is also effective and may ameliorate as much as 30 prism diopters between upgaze and downgaze (Dunlap, 1965). Dunlap advised that displacement without recession or resection could be indicated (1) where a small horizontal deviation exists, (2) when a mixed form of

A–V imbalance exists (eso up, exo down, for example) and the downgaze misalignment requires treatment, (3) as a second procedure after an incomplete response to a first one, and (4) in phoric deviations.

Treatment of *V*-Pattern Esotropia

As the reader will have noted, the surgeon has several options for management of V patterns associated with esotropia. The first step is to determine whether inferior oblique overaction accompanies the esotropia. If so, inferior oblique weakening accompanied by an appropriate amount of movement of the horizontal muscles will collapse 15–25 prism diopters of the V pattern. Note that the V pattern refers to the difference in the amount of deviation of upgaze versus downgaze. Simply weakening the medial recti muscles will collapse a small amount of V esotropia, due to the fact that the medial recti muscles have their greatest effect in downgaze (Urist, 1958).

In the case of V-pattern esotropia caused by bilateral superior oblique palsy, the V pattern can be treated with a bilateral superior oblique tuck procedure. This will correct 15–25 prism diopters of the V pattern. Again, this amount of correction indicates the amount of difference in horizontal misalignment of the eyes between upgaze and downgaze.

In the absence of inferior oblique overaction, the horizontal recti muscles can be transposed. By shifting the horizontal recti muscles inferiorly, approximately 20–25 prism diopters of V esotropia can be corrected. By combining a transposition of recti muscles with inferior oblique weakening, the amount of correction can be augmented to approximately 30 prism diopters.

Treatment of *A*-Pattern Esotropia

It is extremely important to diagnose A patterns. Failure to do so will result in an overcorrection of esotropia in downgaze. Once a diagnosis of A-pattern esotropia is made, the surgeon must then decide on an appropriate treatment plan.

Several rules of thumb can be used in determining management. Superior oblique weakening works when superior oblique overaction is present. The A pattern is collapsed by 30–45 prism diopters, depending on the surgeon (Jampolsky, 1965; Harley and Manley, 1969; Scott et al., 1976). In fact, if patients are followed long enough after surgery, they may show a small exoshift in primary gaze and a more substantial exoshift in upgaze (Fierson et al., 1980). However, there is seldom much horizontal shift of the eyes in primary gaze (Pollard, 1978; Fierson et al., 1980; Diamond and Parks, 1981). Therefore, when performing superior oblique weakening, the underlying "base" amount of esotropia in primary gaze should be managed in the usual way, usually with bilateral medial rectus muscle recessions or recession of the medial rectus muscle accompanied by resection of the lateral rectus muscle or muscles.

The decision to perform superior oblique tenotomies must be partly predicated on the age of the patient and the willingness of the surgeon and patient to tolerate symptoms from the superior oblique weakening procedure. Posterior "seven-eighths" superior oblique tenotomies will cause an esoshift of the eyes in downgaze without much torsional effect. For this reason, this form of the procedure may be desirable to avoid the potentially troubling symptom of torsion. Torsional symptoms are far more likely to occur in older children or adults than in younger children.

Transposition of the medial rectus muscles one-half tendon width upward will collapse approximately 15–20 prism diopters of **A** esotropia (Knapp, 1959). In the absence of superior oblique overaction, tendon transposition works well.

Management of **V**-Pattern Exotropia

A surgeon can expect that weakening of the inferior oblique muscles will eliminate approximately 20 prism diopters of **V** pattern (Table 10.2). The surgery has no effect on the position of the eyes in primary or downgaze (Stager and Parks, 1973). On the other hand, shifting the lateral recti muscles up will correct about 15 prism diopters of **V** pattern. The combination of inferior oblique weakening and vertical transposition of the lateral recti muscles may eliminate as much as 30.00 prism diopters of **V** pattern.

Treatment of **A**-Pattern Exotropia

By weakening the superior oblique muscles, approximately 35 prism diopters of **A**-pattern exotropia can be corrected. On the other hand, shifting the lateral recti muscles downward will only correct 15–20 prism diopters of **A** pattern. Therefore, treatment choice should be based partly on the amount of **A** pattern.

The potential for troublesome side effects from superior oblique weakening procedures, particularly in adults, should be taken into consideration before undertaking this procedure (see below). The surgeon should consider that when superior oblique overaction is also accompanied by inferior oblique overaction, weakening the superior oblique muscles may result in considerably more overaction of the inferior oblique muscles than noted preoperatively. Therefore, the inferior oblique muscles should be weakened at the same time.

TABLE 10.2   Effect of surgical procedures on A- or V-pattern exotropia

Goal	Procedure
V patterns collapse 20 PD	Weaken inferior oblique muscles if they overact
V patterns collapse 15–20 PD; no IO overaction	Transpose lateral recti muscles up
V patterns collapse 30 PD	Weaken inferior oblique muscles and transpose lateral recti muscles up
Monocular surgery (15 PD of V pattern)	Elevate lateral rectus muscle and lower medial rectus muscle
A patterns collapse 15–20 PD	Lower lateral recti muscles
A patterns collapse 35 PD	Weaken superior oblique muscles if they overact
A patterns collapse 40 PD	Lower lateral recti muscles and weaken superior oblique muscles
Monocular surgery 15 PD	Lower lateral rectus muscle and elevate medial rectus muscle

PD = prism diopters; IO = inferior oblique.

COMPLICATIONS OF MANAGEMENT

Complications can be divided into undercorrection, overcorrection, and problems related to superior oblique weakening procedures. The risk of overcorrecting esotropia, particularly in downgaze, when inferior oblique muscles are weakened, is practically zero. Weakening the inferior oblique muscles has no effect on the horizontal misalignment of the eyes in either primary gaze or downgaze (Stager and Parks, 1973). Weakening the superior oblique muscles also seldom substantially affects primary gaze.

Weakening the superior oblique muscles is associated with the risk of causing a secondary overaction of the inferior oblique muscles (Fierson et al., 1980) (Table 10.3). The reverse is not true, in that superior oblique overaction does not result from inferior oblique weakening. The superior oblique tenotomy can be accompanied by symptoms of torsion. Management of this problem is discussed in Chapter 12. Bilateral tenotomies can occasionally cause an asymmetric effect.

TABLE 10.3 Complications of superior oblique weakening

Overaction of inferior oblique (may be delayed)

Fat adherence (more likely with blind sweep of tenotomy hook)

Torsion symptoms

Asymmetric effect

Brown's syndrome

REFERENCES

Adler FH. (Statement made when discussing Friedenwald's paper). In Friedenwald JS. Diagnosis and treatment of anisophoria. Arch Ophthalmol 1936;15:283–307.

Biglan AW. Ophthalmologic complications of meningomyelocele: A longitudinal study. Trans Am Ophthalmol Soc 1990;88:389–462.

Capo H, Mallette RA, Guyton DL. Overacting oblique muscles in exotropia: A mechanical explanation. J Pediatr Ophthalmol Strabismus 1988;25:281–285.

Cheng H, Burdon MA, Shun-Shin GA, Czypionka S. Dissociated eye movements in craniosynostosis: A hypothesis revived. Br J Ophthalmol 1993;77:563–568.

Costenbader FD. Clinical Course and Management of Esotropia. In JH Allen (ed), Strabismus Ophthalmic Symposium II. St. Louis: Mosby, 1965;325.

Diamond GR, Parks MM. The effect of superior oblique weakening procedures on primary position horizontal alignment. J Pediatr Ophthalmol Strabismus 1981;18:35–38.

Duane A. Isolated paralyses of the ocular muscles. Arch Ophthalmol 1897;26:312–334.

Dunlap EA. Vertical displacement of the horizontal recti. J Pediatr Ophthalmol 1965;2:37–40.

Fierson WM, Boger WP III, Diorio PC et al. The effect of bilateral superior oblique tenotomy on horizontal deviation in A-pattern strabismus. J Pediatr Ophthalmol Strabismus 1980;17:364–371.

Fink WH. The A and V syndromes. Am Orthopt J 1959;9:105–110.

France TD. Strabismus in hydrocephalus. Am Orthopt J 1975;25:101–105.

France TD. The Association of A Pattern Strabismus with Hydrocephalus. In S Moore, J Mein (eds), Orthoptics: Past, Present and Future. New York: Grune & Stratton, 1976;287–292.

Goldstein JH. Monocular vertical displacement of the horizontal rectus muscles in the A and V patterns. Am J Ophthalmol 1967;64:265–267.

Harley RD, Manley DR. Bilateral superior oblique tenotomy in A-pattern exotropia. Trans Am Ophthalmol Soc 1969;67:324–338.

Jampolsky A. Oblique muscle surgery of the A–V patterns. J Pediatr Ophthalmol 1965;2:31–36.

Jampolsky A. Surgical Leashes and Reverse Leashes in Strabismus Surgical Management. In Symposium on Strabismus. Transactions of the New Orleans Academy of Ophthalmology. St. Louis: Mosby, 1978;244–268.

Khawam E, Traboulsi EI. A-pattern esotropia with bilateral inferior oblique muscle overaction. Ann Ophthalmol 1988;20:20–22.

Knapp P. Vertically incomitant horizontal strabismus: The so-called "A" and "V" syndromes. Trans Am Ophthalmol Soc 1959;57:666–699.

Kushner BJ. Pseudo inferior oblique overaction associated with Y and V patterns. Ophthalmology 1991;98:1500–1505.

Magee AJ. Minimal values for the A and V syndromes. Am J Ophthalmol 1960;50:753–756.

Maloney A, Weber A, Smith D. A and V patterns of strabismus in meningomyelocele. Am Orthopt J 1977;27:115–118.

Metz HS, Schwartz L. The treatment of A and V patterns by monocular surgery. Arch Ophthalmol 1977;95:251–253.

Miller JE. Vertical recti transplantation in the A and V syndromes. Arch Ophthalmol 1960;64:175–179.

Pollard ZF. Superior oblique tenotomy in A pattern strabismus. Ann Ophthalmol 1978;10:211–215.

Rabinowicz IM. Visual function in children with hydrocephalus. Trans Opthalmol Soc UK 1974;94:356–365.

Rosenberg P, Weseley A, Shippman S, Kelly H. Paradoxical inferior oblique muscle overaction with A-pattern esotropia. Arch Ophthalmol 1983;101:1392–1394.

Scott AB. A and V patterns in exotropia: An electromyographic study of horizontal rectus muscles. Am J Ophthalmol 1968;65:12–19.

Scott AB. Strabismus—Muscle Forces and Innervations. In G Lennerstrand, P Bach-y-Rita (eds), Basic Mechanisms of Ocular Motility and Their Clinical Implications. Proceedings of the International Symposium in Werner-Gren Center. Stockholm: Pergamon, 1978;181–191.

Scott WE, Jampolsky AJ, Redmond MR. Superior oblique tenotomy. Indications and complications. Int Ophthalmol Clin 1976;16:151–159.

Stager DR, Parks MM. Inferior oblique weakening procedures. Effect on primary position horizontal alignment. Arch Ophthalmol 1973;90:15–16.

Urist MJ. The etiology of the so-called A and V syndromes. Am J Ophthalmol 1958;46:835–844.

Urrets-Zavalia A Jr. Paralises bilateral congenital del musculo oblieqo inferior. Arch Oftal Buenos Aires 1948;23:172.

Urrets-Zavalia A Jr. Significance of congenital cyclovertical motor defects of the eyes. Br J Ophthalmol 1955;39:11–20.

Urrets-Zavalia A Jr. Reaction to dissociations and primary insufficiencies of the vertical acting muscles: A discussion of the pathogenesis of the A + V syndromes. Transactions of the American Academy of Ophthalmology and Otolaryngology 1981;91:324.

von Noorden GH. Surgical indications in the A and V patterns. J Pediatr Ophthalmol 1965;2:21–24.

11

Craniofacial Anomalies and Strabismus

Luis C. F. deSa and William V. Good

ETIOLOGY OF SYNDROMES

The association between ocular abnormalities and craniofacial anomalies was noted by Virchow in 1851 and Von Graefe in 1866 (Pemberton and Freeman, 1962). Both described optic nerve involvement in oxycephaly (Pemberton and Freeman, 1962). Since then, a variety of ocular manifestations have been reported in craniofacial abnormalities, including strabismus and ocular motility disturbances, nystagmus, exorbitism, orbital divergence, disk edema, optic atrophy, ocular dermoids, iris and choroidal coloboma, congenital cataract, and retinal detachment (Howell, 1954; Miller and Folk, 1975; Fries and Kastowitz, 1990; Jones et al., 1993; Brazier, 1991).

Ocular motility disturbances occur in 74% of patients with craniofacial anomalies (Diamond and Whitaker, 1984; Morax, 1985). Recognition of the type of craniofacial deformity is helpful, because certain types of strabismus are prone to occur in children with certain craniofacial anomalies. Conditions that affect the orbital bones or eyes are most likely to produce strabismus. Both craniosynostosis and clefting syndromes affect the orbital bones.

Craniosynostosis

Craniosynostosis indicates premature closure of one or more cranial sutures. When this occurs, growth of the cranium is inhibited in the direction that is perpendicular to the axis of the suture (Virchow, 1851). Growth continues parallel to the suture. Different patterns of

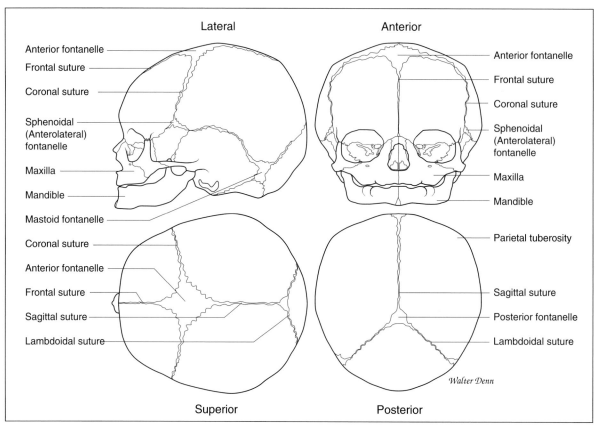

Lateral   Anterior

Anterior fontanelle
Frontal suture   Anterior fontanelle
Coronal suture   Frontal suture
                                                           Coronal suture
Sphenoidal
(Anterolateral)   Sphenoidal
fontanelle   (Anterolateral)
                                                           fontanelle
Maxilla   Maxilla
Mandible   Mandible
Mastoid fontanelle
Coronal suture   Parietal tuberosity
Anterior fontanelle
Frontal suture
Sagittal suture   Sagittal suture
                                                           Posterior fontanelle
Lambdoidal suture   Lambdoidal suture

                                                    Walter Denn

Superior   Posterior

A

FIGURE 11.1   *A. Position of sutures on the skull. B. Coronal suture closure causes brachycephaly. C. In sagittal suture closure, scaphocephaly develops.*

calvarial abnormalities are the result, depending on the suture or sutures involved (Fries and Kastowitz, 1990) (Figure 11.1).

Craniosynostosis has been classified into three groups: simple craniosynostosis, craniofacial dysostosis (Crouzon's disease), and acrocephalosyndactyly (Apert's disease) (Pemberton and Freeman, 1962). A total of 14 craniosynostosis syndromes have been identified, based on clinical and genetic features (Cohen, 1975). Of these 14 types, the most common are Crouzon's disease, Apert's disease, and Pfeiffer's syndrome. Crouzon's disease is one of the most common forms of craniosynostosis (Figure 11.2). It is defined as craniosynostosis, exophthalmos, and hypertelorism (Fries and Kastowitz, 1990). Multiple combinations of suture closure can occur in this syndrome, and thus there is no characteristic calvarial shape (Bertelson, 1958). Virtually any kind of strabismus can occur in Crouzon's disease, but in our experience, V-pattern exotropia is the most common. This type of abnormality may be caused by superior oblique or superior rectus underaction, which can cause

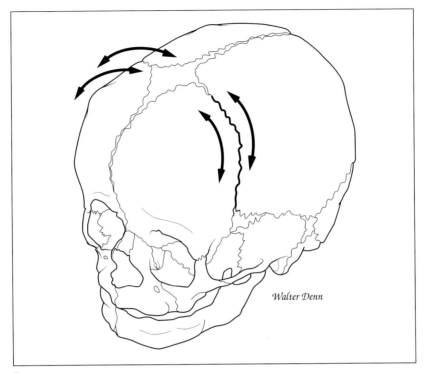

B

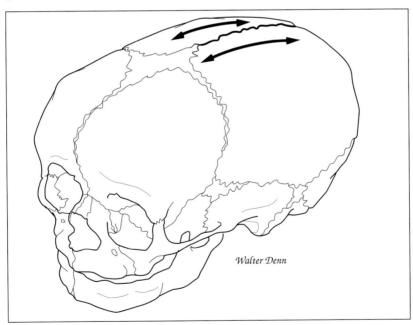

C

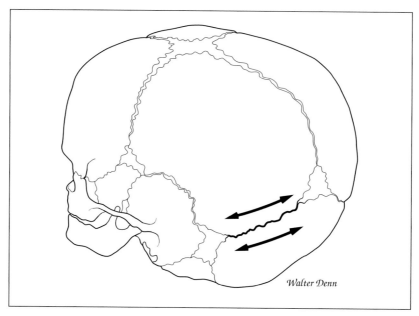

D

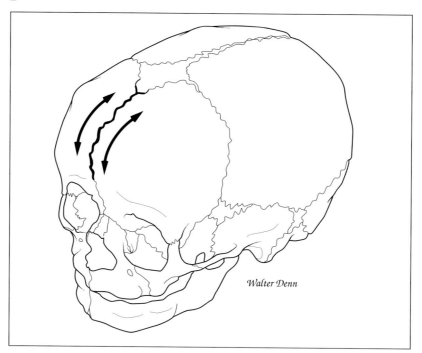

E

FIGURE 11.1 *(continued)   D. Lambdoidal suture closure causes plagiocephaly.
E. Closure of the frontal suture results in trigonocephaly.*

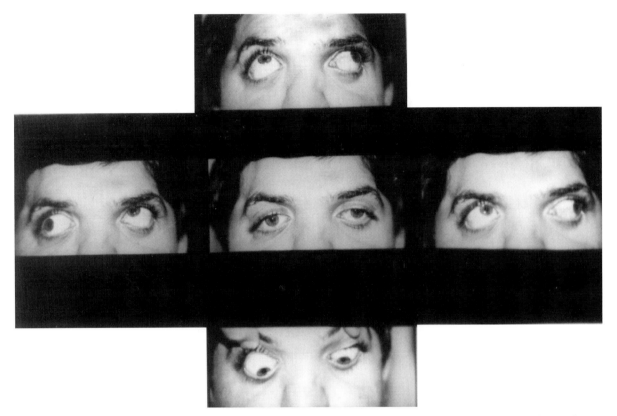

FIGURE 11.2 *This man has Crouzon's disease. Note the marked superior rectus underaction, which leads to inferior oblique overaction. The inferior oblique muscle is the yoke muscle of the superior rectus.*

inferior oblique overaction: If the yoke muscle of an inferior oblique muscle (i.e., the superior rectus) underacts, then Hering's law would provide equal innervation to the inferior oblique muscle, causing apparent overaction (Diamond and Whittaker, 1984; Diamond et al., 1980b).

An association between syndactyly and craniosynostosis (acrocephaly or brachycephaly) is common in patients with craniosynostosis. These patients can be categorized to have yet another type of craniosynostosis known as acrocephalosyndactyly, of which Apert's disease and Pfeiffer's syndrome are the most common. In Apert's disease (Figure 11.3), there is syndactyly of the fingers and toes. In Pfeiffer's syndrome, syndactyly can occur, but broad, large toes and thumbs are most characteristic (Martsolf et al., 1971). Strabismus abnormalities are common and are similar to those seen in Crouzon's disease.

Cleft Syndromes

Fusion of almost all facial fissures and furrows occurs between the sixth and seventh week of gestation (Fries and Kastowitz, 1990). A cleft syndrome results when one or more facial fissures fails to close. The cleft

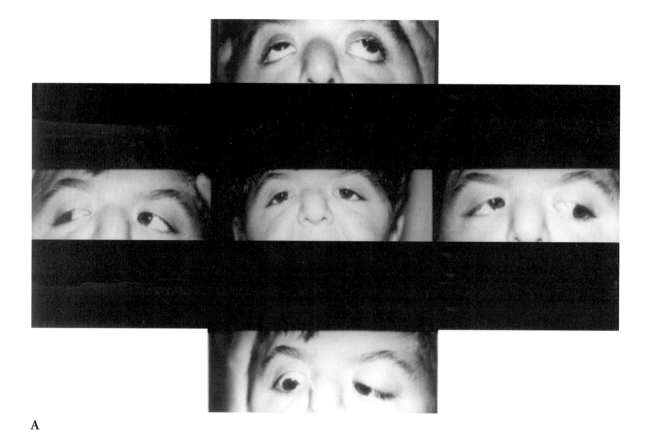

A

B

FIGURE 11.3 *In Apert's disease, craniosynostosis is accompanied by syndactyly (fingers and toes). A. Note this child's V exotropia and superior rectus underaction. B. His fingers after surgical treatment of syndactyly. C. Syndactyly of his toes.*

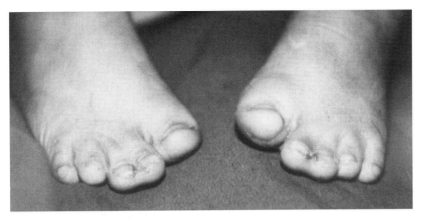

C

can be easily recognized as a cleft lip or palate, but the defect can be difficult to identify in other cases. Tessier (1976) classified the clefting syndromes into 14 types, according to the anatomic area of the cleft.

Clefts can involve the facial midline, causing hypertelorism, or they can occur in the medial canthal and nasolacrimal positions, in the eyelids, or in the lateral canthal and facial positions. A variety of clinical manifestations can occur, depending on the location of the cleft, including nasolacrimal abnormalities; eyelid colobomas; microphthalmos; ear deformities; auricular tags; mandibular and maxillary hypoplasia; parotid, tongue, and soft-palate hypoplasia; and abnormalities of the fifth and seventh cranial nerves (Fries and Kastowitz, 1990). Treacher Collins syndrome and Goldenhar's syndrome are syndromes of interest to ophthalmologists, because they affect lateral canthal clefts.

Treacher Collins syndrome (Figure 11.4) consists of malar hypoplasia, absence of the zygomatic arch, coloboma of the outer third of the lower lid, and external and internal ear abnormalities. The syndrome is dominantly inherited, with almost 100% penetrance. Children show a bird-like facies due to malar hypoplasia. Strabismus is common.

In Goldenhar's syndrome (Figure 11.5), children show limbal dermoids, lid coloboma, preauricular tags, and vertebral abnormalities (Goldenhar, 1952). Strabismus, particularly Duane's syndrome, is common.

ETIOLOGY OF OCULAR MOTILITY DISTURBANCES AND STRABISMUS

Ocular motility disturbances are commonly found in patients with craniofacial abnormalities and may be due to a variety of causes, including (1) visual loss (and unequal sensory input), (2) orbital dystopia, (3) extraocular muscle abnormalities, and (4) cranial nerve involvement.

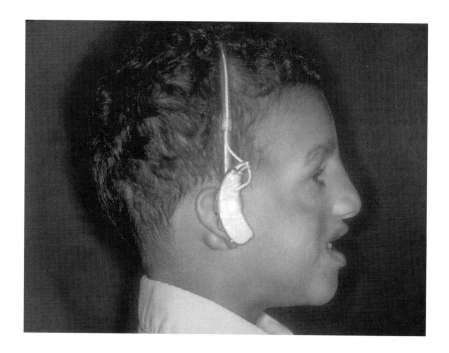

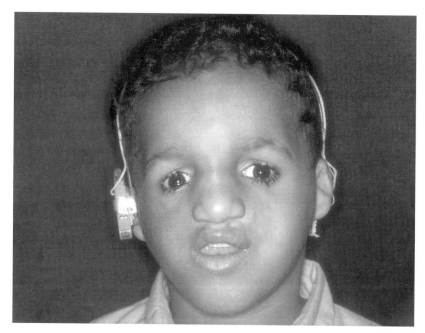

FIGURE 11.4 *Treacher Collins syndrome causes downward displacement of the lateral canthi. Malar hypoplasia leads to a bird-like facial appearance. The cause is clefting in the area of the lateral canthus. (Courtesy of Mahin Golabi, M.D.)*

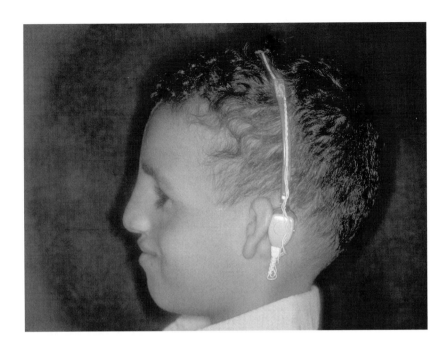

Strabismus Caused by Visual Loss

Poor vision in one or both eyes can occur from diseases of the eyes (microphthalmos, cataracts, coloboma), the ocular adnexa (e.g., proptosis with corneal involvement), or the central nervous system (Miller and Folk, 1975). Optic atrophy is a frequent cause of decreased visual acuity in children with craniofacial defects. In craniosynostosis, optic atrophy may be secondary to raised intracranial pressure and chronic papilledema (Howell, 1954; Blodi, 1957; Renier et al., 1982). Because of early synostosis, the skull cannot keep pace with brain growth, and this results in increased intracranial pressure. Primary optic atrophy may occur in some cases due to stretching and kinking of the optic nerves caused by abnormalities of the skull and optic canals (Howell, 1954; Blodi, 1957).

Strabismus Caused by Orbital Dystopia

Abnormalities of the orbital walls can be associated with strabismus even when no craniofacial anomaly is present. Zaki and Keeney (1957) found a smaller orbital angle (formed by the lateral and medial walls) in 25% of patients with monocular esotropia and a larger angle in 33% of those with monocular exotropia. The facial malformations (including malar hypoplasia or malar hyperplasia) that occur frequently in some ethnic groups were associated with some forms of cyclovertical strabismus (Urrets-Zavalia et al., 1961).

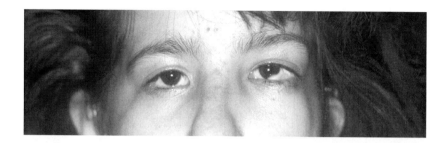

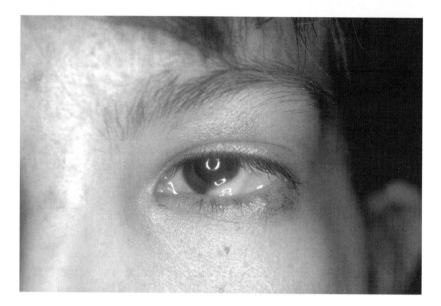

FIGURE 11.5   *This child has Goldenhar's syndrome. Note the limbal dermoids located inferotemporally as well as the ear abnormalities.*

In the presence of a major craniofacial defect, the likelihood of strabismus must be even greater.

Abnormalities of the orbital walls may contribute to ocular motility disturbances by changing the vectors of action of extraocular muscles. Presumably, strabismus occurs as a result of (local) mechanical alterations of extraocular muscles (Kushner, 1985). It is important to remember, however, that orbital realignment following craniofacial reconstruction usually does not alter preexisting strabismus (Diamond et al., 1980a).

Strabismus Caused by Extraocular Muscle Abnormalities
A variety of extraocular muscle abnormalities have been reported in patients with craniofacial anomalies, including absence of muscle,

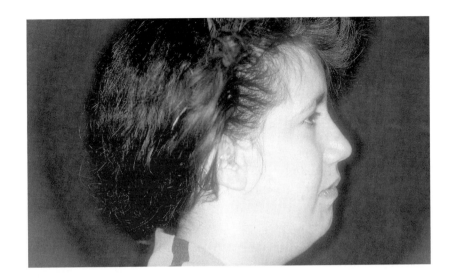

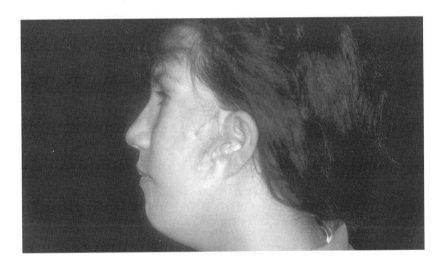

aberrant insertions, and structural alterations. The superior rectus muscle is commonly absent (Weinstock and Hardesty, 1965; Cuttone et al., 1979; Diamond et al., 1980b). Its absence is usually not associated with levator dysfunction or blepharoptosis. Absence of the inferior rectus, superior oblique, and inferior oblique muscles has been reported, but less frequently (Diamond et al., 1980b; Fries and Kastowitz, 1990).

Aberrant muscle insertions, including bifid and displaced insertions, can occur in these patients (Caputo and Lingua, 1980). Alterations in the muscle fibers, myoneural junctions, and intramuscular nerves of extraocular muscles have also been reported in craniosynostosis (Margolis et al., 1977).

Strabismus Caused by Cranial Nerve Involvement

Involvement of the cranial nerves can cause eye motility abnormalities in children with craniofacial defects. Elevated intracranial pressure can produce sixth nerve paralysis, for example.

STRABISMUS

Strabismus is a frequent occurrence in craniofacial syndromes and may present as esotropia, exotropia, hypertropia, or a combination of horizontal and vertical deviations. Often, correlation exists between the craniofacial syndrome and the ocular motor abnormality.

Craniosynostosis

The prevalence of strabismus and ocular motor imbalance in craniosynostosis ranges from 36.5% to 90.0%, depending on the population studied, the severity of the deformities, and the criteria used to classify the ocular motor disturbance (Nelson et al., 1981; Dufier et al., 1986; Carruthers, 1988). The deviation in primary position may be esotropic or exotropic, with or without vertical strabismus. Dufier and colleagues (1986) found esotropia more commonly in Apert's disease and exotropia in Crouzon's disease. Others have noted exotropia more frequently in all craniosynostosis cases at a prevalence of 60.6% and 77.7% (Nelson et al., 1981; Carruthers, 1988).

One of the most consistent findings in patients with craniosynostosis is the presence of a V pattern, which is associated with overaction of the inferior oblique muscles and limitation of movement in the field of the superior rectus muscle (see Figure 11.3).

Inferior oblique overaction may occur secondary to underaction of the superior rectus (see below). The superior rectus muscle may underact due to hypoplasia or agenesis, but some patients have a normal, but underactive, superior rectus muscle. Shortening of the orbital roof may produce underaction of the superior rectus muscle on a mechanical basis, due to the shortened length of the muscle.

Plagiocephaly and "Superior Oblique Palsy"

Plagiocephaly is one of the craniosynostosis syndromes that results from premature closure of one half the coronal sutures. In these patients the skull develops normally on one side and is underdeveloped on the other, producing a flattened face on the affected side.

Bagolini and associates (1982) observed 10 patients with plagiocephaly and torticollis and correlated these phenomena. Typically, these patients present with strabismus on the affected side. Overaction of the inferior oblique muscle, underaction of the superior oblique

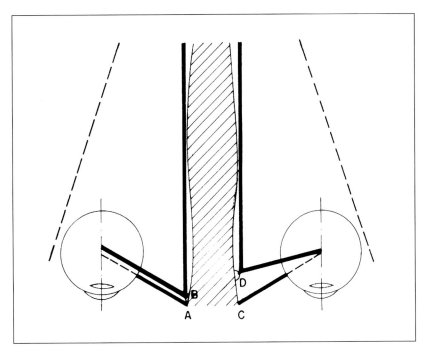

FIGURE 11.6 *The trochlea is displaced to the rear on the affected side in plagiocephaly because the orbital roof is shorter (C to D). The vertical power of the superior oblique muscle is decreased due to shortening of the muscle and its desagittalization; its torsional effect is increased.*

muscle, and a positive Bielschowsky head-tilt test indicate a "superior oblique palsy." According to these authors, the orbital roof on the affected side is shorter because the frontal bone is insufficiently developed; as a consequence, the trochlea is located posteriorly, which decreases the vertical power of the superior oblique muscle, causing superior oblique deficiency (Figure 11.6).

This decreased effect of the superior oblique muscle as a depressor facilitates overaction of the inferior oblique muscle. The inferior oblique muscle is not affected because the orbital floor is normal. A genuine palsy, as opposed to this pseudopalsy, should be excluded, if possible. Forced duction testing has never shown a restriction in this type of patient (to our knowledge), excluding the possibility of a mechanical cause for the strabismus.

Cleft Syndromes

Clefts involving midline (Tessier numbers 0, 1, 13, and 14) or medial and canthal areas (Tessier numbers 2, 3, and 4) produce variable degrees of hypertelorism (Fries and Kastowitz, 1990). Exotropia is the most common type of strabismus associated with hypertelorism (Walsh and Hoyt, 1969). Morax (1984) found that patients with hypertelorism and strabismus usually show exotropia (83.3%), with 16.7% showing esotropia. Exotropia is attributed, in part, to the increased distance between the orbits, which changes the angle between the origin and the insertion of the extraocular muscles (Morax, 1984). The greatest separation occurs more anteriorly, but the intraorbital distance at the level of the optic foramen is normal (Tessier, 1972).

In Goldenhar's syndrome and hemifacial microsomia, which are related to lateral canthal clefts, many forms of motility disturbances have been reported, including Duane's syndrome, isolated duction deficiencies, esotropia, and exotropia (Feingold and Gellis, 1969; Baum and Feingold, 1973).

MANAGEMENT

General Considerations

Amblyopia should be investigated and managed in the usual manner. It may occur due to a variety of causes, including strabismus, ptosis, anisometropia, cataract, corneal opacities, and even corneal exposure, requiring frequent ointment, occlusion, or tarsorrhaphy (Figure 11.7).

SURGERY

Anomalous Insertions of Extraocular Muscles

When strabismus surgery is indicated and the craniofacial anomaly is mild and does not require craniofacial reconstruction, surgery for strabismus follows the basic principles used in other strabismus cases. However, when the craniofacial defect is severe, special considerations should be given to extraocular muscle anatomy. Absence and hypoplasia of extraocular muscles have been reported (Weinstock and Hardesty, 1965; Cuttone et al., 1979; Diamond et al., 1980b). The superior rectus muscle is most commonly reported to be absent. This absence may occur with or without ptosis or levator muscle dysfunction (Diamond et al., 1980b). When an absence of extraocular muscles is suspected and detected, the surgeon should plan the surgery to avoid the possibility of anterior segment ischemia (Hayreh and Scott, 1978).

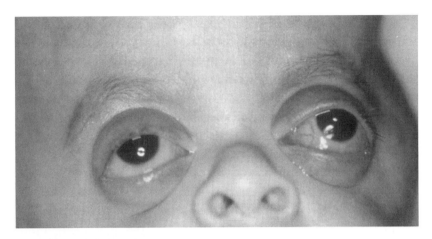

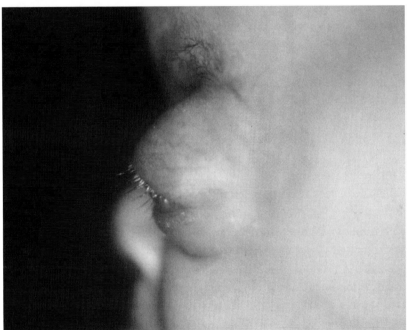

FIGURE 11.7   *This child has Pfeiffer's syndrome and marked proptosis. Even after skull advancement, he began to develop unilateral keratopathy due to exposure. Constant lubrication blurred his vision and may have contributed to his developing nystagmus.*

First, the number of extraocular muscles and their relationship and orientation to the globe should be determined. Underaction of the hypoplastic superior rectus muscle can be "matched" by weakening the yoke inferior oblique muscle (in the other eye). Other underacting muscles can also be matched. For example, a weak inferior rectus muscle can be matched by placing a Faden suture in the fellow inferior rectus muscle. If fewer than normal extraocular muscles are discovered, at least one should be left unoperated.

Abnormalities at the insertion of extraocular muscles may occur, including bifid or displaced insertions (Caputo and Lingua, 1980). In some cases, the extraocular muscle insertions appear to be rotated by 30 degrees. For example, the medial rectus insertion is at an angle and superiorly displaced (Kushner, 1985), which can potentially cause the eye to elevate in adduction, simulating inferior oblique overaction. Imaging modalities such as computed tomography and magnetic resonance imaging may be helpful in evaluating the possibility of extraocular muscle abnormalities. If the medial rectus muscle is rotated superonasally, its effect will be to rotate the eye in and up, simulating inferior oblique overaction. Therefore, its recession could correct the pseudoinferior oblique overaction.

Timing of Surgery

When both strabismus surgery and craniofacial reconstruction are indicated, one must decide which to perform first. Craniofacial surgery with upper facial mobilization was once assumed to change postoperative visual axis alignment and cause realignment or disruption of any preexisting binocularity, or both. Therefore, strabismus surgery was usually postponed until craniofacial reconstruction was completed. Diamond et al. (1980a) reported the results of craniofacial reconstruction on ocular alignment of 160 children undergoing surgery. Only nine (6.4%) showed a shift in primary position, and only three (2.1%) had a shift greater than 10 prism diopters. In one of these nine cases the strabismus did not exist preoperatively (Diamond et al., 1980a). The investigators of a retrospective evaluation of a large number of patients came to the same conclusion (Diamond and Whitaker, 1984). Diamond and colleagues (1980a) advocated early strabismus surgery before major craniofacial reconstruction, because earlier strabismus surgery is more likely to achieve binocularity. According to these authors, motility surgery performed after orbital manipulation is less than optimal because hemorrhage may be more profuse and soft tissues are more friable.

Carruthers (1988) also studied 10 patients with craniosynostosis who underwent craniofacial reconstruction. None of her patients developed any change in ocular alignment after craniectomy. On the other hand, Morax (1984) noted a trend toward esodeviation in the postoperative period in hyperteloric patients undergoing Tessier Monobloc osteotomy repair. He advocates deciding which surgical procedure to perform first based on the craniofacial anomaly and its timing of the repair. If the craniofacial anomaly is severe, it should be corrected first. However, if correction of the anomaly is postponed, there is no reason not to proceed with strabismus surgery. If the anomaly is seen and operated on in adulthood, strabismus surgery should be performed after craniofacial reconstruction only for cosmetic purposes.

Buncic (1984) found an effect of orbital surgery on ocular alignment, and he attributed this result to the degree of orbital relocation. In conservative surgical alterations of the orbits, little or no strabismus change is produced, whereas greater amounts of orbital relocation have a greater effect. In infants with simple strabismus, and if craniofacial reconstruction is not imminent, good results can be achieved by early strabismus surgery. In more complex cases, which may need more than one surgery, strabismus surgery should be delayed until after orbital reconstruction and good visual acuity is achieved in each eye with amblyopia therapy.

CONCLUSION

The management of strabismus or ocular motility disturbances, or both, in patients with craniofacial syndromes should follow basic principles of infantile strabismus. Amblyopia should be investigated and treated first, when necessary. The decision to perform strabismus surgery or craniofacial reconstruction should depend on the age of the patient, sensory and motor status, and type and degree of craniofacial syndrome. These patients should be evaluated and managed by a team of other specialists, including plastic surgeons, neurosurgeons, otolaryngologists, psychiatrists, anesthesiologists, and geneticists. The decision to operate on such patients should be discussed with other members of the team, who can provide expertise in the management of such complex patients.

REFERENCES

Bagolini B, Campos EC, Chiesi C. Plagiocephaly causing superior oblique deficiency and ocular torticollis. A new clinical entity. Arch Ophthalmol 1982;100:1093–1096.

Baum JL, Feingold M. Ocular aspects of Goldenhar's syndrome. Am J Ophthalmol 1973;75:250–257.

Bertelson TI. The premature synostosis of the cranial sutures. Acta Ophthalmol (Copenh) 1958;51(Suppl):47–174.

Blodi FC. Developmental anomalies of the skull affecting the eye. Arch Ophthalmol 1957;57:593–610.

Brazier J. Craniofacial Abnormalities. In D Taylor (ed), Pediatric Ophthalmology. Boston: Blackwell Scientific, 1991;213–222.

Buncic JR. Ocular motility in craniofacial reconstruction (comment). Plast Reconstr Surg 1984;73:36–37.

Caputo AR, Lingua RW. Aberrant muscular insertions in Crouzon's disease. J Pediatr Ophthalmol Strabismus 1980;17:239–241.

Carruthers JD. Strabismus in craniofacial dysostosis. Graefe's Arch Clin Exp Ophthalmol 1988;226:230–234.

Cohen MM Jr. An etiologic and nosologic overview of craniosynostosis syndromes. Birth Defects 1975;11:137–189.

Cuttone JM, Brazis PT, Miller MT, Folk ER. Absence of the superior rectus muscle in Apert's syndrome. J Pediatr Ophthalmol Strabismus 1979;16:349–354.

Diamond GR, Katowitz JA, Whitaker L et al. Ocular alignment after craniofacial reconstruction. Am J Ophthalmol 1980a;90:248–250.

Diamond GR, Katowitz JA, Whitaker LH et al. Variations in extraocular muscle number and structure in craniofacial dysostosis. Am J Ophthalmol 1980b;90:416–418.

Diamond GR, Whitaker LH. Ocular motility in craniofacial reconstruction. Plast Reconstr Surg 1984;73:31–37.

Dufier JL, Vinurel MC, Renier D, Marchac D. Les complications ophthalmologiques des craniofaciostenoses. A propos de 244 observations. J Fr Ophthalmol 1986;9:273–280.

Feingold M, Gellis SS. Ocular abnormalities associated with first and second arch syndromes. Surv Ophthalmol 1969;14:30–42.

Fries PD, Katowitz JA. Congenital craniofacial anomalies of ophthalmic importance. Surv Ophthalmol 1990;35:87–119.

Goldenhar M. Associations malformatives de l'oeil et de l'oreille; en particulier le syndrome dermoide epibulbaire-appendices auricullaires-festula auris congenitas et ses relations avec la dysostose mandibulo-faciale. J Genet Hum 1952;1:243–283.

Hayreh SS, Scott WE. Fluorescein iris angiography. II. Disturbances in iris circulation following strabismus operation on the various recti. Arch Ophthalmol 1978;96:1390–1400.

Howell SC. The craniostenoses. Am J Ophthalmol 1954;37:359–379.

Jones MR, de Sa LC, Good WV. Atypical iris coloboma and Pfeiffer syndrome. J Pediatr Ophthalmol Strabismus 1993;30:266–267.

Kushner BJ. The role of ocular torsion on the etiology of A and V patterns. J Pediatr Ophthalmol Strabismus 1985;22:171–179.

Margolis S, Pachter BR, Breinin GM. Structural alterations of extraocular muscle associated with Apert's syndrome. Br J Ophthalmol 1977;61:683–689.

Martsolf JT, Cracco JB, Carpenter GG, O'Hara AE. Pfeiffer syndrome. An unusual type of acrocephalosyndactyly with broad thumbs and great toes. Am J Dis Child 1971;121:257–262.

Miller M, Folk E. Strabismus associated with craniofacial anomalies. Am Orthop J 1975;25:27–37.

Morax S. Change in eye position after cranio-facial surgery. J Maxillofac Surg 1984;12:47–55.

Nelson LB, Ingoglia S, Breinin GM. Sensorimotor disturbances in craniostenosis. J Pediatr Ophthalmol Strabismus 1981;18:32–41.

Pemberton JW, Freeman JM. Craniosynostosis. A review of experience with forty patients with particular reference to ocular aspects and comments on operative indications. Am J Ophthalmol 1962;54:641–650.

Renier D, Sainte-Rose C, Marchac D, Hisch JF. Intracranial pressure in craniostenosis. J Neurosurg 1982;57:370–377.

Tessier P. Orbital hypertelorism. I. Successive surgical attempts. Material and methods. Causes and mechanisms. Scand J Plast Reconstr Surg 1972;6:135–155.

Tessier P. Anatomical classification of facial, cranio-facial and latero-facial clefts. J Maxillofac Surg 1976;4:69–94.

Urrets-Zavalia A, Solares-Zamorra J, Olmos HR. Anthropological studies on the nature of cyclovertical squint. Br J Ophthalmol 1961;45:578–596.

Virchow R. Ueber den cretinismus namentlich in franken und über pathologische Schädelformen. Verhandl Phys-Med Gesellsch 1851;2:230–271.

Walsh FB, Hoyt WF. Clinical Neuro-Ophthalmology (3rd ed). Vol. 1. Baltimore: Williams & Wilkins, 1969;684–704.

Weinstock FJ, Hardesty HH. Absence of superior recti in craniofacial dysostosis. Arch Ophthalmol 1965;74:152–153.

Zaki HAA, Keeney AH. The bony orbital walls in horizontal strabismus. Arch Ophthalmol 1957;57:418–424.

IV

Vertical Strabismus

12

Superior Oblique Palsy

ETIOLOGY

Most cases of superior oblique palsy (SOP) are traumatically induced. The trochlear nerves exit the dorsal midbrain and can be damaged by contrecoup forces that are transmitted to the free tentorial edge. Very slight head trauma can cause SOP, but only in the presence of an underlying problem—for example, an arteriovenous malformation (Jacobson et al., 1988). Otherwise, the etiologic trauma is a forceful blow to the head. Many cases undoubtedly are congenital, but the etiology is also often presumed to be trauma in these cases.

Another cause of SOP is ischemia, which can occur in patients with hypertension or diabetes mellitus. The palsy may be isolated or may occur in conjunction with other neurologic problems.

Occasionally, an acquired SOP will occur because of underlying and serious neurologic disease. A contralateral Horner's sign accompanied by SOP may indicate intrinsic midbrain disease (Guy et al., 1989). When the trochlear nerve is damaged along its course to the superior oblique muscle, other localizing signs are almost always present. For example, an intracavernous sinus aneurysm can produce SOP, but other contiguous structures are also involved (e.g., oculomotor nerves, fifth cranial nerve).

DIAGNOSIS

Congenital Versus Acquired Superior Oblique Palsy

Congenital cases can be distinguished from acquired cases by a number of features: The patient may have had a head tilt since early childhood, which can be documented by childhood photographs; and patients with long-standing superior oblique palsies tend to have large fusional amplitudes, as much as 15 prism diopters or more (as compared to newly acquired SOP, where there is very little fusion amplitude).

Diplopia

Superior oblique palsy causes vertical, some degree of horizontal, and torsional diplopia. The last symptom is often most pronounced on downgaze, in the field of action of the superior oblique muscle. Vertical diplopia is usually worse in gaze directed toward the uninvolved eye, due to inferior oblique overaction (IOOA), or on head tilt to the involved side.

Three-Step Test

Park's three-step test is especially valuable for diagnosing paralysis of vertically acting extraocular muscles and has been shown to be invaluable in the diagnosis of SOP (Parks, 1958). The patient's ocular deviation is first measured in primary gaze, then left and right gaze, and finally with a head tilt to the right and left (Figure 12.1). For example, in the first step of the test, vertical deviation in primary gaze is noted. If the patient has left hypertropia, this indicates that there is underaction (paralysis) of the left eye depressors or right eye elevators. (The depressors are the superior oblique and inferior rectus muscles; the elevators are the inferior oblique and superior rectus muscles).

In the second step, deviation to the right and left is measured. If the defect worsens in left gaze, this indicates a problem with muscles of the left eye, whose greatest vertical action occurs during abduction (e.g., superior and inferior rectus muscles), or a problem with muscles of the right eye, whose greatest vertical action occurs in adduction (e.g., superior and inferior oblique muscles).

In the third step, vertical deviation with head tilt to either side is measured. If the problem worsens with head tilt to the left, the muscles responsible for left incyclotorsion or right excyclotorsion are implicated. (The left incyclotorters are the left superior rectus and superior oblique muscles. The right excyclotorters are the right inferior rectus and right inferior oblique muscles.) By observing the patient's eye movements in these fields of gaze, diagnosis of the exact problematic muscle can be made.

An additional physical finding is that of IOOA (see Figures 4.1 and 10.1). The overactive inferior oblique muscle elevates (and abducts) the involved eye farther than its yoke superior rectus muscle. The involved superior oblique muscle may also underact, and this can be observed by having the patient look into the field of action of the particular superior oblique muscle—i.e., down and in.

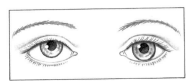

Step 1: Which eye is higher?

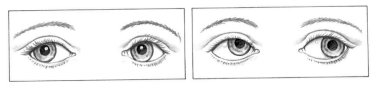

Step 2: Is the hypertropia worse in gaze left or right?

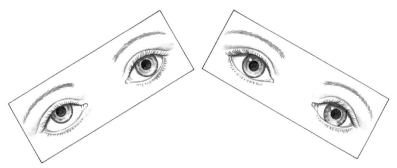

Step 3: Is the hypertropia worse in right or left head tilt?

FIGURE 12.1   *Park's three-step test. The patient has a right superior oblique palsy.*

Paralysis of the superior oblique muscle may also cause symptoms of excyclotorsion. This can be measured with a double Maddox rod or with Bagolini striated lenses. Unilateral SOP typically causes less than 8 degrees of excyclotorsion (see below).

Bilateral Superior Oblique Palsy

The features of bilateral SOP are the following:

1. Vertical deviation in primary gaze may or may not be present.
2. Right hypertropia occurs in left gaze and left hypertropia in right gaze.
3. IOOA may occur on both sides.
4. V-pattern esotropia occurs with the patient frankly esotropic in downgaze, and occasionally exotropic in upgaze.

The underacting superior oblique muscle and overacting inferior oblique muscle cause the V pattern. Excyclotorsion usually measures greater than 8–10 degrees and may cause prominent symptoms for the patient. Head tilt testing shows right hypertropia on right tilt and left hypertropia on left tilt.

Masked Bilateral Superior Oblique Palsy

Not every patient fits neatly into the category of unilateral or bilateral SOP. Sometimes patients are initially diagnosed with unilateral palsy, but when they undergo surgery, a contralateral palsy emerges (Kraft and Scott, 1986). In one study, 8.7% of patients showed bilateral SOP only after diagnosis and treatment for unilateral SOP (Kraft and Scott, 1986), but the rate may be as high as 30% in some patients (Souza-Diaz, 1976; Hermann, 1981; Scott, 1978; Reynolds et al., 1984).

Are there any clues to the possibility of masked bilateral SOP? When a history of head trauma is elicited, particularly with loss of consciousness, bilaterality is more likely (Sydnor et al., 1982; Mittleman and Folk, 1976; Chapman et al., 1970). In cases of *idiopathic* SOP (i.e., non-traumatic and nonneurologic), the risk of bilaterality is less (Helveston and Ellis, 1980; von Noorden et al., 1986), but bilateral cases still occur. Idiopathic (and unilateral) cases are more common in the left eye, for unknown reasons (Robb, 1990).

Even a slight reversal of the hypertropia or alternating head tilt testing is suggestive of bilaterality (Jampolsky, 1971; Kraft and Scott, 1986). The amount of excyclotorsion may be useful when no other physical findings of bilaterality are present. Excyclotorsion greater than 12 degrees suggests bilaterality (Sydnor et al., 1982; Ellis and Helveston, 1976; Lyle, 1964; Mitchell and Parks, 1982). However, even this type of testing has its pitfalls, and the real amount of excyclotorsion may be obscured by the patient's subjective responses to double Maddox rod testing (von Noorden, 1984).

Robb (1990) emphasized the distinction between unmasking a bilateral SOP and overcorrecting a unilateral SOP. Some cases of "unmasked" bilateral SOP may represent an overcorrection, particularly when two muscles have been operated on (e.g., inferior oblique weakening and *contralateral* inferior rectus recession or ipsilateral superior rectus recession).

DIFFERENTIAL DIAGNOSIS

Divergent vertical deviation (DVD) can emulate IOOA: Alternating cover test in DVD fails to demonstrate a true hypertropia.

Inferior oblique overaction frequently accompanies horizontal strabismus. Head tilt testing usually fails to lateralize any problem, and IOOA develops *after* the onset of horizontal strabismus.

Skew deviation is a vertical strabismus problem caused by a disturbance or asymmetry of supranuclear input (Leigh and Zee, 1991; Keane, 1975, 1985). Some patients will experience torsional symptoms. The hypertropia is oftentimes concomitant, but it may vary in different gaze positions. An alternating skew deviation has been described in which the hyperdeviation changes from side to side (Moster et al., 1988). Some patients have a head tilt referred to as the ocular tilt reaction (Westheimer and Blair, 1975; Hedges and Hoyt, 1982). This tends to occur with lesions in the upper brain stem, but has also been reported in medullary lesions (Brandt, 1987). Ocular tilt consists of vertical divergence of the eyes, accompanied by torsion of the eyes and head tilt.

Skew deviation is a vertical, comitant strabismus that can occur with brain stem infarcts, multiple sclerosis, increased intracranial pressure, and even pseudotumor cerebri. Hoyt and colleagues (1980) noted skew deviation in the immediate postnatal period and found it to be a transient supranuclear disorder of normal newborn children. Lesions of the vestibular organ can cause a skew deviation. Cerebellar lesions can cause either ipsilateral or alternating skew deviation. Skew deviations frequently accompany lesions of the medial longitudinal fasciculus, in which case the eye with hypertropia is usually on the side of the lesion. Lesions in the interstitial nucleus of Cajal can also cause skew deviation.

MANAGEMENT

The following classification scheme is rather complicated at first review, but there are several principles involved in the management of superior oblique palsies that are straightforward. First, the amount of vertical deviation that can be corrected with an inferior oblique weakening procedure is 15 prism diopters or less. This means that deviations greater than 15 prism diopters usually should be approached with surgery on at least two muscles.

Second, weakening the inferior oblique muscle affects the vertical alignment of the eyes in primary gaze, adduction of the involved eye, and elevation. However, a vertical deviation that exists in downgaze may not be adequately affected by an inferior oblique weakening procedure. Therefore, measurements of the vertical deviation in downgaze are an important part of the preoperative evaluation. If significant deviation is present, this can be managed with a contralateral inferior rectus recession (or ipsilateral superior oblique tuck, if the superior oblique muscle underacts). In the event that the involved eye does not rotate down completely (–1 or –2 underaction of the ipsilateral inferior rectus or superior oblique muscle), then consideration should be given to recessing the ipsilateral superior rectus muscle if it is tight or tucking the ipsilateral superior oblique muscle. Unfortunately, a combined inferior oblique weakening and ipsilateral superior rectus recession often has greater effect than one would predict. For that reason, care should be taken when planning this type of procedure, and adjustable sutures are advisable.

When the SOP has become concomitant, then rectus muscle recession is indicated. An inferior rectus recession or superior rectus recession will usually be effective. Next, if the vertical deviation is actually greater in fields of gaze toward the involved eye, an ipsilateral superior rectus weakening procedure may be indicated.

Bilateral superior oblique palsies are notoriously difficult to manage, despite the substantial amount of literature on the subject. The patient may not improve from surgery, or the improvement may be modest with variable strabismus in various fields of gaze. As always, the goal should be to correct the deviation in primary gaze and downgaze.

Superior oblique palsies have been categorized in a number of ways to determine what treatment is most effective in what setting. Scott and Kraft (1986a, b) have classified unilateral SOP into eight types (and bilateral SOP into four categories), and we will follow their classification scheme, more or less, because it encompasses every possible strabismus scenario encountered in SOP. Knapp (1974) has also provided a logical classification scheme.

Overacting Inferior Oblique Muscle: Superior Oblique Muscle Does Not Underact

In type 1 unilateral SOP, according to Scott and Kraft (1986a, b), the physical findings are less than 15 prism diopters of hypertropia in primary gazes with +2 to +3 overaction of the inferior oblique muscle. Scott and Kraft's type 1 nearly corresponds to Knapp's type 1 (Knapp, 1974). The strabismus deviation should be the greatest in the field of action of the overacting inferior oblique muscle. In this setting, most authorities would recommend weakening the inferior oblique muscle with the expectation that there would be a good outcome.

Overacting Inferior Oblique Muscle: Underacting Superior Oblique Muscle

In type 2 unilateral SOP, there are less than 15 prism diopters of hypertropia in primary gaze, but there is +3 to +4 IOOA. The superior oblique muscle may underact as much as −2. The amount of vertical deviation in gaze toward the uninvolved eye is greater than the

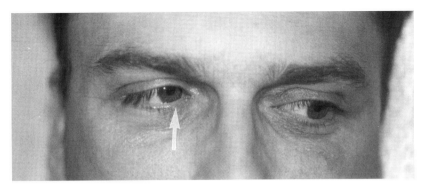

FIGURE 12.2 *Right superior oblique underaction (arrow). Note how the left eye drops as the patient looks to the left, demonstrating a "fallen eye syndrome."*

amount of deviation in gaze toward the involved side, and gaze into the field of action of the paretic superior oblique muscle is particularly bad. In this situation, Knapp (1974) would have recommended a tuck of the superior oblique muscle, if the patient had significant torsion symptoms (Knapp, 1974; Knapp and Moore, 1976), or recession of the yoke inferior rectus muscle otherwise. Scott and Kraft would recommend inferior oblique weakening, with a good chance for satisfactory outcome.

Superior Oblique Muscle Underacts: Inferior Oblique Muscle Does Not Overact

Scott and Kraft's type 3A unilateral SOP still involves less than 15 prism diopters of hypertropia in primary gaze. However, the inferior oblique muscle overacts very little and the superior oblique muscle underacts at –2 (Figure 12.2).

Type 3B is similar to type 3A, except for a much more marked underaction of the superior oblique muscle. In type 3A, Scott and Kraft would recommend weakening the contralateral inferior rectus muscle or doing a superior oblique tuck of the involved superior oblique muscle. In type 3B, these authors would recommend weakening the contralateral inferior rectus muscle or actually performing a Harada-Ito procedure while weakening the contralateral inferior rectus muscle. In types 3A and 3B, the results are still usually excellent, although a few cases do not respond so well.

Inferior Oblique Overaction—Superior Oblique Underaction: Primary Gaze Deviation Exceeds 15 Prism Diopters

Type 4 SOP involves greater than 15 prism diopters of hypertropia in primary gaze with marked IOOA, and superior oblique underaction is

−2 or less. The deviation is greater in upgaze than in downgaze in type 4. The recommendation by Scott and Kraft would be to weaken the inferior oblique muscle as well as the ipsilateral superior rectus muscle. Here the results also are usually excellent. However, approximately 33% of cases that respond to treatment do so partially or poorly.

Deviation Is Greatest in Downgaze

Type 5 SOP, according to Scott and Kraft, shows greater than 15 prism diopters of hypertropia in primary gaze with mild to moderate IOOA, mild to moderate superior oblique underaction, and deviation greater in downgaze than in upgaze. For this type of palsy, an ipsilateral inferior oblique weakening procedure combined with a contralateral inferior rectus recession would be indicated. However, if the ipsilateral (involved) eye could not rotate down completely, an ipsilateral superior rectus recession would replace the contralateral inferior rectus recession. Here the results are mixed. Approximately 50% of patients respond very well and approximately 30% respond poorly or have a fair outcome.

Knapp (1974) would characterize this problem as class 2, with a so-called L-shaped spread of deviation into downgaze, but including all fields of downgaze. He recommended an ipsilateral superior oblique tuck and a contralateral superior oblique tenotomy. Although this procedure worked for him, it runs the risk of creating bilateral SOP problems.

Large Primary Gaze Deviation with Superior Rectus Underaction

Type 6 palsy shows greater than 30 prism diopters of hypertropia in primary gaze with marked inferior oblique overaction, marked superior oblique underaction, and mild contralateral superior rectus underaction. Scott and Kraft would recommend weakening the inferior oblique muscle and also doing an ipsilateral superior rectus recession and inferior rectus resection. Knapp, according to his classification scheme, would have recommended a tuck of the superior oblique muscle and combined that with an inferior oblique weakening procedure if vertical deviation was greater than 25 prism diopters.

Concomitant Vertical Deviation

Type 7 palsy shows a concomitant hypertropia and only mild oblique dysfunction. For less than 15 prism diopters of hypertropia, Scott and Kraft would recommend an ipsilateral superior rectus recession. If the deviation was greater, they would recess the ipsilateral superior rectus muscle and resect the ipsilateral inferior rectus muscle, or recess the contralateral inferior rectus muscle.

Fallen Eye Syndrome

The fallen eye syndrome was categorized as type 8 SOP (see Figure 12.2). In this situation, the contralateral eye drops as the patient moves his or her eyes across the horizontal toward the contralateral eye. The etiology of the fallen eye has to do with Hering's law. The overacting inferior oblique muscle engenders less innervation to the yoke superior rectus muscle. The result is that adduction of the paretic eye causes the nonparetic eye to become more hypotropic. Eventually the contralateral inferior rectus muscle becomes tightened, and an elevation deficiency may occur on account of this. In this situation, it is obviously important to recess the tight inferior rectus muscle, possibly combined with an inferior oblique muscle weakening procedure on the affected eye.

Bilateral Superior Oblique Palsy

Bilateral superior oblique palsies were divided into five categories by Scott and Kraft (1986a, b). Type 1 shows alternating hypertropia on side gaze. The patient shows no significant hypertropia in primary gaze and no symptoms of torsion but a significant bilateral IOOA. This type of bilateral palsy can be treated with bilateral inferior oblique weakening.

Type 2 also shows no significant vertical deviation in primary gaze but marked underaction of the superior oblique muscle. This abnormality can be treated with the strengthening procedure of both superior obliques (tuck) (Figure 12.3).

In type 3, all of the oblique muscles are dysfunctional: The inferior oblique muscles overact, and the superior oblique muscles underact. All four muscles should be operated on—the inferior obliques via weakening and the superior obliques via strengthening.

In type 4, all oblique muscles are dysfunctional, but there is also a vertical deviation in primary gaze. This type of problem has to be treated in a specific manner. For example, if one inferior oblique muscle overacts more than the other, then a unilateral inferior oblique recession should be performed, accompanied by bilateral superior oblique strengthening procedures.

Type 5 is also referred to as "masked bilateral SOP." This is a clinical problem in which a bilateral SOP presents, at least in terms of the motility examination, as a unilateral problem (see above). It is only after surgery is performed that the bilaterality becomes apparent, because the patient shows SOP of the fellow eye. The incidence of masked bilateral SOP is estimated to be 10% of all cases of unilateral SOP, although this is debated (Robb, 1990). Treatment needs to be tailored to the ocular motor defect, as described above.

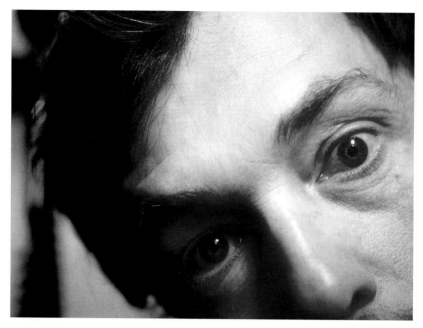

A

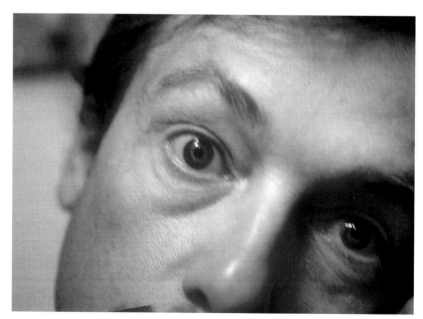

B

FIGURE 12.3 *Bilateral SOP causes V patterns with right hypertropia in left gaze and left hypertropia in right gaze. Patients may also show right hypertropia on right tilt and left hypertropia on left tilt, as shown here.*

TABLE 12.1 Complications of superior oblique tuck

Brown's syndrome
Under- or overcorrection
Asymmetric correction (for bilateral tucks)
Damage to superior rectus muscle

COMPLICATIONS

The complications related to superior oblique tuck procedures (Table 12.1) are discussed here. It is difficult to measure the amount of superior oblique tuck in terms of the effect of the procedure on ocular deviation. For that reason, the tuck may under- or overcorrect the patient's deviation. A second complication is the development of Brown's vertical retraction syndrome. The patient may have difficulty elevating his or her eye in adduction. A moderate amount of Brown's syndrome is actually inevitable after tucking the superior oblique muscle. However, marked superior oblique restriction is not desirable and occasionally is an indication for taking down the superior oblique tuck. If the tuck is deemed to be too strong—i.e., causes a troublesome strabismus—then it should be taken down promptly. Failure to do so can lead to difficulty in identifying the superior oblique tendon, sutures used for the tuck, etc. There is no reason to wait to take down the tuck, because Brown's syndrome is not going to improve over time, in most cases.

TORSION

Etiology

The oblique and vertical rectus muscles may act as incyclotorters or excyclotorters of the eye. The superior oblique and superior rectus muscles cause incyclotorsion; the inferior oblique and inferior rectus muscles cause excyclotorsion. Paralysis of one of these muscles has the opposite effect. For example, paralysis of the superior oblique or superior rectus muscle will cause excyclotorsion of the fundus. The reverse is true for paralysis of the inferior oblique or inferior rectus muscle.

Trobe (1984) studied cyclodeviation in acquired vertical strabismus. Excyclotorsion occurred in nearly every case of SOP and in about 50% of cases of thyroid ophthalmopathy. Most other cases of Graves' disease showed no ocular torsion. Fifty percent of cases where there were causes of restrictive ophthalmopathy other than Graves' disease also showed torsion. In myasthenia gravis, cyclodeviation of the eye was rare. Trobe's study was very helpful in clarifying that patients usually do not tilt their heads to compensate for cyclodeviation. Rather, they appear to tilt their heads to compensate for the vertical strabismus problem. The amount of cyclodeviation in Trobe's study did not vary according to how much the patients tilted their heads.

Kraft and colleagues (1993) studied torsion as a way of distinguishing unilateral from bilateral superior oblique palsies. Unilateral SOP could be diagnosed easily with 6 degrees of excyclotorsion. Bilateral SOP could be diagnosed reliably with 20 degrees of excyclotorsion. With excyclotorsion between 6 and 20 degrees, other criteria for diagnosis of unilateral versus bilateral SOP should by relied on.

Diagnosis

Torsion can be measured in one of several ways. The double Maddox rod test can be used as a way of distinguishing torsion, or Bagolini lenses can also be used to diagnose torsion. The patient should be asked to identify torsion in several fields of gaze, particularly primary gaze and downgaze. Excyclotorsion of the eye may worsen with downgaze in SOP, and this problematic fact can be overlooked in routine measurements of excyclotorsion.

Cyclodeviation of the eyes certainly can prevent fusion, particularly in bilateral superior oblique palsies (Pratt-Johnson and Tillson, 1987). Patients who complain of double vision, but who only have a few prism diopters of vertical deviation, may have torsion interfering with fusion. Many patients will have suffered head trauma and therefore may be mistaken as having disruption of fusion (Kushner, 1992). The goal in treating torsion is not necessarily to eliminate it entirely, though. Most people are able to tolerate up to 7 degrees of incyclotorsion or excyclotorsion. If a larger amount of torsion can be reduced, this may be enough to provide symptomatic relief.

Finally, it should be mentioned that a type of paradoxical torsion can exist in the normal fellow eye in cases of inferior rectus palsy (von Noorden and Hansell, 1991) and in cases of unilateral SOP (Olivier and von Noorden, 1982).

In cases of congenital torsion, patients are usually asymptomatic. There is probably some value in waiting 3–6 months after the onset of acquired torsion to determine whether the patient can adjust to it. If not, then the only real option for successful management is surgery. Surgical management takes advantage of the fact that a variety of extraocular muscles tort the eyes. The superior oblique and superior rectus muscles are incyclotorters. The inferior oblique and inferior rectus muscles are excyclotorters. Weakening the superior rectus or superior oblique muscle will have the effect of creating excyclotorsion. On the other hand, strengthening these muscles will create some incyclotorsion. Weakening the inferior oblique or inferior rectus muscle will cause incyclotorsion, and strengthening them will have the opposite effect.

Management

Harada-Ito Procedure
This procedure involves splitting the superior oblique tendon and moving the anterior half of the tendon anteriorly and temporally (Figure 12.4). The effect of this change in position is to incyclotort the eye. The procedure can be performed unilaterally or bilaterally. The Harada-Ito procedure probably has no other utility than to help in the management of excyclotorsion.

Inferior Oblique Weakening
In theory, the inferior oblique muscle is an excyclotorter. In reality, weakening it may have little effect on the torsional position of the eye. In cases of bilateral SOP, inferior oblique weakening procedures usually will not eliminate symptoms of torsion.

Superior Oblique Tuck
Superior oblique tuck procedures can also alleviate excyclotorsion in cases of unilateral or bilateral SOP. The tuck procedure can be performed on either the temporal or nasal side of the superior rectus muscle. The tuck procedure has the side effect of causing Brown's syndrome in virtually every case. The amount of Brown's syndrome can be titrated somewhat at the time of surgery and based on the amount of tendon that is actually tucked. Superior oblique tucking probably is the most effective treatment for excyclotorsion, although many authorities prefer the Harada-Ito procedure to manage torsion (von Noorden and Chu, 1990).

Vertical Rectus Muscle Transposition
von Noorden and colleagues have commented on the value of altering the position of the vertical rectus muscles to manage torsional symptoms (von Noorden and Chu, 1990; von Noorden et al., 1993). Shifting the inferior rectus muscle nasally reduces its incyclotorsional effect, and shifting it temporally increases its effect. Likewise, shifting the superior rectus muscle nasally weakens its incyclotorsional effect, and shifting it temporally increases its incyclotorsional effect.

Excyclotorsion could be treated via temporal transposition of the superior rectus muscle or nasal transposition of the inferior rectus muscle, or both. Incyclotorsion could be treated by nasal transposition of the superior rectus muscle or temporal transposition of the inferior rectus muscle, or both.

Thyroid myopathy is an example of a condition where movement of the vertical rectus muscles will occasionally create marked symp-

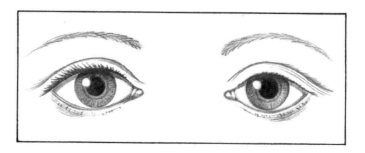

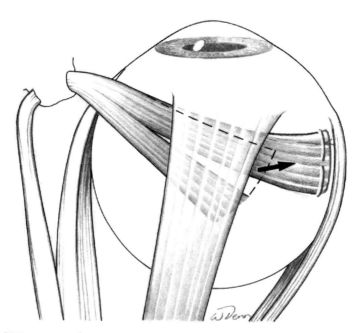

FIGURE 12.4 *The Harada-Ito procedure splits the superior oblique tendon and moves the anterior half toward the lateral rectus muscle.*

toms of torsion (Garrity et al., 1992). Even before surgery, excyclodeviation of the eye in thyroid myopathy may be detected in up to 50% of patients. This presumably is caused by tightening and restriction of the inferior rectus muscle, which cause the eyes to excyclotort (due to the excyclotorting effect of the inferior rectus muscle). Occasionally a patient with thyroid myopathy will have symptoms of incyclotorsion prior to surgery (Trobe, 1984).

After surgery, inferior rectus recessions may cause a patient to experience incyclotorsion symptoms. In our experience, if all else is well in terms of horizontal and vertical alignment, patients will adapt and adjust to this problem. When accompanied by persisting vertical or horizontal strabismus, the torsional symptoms remain bothersome and can be managed by readvancing an inferior rectus muscle, or by recessing an ipsilateral superior rectus muscle to deal with incyclotorsion. It may also be possible to reduce excyclotorsion by advancing the superior half of the medial rectus muscle while recessing the inferior half (Fink, 1951).

REFERENCES

Brandt T, Dieterich M. Pathological eye–head coordination in role: tonic ocular tilt reaction in mesencephalic and medullary lesions. Brain 1987;110:649–666.

Chapman LI, Urist MJ, Folk ER, Miller MT. Acquired bilateral superior oblique muscle palsy. Arch Ophthalmol 1970;84:137–142.

Ellis FD, Helveston EM. Superior oblique palsy: diagnosis and classification. Int Ophthalmol Clin 1976;16:127–135.

Fink WH. Surgery of the Oblique Muscles of the Eye. St. Louis: Mosby, 1951;296.

Garrity JA, Saggau DD, Gorman CA et al. Torsional diplopia after transantral orbital decompression and extraocular muscle surgery associated with Graves' orbitopathy. Am J Ophthalmol 1992;113:363–373.

Guy J, Day AL, Mickle JP, Schatz NJ. Contralateral trochlear nerve paresis and ipsilateral Horner's syndrome. Am J Ophthalmol 1989;107;73–76.

Hedges TR 3d, Hoyt WF. Ocular tilt reaction due to an upper brainstem lesion: Paroxysmal skew deviation, torsion, and oscillation of the eyes with head tilt. Ann Neurol 1982;11:537–540.

Helveston EM, Ellis FD. Pediatric Ophthalmology Practice. St. Louis: Mosby, 1980;46.

Hermann JS. Masked bilateral superior oblique paresis. J Pediatr Ophthalmol Strabismus 1981;18:43–48.

Hoyt CS, Mousel DK, Weber AA. Transient supranuclear disturbances of gaze in healthy neonates. Am J Ophthalmol 1980;89:708–713.

Jacobson DM, Warner JJ, Choucair AK, Ptacek LJ. Trochlear nerve palsy following minor head trauma. A sign of structural disorder. J Clin Neuro-Ophthalmol 1988;8:263–268.

Jampolsky A. Vertical Strabismus Surgery. In Symposium on Strabismus. Transactions of the New Orleans Academy of Ophthalmology. St. Louis: Mosby, 1971;366–385.

Keane JR. Alternating skew deviation: 47 patients. Neurology 1985;35:725–728.

Keane JR. Ocular skew deviation: analysis of 100 cases. Arch Neurol 1975;32:185–190.

Knapp P. Classification and treatment of superior oblique palsy. Am Orthop J 1974;24:18–22.

Knapp P, Moore S. Diagnosis and surgical options in superior oblique surgery. Int Ophthalmol Clin 1976;16:137–149.

Kraft SP, O'Reilly C, Quigley PL et al. Cyclotorsion in unilateral and bilateral superior oblique paresis. J Pediatr Ophthalmol Strabismus 1993;30:361–367.

Kraft SP, Scott WE. Masked bilateral superior oblique palsy: clinical features and diagnosis. J Pediatr Ophthalmol Strabismus 1986;23:264–267.

Kushner BJ. Unexpected cyclotropia simulating disruption of fusion. Arch Ophthalmol 1992;110:1415–1418.

Leigh RJ, Zee DS. The Neurology of Eye Movements (2nd ed). Philadelphia: FA Davis, 1991;410–412, 432–437.

Lyle TK. Torsional diplopia due to cyclotropia and its surgical treatment. Trans Am Acad Ophthalmol Otolaryngol 1964;68:387–411.

Mitchell PR, Parks MM: Surgery for bilateral superior oblique palsy. Ophthalmology 1982;89:484–448.

Mittelman D, Folk ER. The evaluation and treatment of superior oblique muscle palsy. Trans Am Acad Ophthalmol Otolaryngol 1976;81:893–898.

Moster ML, Schatz NJ, Savino PJ et al. Alternating skew on lateral gaze (bilateral abducting hypertropia). Ann Neurol 1988;23:190–192.

Olivier P, von Noorden GK. Excyclotropia of the nonparetic eye in unilateral superior oblique muscle paralysis. Am J Ophthalmol 1982;93:30–33.

Parks MM. Isolated cyclovertical muscle palsy. Arch Ophthalmol 1958;60:1027–1035.

Pratt-Johnson JA, Tillson G. The investigation and management of torsion preventing fusion in bilateral superior oblique palsies. J Pediatr Ophthalmol Strabismus 1987;24:145–150.

Reynolds JD, Biglan AW, Hiles DA. Congenital superior oblique palsy in infants. Arch Ophthalmol 1984;102:1503–1505.

Robb RM. Idiopathic superior oblique palsies in children. J Pediatr Ophthalmol Strabismus 1990;27:66–69.

Scott WE. Differential Diagnosis of Vertical Muscle Palsies. In Symposium on Strabismus. Transactions of the New Orleans Academy of Ophthalmology. St. Louis: Mosby, 1978;118–134.

Scott WE, Kraft SP. Classification and Surgical Treatment of Superior Oblique Palsies: I. Unilateral Superior Oblique Palsies. In Pediatric Ophthalmology and Strabismus. Transactions of the New Orleans Academy of Ophthalmology. New York: Raven, 1986;15–38.

Scott WE, Kraft SP. Classification and Treatment of Superior Oblique Palsies. II. Bilateral Superior Oblique Palsies. In Pediatric Ophthalmology and Strabismus. Transactions of the New Orleans Academy of Ophthalmology. New York: Raven, 1986;265–291.

Souza-Dias C. Surgical Management of Superior Oblique Paresis. In S Moore, J Mein, L Stockbridge (eds), Orthoptics: Past, Present and Future. Miami: Symposia Specialists, 1976;379–391.

Sydnor CF, Seaber JH, Buckley EG. Traumatic superior oblique palsies. Ophthalmology 1982;89:134–138.

Trobe JD. Cyclodeviation in acquired vertical strabismus. Arch Ophthalmol 1984;102:717–720.

von Noorden GK, Chu MW. Surgical treatment options in cyclotropia. J Pediatr Ophthalmol Strabismus 1990;27:291–293.

von Noorden GK. Clinical and theoretical aspects of cyclotropia. J Pediatr Ophthalmol Strabismus 1984;21:126–132.

von Noorden GK, Jenkins RH, Rosenbaum AL. Horizontal transposition of the vertical rectus muscles for treatment of ocular torticollis. J Pediatr Ophthalmol Strabismus 1993;30:8–14.

von Noorden GK, Hansell R. Clinical characteristics and treatment of isolated inferior rectus paralysis. Ophthalmology 1991;98:253–257.

von Noorden GK, Murray E, Wong SY. Superior oblique paralysis. A review of 270 cases. Arch Ophthalmol 1986;104:1771–1776.

Westheimer G, Blair SM. The ocular tilt reaction—a brainstem oculomotor routine. Invest Ophthalmol 1975;14:833–839.

13

Double Elevator Palsy

ETIOLOGY

Double elevator palsy refers to the inability to elevate one eye (Figure 13.1). The problem usually is monocular; seldom are both eyes involved except in cases of bilateral congenital inferior rectus fibrosis. The term *double elevator palsy* is probably a misnomer, since the usual etiology of this condition may not be supranuclear (Scott and Jackson, 1977), and therefore may not involve both elevator muscles.

The eye has two muscles that can elevate it: The superior rectus provides most of the generation of upward gaze, but the inferior oblique muscle also contributes. Collins and colleagues (1983) have shown that the inferior oblique muscle provides an elevation force to midline, beyond which it contributes little or nothing to upgaze. Above midline, the superior rectus muscle provides most elevation force.

White (1942) coined the term *double elevator palsy*. At that time, authorities believed that the origin of the upgaze abnormality in double elevator palsy was in the central nervous system—i.e., supranuclear. Unilateral upgaze palsy has been noted in cases with documented supranuclear pathology (Lessell, 1975; Ford et al., 1984), either ipsilateral to the palsy or contralateral to it (Jampel and Fell, 1968). Kirkham and Kline (1976) suggested that upgaze is "compartmentalized" in the central nervous system, with upgaze starting from above and/or below the midline, controlled by different centers. Ziffer and associates (1992) have revived the concept that at least some cases of double elevator palsy are supranuclear in origin. They showed that some patients have a normal upward saccadic trajectory below, but not above, the midline.

158

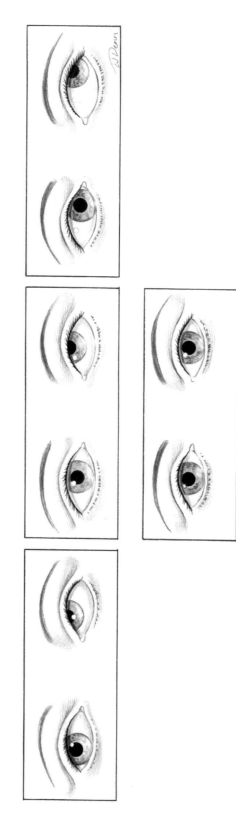

FIGURE 13.1 *In double elevator palsy, the eye fails to rotate up in abduction and adduction.*

The fact that most cases of double elevator palsy are probably caused by a tight or contracted inferior rectus muscle has been demonstrated in several studies (Scott and Jackson, 1977; Metz, 1979). Some cases of double elevator palsy are caused by a hypoplastic or ineffective superior rectus muscle, and some cases are likely caused by both conditions. Long-standing hypotropia (e.g., with superior rectus paresis) will eventually cause a tight ipsilateral inferior rectus muscle.

Nearly all cases of double elevator palsy occur sporadically. Bell and colleagues (1990) invoked a supranuclear hypothesis in describing double elevator palsy in identical twins. However, the exact mechanism of upgaze deficiency in these children cannot be determined on the basis of data supplied in their report.

DIAGNOSIS

In many cases, the diagnosis of double elevator palsy is obvious. The child is unable to elevate an eye, and as long as he or she cooperates with the examination, this can be seen without difficulty. The abnormality of upgaze persists across the horizontal plane, from abduction to adduction (see Figure 13.1). This elevation deficit may be profound, leading to a –5 or –6 inability to elevate the eye. Occasionally the problem is less severe. Up to 33% of patients with double elevator palsy may even demonstrate orthotropia in primary gaze (Metz, 1979).

A chin-up position for fusion is an occasional presenting sign in double elevator palsy. The child with good fusion potential but difficulty raising one eye will elevate his or her chin and look down on objects of interest, presumably to avoid double vision.

Eyelid position abnormalities can also be helpful in diagnosing double elevator palsy (White, 1942). A hypoplastic or inactive superior rectus muscle will often be found in conjunction with ptosis of the upper eyelid. Pseudoptosis occurs with hypotropia and is diagnosed after correction of the strabismus—that is, the ptosis resolves. Prior to surgery, in the absence of true ptosis, the upper lid should assume a normal position when the eye is elevated (if it can be elevated).

We have noted abnormalities in the lower lid in cases in which a restricted or tightened inferior rectus muscle is the cause. Lower lid retractors may be trapped or incorporated into a tight inferior rectus muscle, causing entropion of the lower lid or an extra skin fold 2–3 mm below the lower eyelid margin (Figure 13.2). The presence of lower lid abnormalities can be used to help distinguish restriction of the inferior rectus muscle (where the lower lid abnormality may be seen) from hypoplasia of the superior rectus muscle or a supranuclear disturbance.

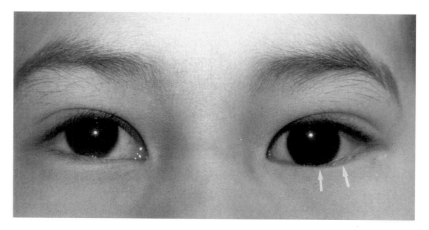

FIGURE 13.2   *In cases in which the cause of the double elevator palsy is a tight (fibrotic) inferior rectus muscle, a lid crease (arrows) below the lower lid margin may be present. This crease may help distinguish restrictive strabismus (inferior rectus) from strabismus caused by a hypoplastic or paralyzed superior rectus muscle.*

Forced duction testing in patients with double elevator palsy is helpful. If the examiner has difficulty elevating the eye on forced duction testing, this implies a tight inferior rectus muscle. Conversely, if the eye can be easily elevated passively, but does not elevate actively, this implies an underacting superior rectus muscle. The distinction between these two is paramount, because treatment may be different for each entity.

DIFFERENTIAL DIAGNOSIS

Other conditions that may completely or partially restrict elevation of an eye should be considered in the differential diagnosis of double elevator palsy. Brown's syndrome consists of difficulty elevating the eye in the adducted position. There may also be some restriction of elevation in primary gaze, and lesser amounts of restricted elevation in abduction. A forced duction test is positive when the eye is rotated up and in, but normal when the eye is rotated up and out. Other distinguishing features of Brown's syndrome include pain on elevation, a click near the area of the trochlea, the presence of a V pattern strabismus, occasional superior oblique overaction, head tilting, a history of trauma, endocrine disease, or Marfan's syndrome (Good and Corbett, 1991).

Graves' ophthalmopathy can cause restriction of the inferior rectus muscle. The result is almost a reverse Brown's syndrome with greater restricted upgaze in abduction. In cases of double elevator palsy, the abnormality is congenital. Graves' disease is acquired. Eye movement abnormalities of Graves' disease are rarely encountered in children. Nevertheless, the child who presents with progressive chin-up position for fusion should undergo a careful endocrine assessment and computed tomographic and magnetic resonance imaging scanning of the orbit for assessment of the size of the extraocular muscles.

A blowout fracture as a result of strabismus is also in the differential diagnosis of double elevator palsy. When the inferior rectus muscle becomes trapped in an orbital floor fracture, restriction of upgaze can occur. Other ocular motility abnormalities may coexist and help to distinguish blowout fracture–induced strabismus from double elevator palsy. For example, paralysis of the inferior rectus muscle secondary to blowout fracture can cause poor downgaze in addition to restricted upgaze. A fracture affecting the rectus muscle can cause ipsilateral hypertropia, but also deficient elevation or depression. Other distinguishing features of blowout fractures include enophthalmos and abnormalities on x-ray or computed tomography scanning.

In cases of fourth nerve palsy where the patient fixes with the paretic eye, the uninvolved eye may appear to have an elevation deficiency. Ductions of the uninvolved eye should be normal if tested properly. Forced head tilt testing should be lateralizing in cases of fourth nerve palsy. In double elevator palsy, the forced head tilt test is not helpful diagnostically.

Elevation weakness in an eye is also occasionally encountered following cataract surgery (Rao and Kawatra, 1988). One possible cause is the myotoxic effects of local anesthetic agents (Rainin and Carlson, 1985). The clinical course in myotoxin is usually one of immediate paralysis followed by a gradual recovery.

MEDICAL AND SYSTEMIC EVALUATION

Unless there is concern about differential diagnostic possibilities, no systemic or radiologic evaluation is necessary. We are aware of only one association between double elevator palsy and systemic disease—polycythemia vera (Hoyt, 1978). Cases of acquired monocular upgaze deficiency caused by a supranuclear disturbance are rare and may be accompanied by evidence of other central nervous system disease.

SURGICAL MANAGEMENT

In cases in which fusion in the primary gaze has been compromised or a chin-up position is required to maintain fusion, surgical intervention should be considered. Other possible interventions include base-up prism over the involved eye. To our knowledge, botulinum neurotoxin has not been studied in this condition; its use in children remains experimental. Our experience has shown that prism glasses are ineffective in the management of double elevator palsy.

Double Elevator Palsy Associated with a Tight Inferior Rectus Muscle

If the forced duction test indicates difficulty in passively rotating the eye up in abduction and adduction, tightness of the inferior rectus muscle is diagnosed. Surgical management, then, consists of recessing the involved inferior rectus muscle. The muscle may be found to be tight and fibrotic. Care should be taken to avoid losing this muscle when grasping it with muscle hooks, because it can be *avulsed* easily. The amount of recession depends on the amount of preoperative deviation and the monitoring of forced ductions intraoperatively (see below). As a rule of thumb, the effect of the inferior rectus recession is 2.5 prism diopters per millimeter of recession. However, with tightened and fibrotic muscles, the effect of a recession is more unpredictable and may be greater than expected.

The inferior rectus muscle can be recessed to a desired position and then be checked with intraoperative forced duction testing (Jampolsky, 1975). The forced duction in the involved eye is compared with that of the fellow eye, and if the tests are roughly matched (i.e., the recession eliminates the positive forced duction), the amount of recession is probably correct. If there is a great discrepancy, then a change in surgery should be considered. For example, if passive resistance to elevation at the time of surgery remains very positive, even with a 4- or 5-mm inferior rectus recession, the surgeon should consider recessing this inferior rectus muscle several more millimeters.

Double Elevator Palsy with Underaction of the Superior Rectus Muscle

When the forced duction test indicates no or slight restriction of the inferior rectus muscle, the surgeon's treatment must somehow include elevating the eye with other mechanical forces, a goal that the Knapp procedure has been designed to accomplish. The procedure consists of elevation and transposition of the medial and lateral rectus muscles to the sides of the superior rectus muscle (Knapp, 1969) (Figure 13.3).

As long as the inferior rectus muscle is unoperated, the surgeon can anticipate a correction of approximately 20 prism diopters of hypotropia with this procedure, regardless of the preoperative deviation (Burke et al., 1992). If the inferior rectus muscle is recessed, this procedure is more effective and yields approximately 35 prism diopters of correction (Burke et al., 1992).

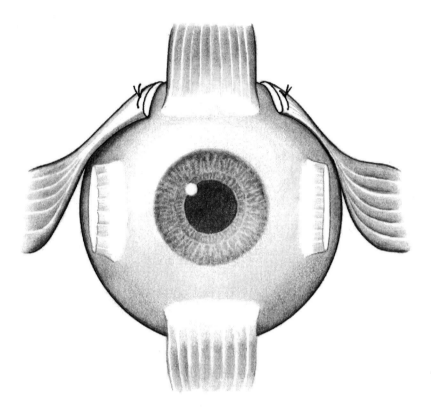

FIGURE 13.3 *The Knapp procedure consists of transposition of the lateral and medial rectus muscles to the sides of the superior rectus muscle.*

Double Elevator Palsy with a Mildly Abnormal Forced Duction Test and an Abnormal Forced Generation Test of Upgaze

Long-standing hypotropia due to underaction of the superior rectus muscle can lead to restriction of the inferior rectus muscle. In cases where this diagnosis is made, the surgeon may need to operate on three muscles in the same eye. The medial and lateral rectus muscles are elevated via a Knapp procedure. Simultaneously, the inferior rectus muscle is recessed. The risk of causing anterior segment ischemia with three-muscle surgery in children is only slight. In some cases, it is possible to cripple the superior rectus muscle in the fellow eye. The amount of recession of the superior rectus muscle necessary to restrict upgaze is enormous. Even a 15-mm recession may only produce a 30% elevation deficit.

Double Elevator Palsy and Ptosis

When ptosis accompanies double elevator palsy, the strabismus should be corrected first (Callahan, 1981). Afterward, any residual ptosis can be managed, usually by levator resection.

COMPLICATIONS OF SURGERY FOR
DOUBLE ELEVATOR PALSY

Undercorrection

In cases where hypotropia persists after inferior rectus recession, several treatment options are available. Prisms can be tried but are often unsatisfactory. With orthotropia in primary gaze but progressive hypotropia in upgaze, the contralateral superior rectus muscle can be recessed. In persistent primary gaze hypotropia and positive forced duction testing, further recession of the ipsilateral inferior rectus muscle is advisable. With negative forced duction testing, a Knapp procedure may be most effective.

Overcorrection

Overcorrection manifests as hypertropia in primary gaze or downgaze, or both. Overcorrections noted following the Knapp procedure are stable or may even progress (Burke et al., 1992). For treatment of primary gaze overcorrection, readvancement of the inferior rectus muscle may be advisable. If accomplished promptly (within 6 weeks of initial inferior rectus recession), the effect may be approximately the same as was obtained with the recession—i.e., 1 mm of readvancement equals 1 mm of recession. After a few months, the length-tension dynamics of the operated muscle change sufficiently to make readvancement less predictable. Nevertheless, this may still be the appropriate procedure.

For (ipsilateral) hypertropia only in downgaze, a Faden operation on the inferior rectus muscle of the fellow eye is appropriate. This procedure does not alter the alignment in primary gaze but restricts the eye's downward rotation.

REFERENCES

Bell JA, Fielder AR, Viney S. Congenital double elevator palsy in identical twins. J Clin Neuro-Ophthalmol 1990;10:32–34.

Burke JP, Ruben JB, Scott WE. Vertical transposition of the horizontal recti (Knapp procedure) for the treatment of double elevator palsy: effectiveness and long-term stability. Br J Ophthalmol 1992;76:734–737.

Callahan MA. Surgically mismanaged ptosis associated with double elevator palsy. Arch Ophthalmol 1981;99:108–112.

Carlson BM, Rainin EA. Rat extraocular muscle regeneration. Repair of local anesthetic–induced damage. Arch Ophthalmol 1985;103:1373–1377.

Collins CC, Jampolsky A, Magoon EH. Vertical action of the inferior oblique muscle. Invest Ophthalmol Vis Sci 1983;24(Suppl):36.

Ford CS, Schwartze GM, Weaver RG, Troost BT. Monocular elevation paresis caused by an ipsilateral lesion. Neurology 1984;34:1264–1267.

Good WV, Corbett TD. Acquired Brown's syndrome in association with Marfan's syndrome. Binoc Vis Eye Muscle Surg Q 1991;6:101–102.

Hoyt CS. Acquired "double elevator" palsy and polycythemia vera. J Pediatr Ophthalmol Strabismus 1978;15:362–365.

Jampel RS, Fells P. Monocular elevation paresis caused by a central nervous system lesion. Arch Ophthalmol 1968;80:45–57.

Jampolsky A. Strabismus reoperation techniques. Trans Am Acad Ophthalmol Otolaryngol 1975;79:704–717.

Kirkham TH, Kline LB. Monocular elevator paresis, Argyll Robertson pupils and sarcoidosis. Can J Ophthalmol 1976;11:330–335.

Knapp P. The surgical treatment of double-elevator paralysis. Trans Am Ophthalmol Soc 1969;67:304–323.

Lessell S. Supranuclear paralysis of monocular elevation. Neurology 1975;25:1134–1143.

Metz HS. Double elevator palsy. Arch Ophthalmol 1979;97:901–903.

Rainin EA, Carlson BM. Postoperative diplopia and ptosis. A clinical hypothesis based on the myotoxicity of local anesthetics. Arch Ophthalmol 1985;103:1337–1339.

Rao VA, Kawatra VK. Ocular myotoxic effects of local anesthetics. Can J Ophthalmol 1988;23:171–173.

Scott WE, Jackson OB. Double elevator palsy: the significance of inferior rectus restriction. Am Orthop J 1977;27:5–10.

White JW. Paralysis of the superior rectus and the inferior oblique muscle of the same eye. Arch Ophthalmol 1942;27:366–371.

Ziffer AJ, Rosenbaum AL, Demer JL, Yee RD. Congenital double elevator palsy: vertical saccadic velocity utilizing the scleral search coil technique. J Pediatr Ophthalmol Strabismus 1992;29:142–149.

14

Brown's Syndrome

THEORY AND ETIOLOGY

Brown's syndrome occurs when the distance between the insertion of the superior oblique tendon and the trochlea cannot be shortened. Patients with Brown's syndrome are therefore unable to adequately elevate their affected eye in the adducted position. This deficiency in elevation is less severe or not present in abduction.

The evolution of understanding of the etiology of Brown's syndrome is noteworthy. Brown (1950) described the syndrome and termed it the *superior oblique tendon syndrome*. His initial theory was that the anterior sheath of the superior oblique tendon was shortened due to a palsy of the ipsilateral inferior oblique muscle (Brown, 1957). Later it was shown that disease in the tendon and superior oblique trochlea is usually etiologic (Wilson et al., 1989). Thickening of tissue in and around the trochlea prevents the superior oblique tendon from sliding passively through the trochlea. Undoubtedly, Brown's syndrome may also be caused by inflammation or thickening of the tendon sheath of the superior oblique tendon, away from the actual region of the trochlea.

Brown's syndrome is usually acquired, with no known cause. Acquired cases may relapse and remit, whereas congenital cases tend to remain stable or progress slowly.

A variety of other conditions can occasionally produce Brown's syndrome (Table 14.1). Inflammatory diseases are well known causes of Brown's syndrome. Rheumatoid arthritis can cause this syndrome (Smith, 1965), but so can other conditions that cause joint or cartilage disease, including Marfan's syndrome (Good and Corbett, 1991 (Figure 14.1).

TABLE 14.1   Conditions that cause Brown's syndrome

Idiopathic
Congenital
Trauma
Tumor metastases of trochlea
Ethmoid/sinus surgery
Marfan's syndrome
Rheumatoid arthritis
Acromegaly
Dental extraction
Retinal detachment surgery
Glaucoma exoplant surgery

Brown's syndrome may occur after superior oblique tucking procedures (Helveston and Ellis, 1983), retinal detachment surgery (Parks and Brown, 1975), and glaucoma exoplant surgery (Ball et al., 1992). Trauma is also a known cause (Baldwin and Baker, 1988).

DIAGNOSIS

The most important feature of Brown's syndrome is difficulty elevating the eye in the adducted position. This finding must be accompanied by a positive forced duction test in the field of action of the inferior oblique muscle (i.e., in elevation and adduction) (Figure 14.2). The forced duction test can be performed either preoperatively on cooperative patients or intraoperatively. The eye is grasped in two positions, usually at 3 o'clock and 9 o'clock, and an attempt is made to elevate the eye in adduction. Comparison of restriction should be made between the involved eye and the uninvolved eye.

When the eye is retroplaced, the superior oblique tendon is stretched and the forced duction test is accentuated (Metz, 1979a, b). Guyton (1981) described a provocative test to elicit an abnormal forced duction finding. The eye is grasped in two positions (again, usually 3 o'clock and 9 o'clock) and extorted, and then an attempt is made to raise and adduct it. The extortion of the eye stretches the superior oblique tendon farther and will accentuate the forced duction test.

Many patients with Brown's syndrome cannot elevate their eye adequately in the primary field of gaze. As a result, they may show hypotropia in primary gaze (Brown, 1973). If the patient is able to fuse, he or she will often elevate the chin and assume an abnormal head position to compensate for the hypotropia (Nutt and Mein, 1963). The eye can be elevated without difficulty when it is abducted. This clinical fea-

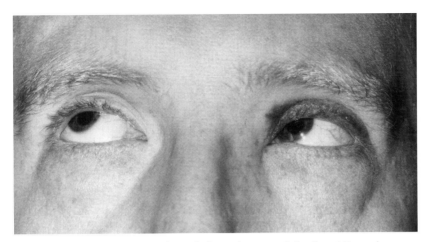

FIGURE 14.1 *This man had Marfan's syndrome and developed Brown's syndrome in his left eye. An attempt to treat his problem with steroid injection failed and caused a small hematoma. After treatment with a left superior oblique tenotomy and inferior oblique myectomy, he was orthotropic in primary gaze. He gradually developed symptomatic left hypertropia in downgaze. After unsuccessful treatment with prisms, he was successfully managed with a small right inferior rectus recession.*

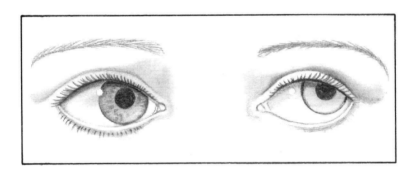

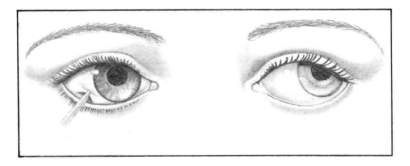

FIGURE 14.2 *In Brown's syndrome, the affected eye fails to rotate up when adducted (right eye). Attempts to move the eye up with forced duction testing meet with resistance.*

ture is helpful when assessing the differential diagnosis. Additional findings include no superior oblique overaction on the involved side. Patients often show a V pattern, and attempted elevation results in some abduction, inducing exotropia in upgaze. Some patients with Brown's syndrome will report pain in the superonasal orbit, the region of the superior oblique trochlea. A click or abnormal sensation in this region may occur when the eye is elevated and adducted.

Brown's syndrome has been classified by Wilson and colleagues (1989) according to its severity. In mild cases, there is restricted elevation in adduction. In moderate cases this restricted elevation is accompanied by a downshoot of the eye when the eye is adducted across the horizontal plane. No hypotropia is present. In severe cases, hypotropia in primary gaze accompanies the finding of restricted elevation and a downward movement of the eye in adduction.

DIFFERENTIAL DIAGNOSIS

A number of conditions can mimic Brown's syndrome and should be considered in the differential diagnosis (Table 14.2). In inferior oblique palsy (see Chapter 16), the eye may also fail to rotate up and in, but forced duction testing is normal. Superior oblique overaction may be present, and forced head tilt testing may show worsening of the hypertropia when the head is tilted away from the involved eye.

Congenital fibrosis syndrome (see Chapter 18) can produce a tight inferior rectus muscle, simulating Brown's syndrome. The forced duction test should be positive in all fields of upgaze. If a tight inferior rectus muscle is accompanied by a tight medial rectus muscle, the forced duction test may dramatically mimic Brown's syndrome. Performance of the forced duction test, with retroplacement of the globe, and the Guyton enhanced forced duction test should help clarify the underlying condition at the time of surgery. In cases where sensory fusion still exists but requires an awkward head position, surgical exploration of potentially involved muscles is advisable. Amblyopia is uncommon in Brown's syndrome (Clarke and Noel, 1983); its presence probably does not help establish a diagnosis of congenital fibrosis.

Double elevator palsy (see Chapter 13) also can mimic Brown's syndrome. In this condition, restriction of the inferior rectus muscle, or supranuclear disturbance of monocular elevation, inhibits elevation in adduction and abduction. Occasional cases of double elevator palsy are caused by underaction of the superior rectus muscle. The same deficiency in active elevation of the eye should be noted. Forced duction testing is normal early on, but prolonged hypertropia may eventually result in tightening of the ipsilateral inferior rectus muscle.

TABLE 14.2   Differential diagnosis of Brown's syndrome

Inferior oblique palsy
Congenital fibrosis syndrome
Double elevator palsy
Blowout fracture
Thyroid myopathy
Fat adherence syndrome

A history of trauma to the eye suggests a diagnosis of blowout fracture (see Chapter 20). Enophthalmos might also be present, and restricted elevation in abduction and adduction is often present. Some patients with blowout fracture cannot depress the involved eye due to paralysis or underaction of the inferior rectus muscle. Imaging studies of the orbit may confirm the diagnosis.

Patients with thyroid myopathy (see Chapter 19) and inferior rectus restriction show deficient eye elevation, which is most pronounced in abduction. Other signs of thyroid ophthalmopathy may be present, including proptosis. Imaging studies of the orbit show enlarged extraocular muscles.

MANAGEMENT

Treatment of the Underlying Cause of Brown's Syndrome

Treatment of the underlying cause of Brown's syndrome can be therapeutic. Effective management of sinusitis can be curative (Clark, 1966; Parks and Brown, 1975). Juvenile rheumatoid arthritis can be treated with anti-inflammatory medication (Wang et al., 1984). Systemic corticosteroids have been used to resolve Brown's syndrome in a child with juvenile rheumatoid arthritis (Moore and Morin, 1985) as well as in adults with Brown's syndrome and rheumatoid arthritis (Beck and Hickling, 1980).

Steroid Injections for the Management of Brown's Syndrome

In cases of acquired Brown's syndrome, injection of corticosteroids in the vicinity of the trochlea may be therapeutic (Sandford-Smith, 1973; Hermann, 1978), especially when there are signs of local inflammation (e.g., redness, tenderness) or systemic inflammatory disease (e.g., juvenile rheumatoid arthritis). A long-acting steroid (e.g., methylprednisolone) can be injected into the superonasal quadrant using a short (⅝ in.), 25-gauge needle. Patients should be observed afterward for increases in intraocular pressure.

In our experience, the use of steroid injections effectively relieves Brown's syndrome temporarily. Many patients suffer recurrences but can be managed with repeated steroid injections.

Brown's Syndrome with Hypotropia in Primary Gaze and/or Head Posture

Surgery is indicated when the patient has hypotropia in primary gaze (Nutt and Mein, 1963). Sheathectomies of the superior oblique tendon fail to correct symptomatic cases of Brown's syndrome (Folk, 1957; Girard, 1956). Combining a sheathectomy with a traction suture (to elevate the eye for several days after surgery) also usually fails (Crawford, 1976; Parks, 1978). Sheathectomy in combination with inferior oblique tuck or superior rectus resection also yields disappointing results (Brown, 1973, 1974).

On the other hand, a weakening procedure of the superior oblique tendon—either tenotomy or tenectomy—is effective in eliminating Brown's syndrome (Berke, 1946; Crawford et al., 1976; Eustis et al., 1987). Examination of the superior oblique tendon may help in the management (Parks and Helveston, 1970). Most patients will be able to elevate the involved eye after superior oblique weakening, but many patients develop a slowly evolving superior oblique palsy (Crawford, 1980).

A combined procedure of superior oblique tenotomy and inferior oblique weakening has been advocated by Parks and Eustis (1987) to manage superior oblique palsy. The addition of the inferior oblique weakening procedure may cause underaction of the inferior oblique muscle and contribute to the preexisting hypotropia. The surgeon can inspect the position of the fovea relative to the optic nerve and attempt to evaluate the presence of excyclotorsion following weakening of the superior oblique tendon (Guyton, 1983). Excyclotorsion that is visible ophthalmoscopically indicates the need to perform an inferior oblique weakening procedure.

Hypertropia in downgaze can also occur after weakening the superior oblique muscle. Some patients tolerate this; others may require an additional operation. Correction of this problem can be accomplished by placing a Faden suture in the inferior rectus muscle of the fellow eye.

REFERENCES

Baldwin L, Baker RS. Acquired Brown's syndrome in a patient with an orbital roof fracture. J Clin Neuro-Ophthalmol 1988;8:127–130.

Ball SF, Ellis GS Jr, Herrington RG, Liang K. Brown's superior oblique tendon syndrome after Baerveldt glaucoma implant [letter]. Arch Ophthalmol 1992;110:1368.

Beck M, Hickling P. Treatment of bilateral superior oblique tendon sheath syndrome complicating rheumatoid arthritis. Br J Ophthalmol 1980;64:358–361.

Berke RN. Tenotomy of the superior oblique for hypertropia; preliminary report. Trans Am Ophthalmol Soc 1946;44:304–342.

Brown HW. Congenital Structural Muscle Anomalies. In Symposium on Strabismus. Transactions of the New Orleans Academy of Ophthalmology. St. Louis: Mosby, 1950;205–236.

Brown HW. Isolated inferior oblique paralyses. Trans Am Ophthalmol Soc 1957;55:415–454.

Brown HW. True and simulated superior oblique tendon sheath syndromes. Doc Ophthalmol 1973;34:123–136.

Brown HW. True and simulated superior oblique tendon sheath syndromes. Aust J Ophthalmol 1974;2:12–19.

Clark E. A case of apparent intermittent overaction of the left superior oblique. Br Orthop J 1966;23:116–117.

Clarke WN, Noel LP. Brown's syndrome: fusion status and amblyopia. Can J Ophthalmol 1983;18:118–123.

Crawford JS. Surgical treatment of true Brown's syndrome. Am J Ophthalmol 1976;81:289–295.

Crawford JS, Orton RB, Labow-Daily L. Late results of superior oblique muscle tenotomy in true Brown's syndrome. Am J Ophthalmol 1980;89:824–829.

Eustis HS, O'Reilly C, Crawford JS. Management of superior oblique palsy after surgery for true Brown's syndrome. J Pediatr Ophthalmol Strabismus 1987;24:10–16.

Folk ER. Superior oblique tendon sheath syndrome. Arch Ophthalmol 1957;57:39–40.

Girard LJ. Pseudoparalysis of the inferior oblique muscle. South Med J 1956;49:342–346.

Good WV, Corbett T. Brown's syndrome occurring in Marfan's syndrome. Binoc Vis Q 1991;6:101–102.

Guyton DL. Exaggerated traction test for the oblique muscles. Ophthalmology 1981;88:1035–1040.

Guyton DL. Clinical assessment of ocular torsion. Am Orthop J 1983;33:7–15.

Helveston EM, Ellis FD. Superior oblique tuck for superior oblique palsy. Aust J Ophthalmol 1983;11:215–220.

Hermann JS. Acquired Brown's syndrome of inflammatory origin. Response to locally injected steroids. Arch Ophthalmol 1978;96:1228–1232.

Metz HS. Restrictions in the diagnosis and management of strabismus problems. J Pediatr Ophthalmol Strabismus 1979a;16:108–112.

Metz HS. Saccadic velocity measurements in Brown's syndrome. Ann Ophthalmol 1979b;11:636–638.

Moore AT, Morin JD. Bilateral acquired inflammatory Brown's syndrome. J Pediatr Ophthalmol Strabismus 1985;22:26–30.

Nutt AB, Mein J. The significance and management of abnormal head postures. Trans Ophthalmol Soc Aust 1963;23:57–71.

Parks MM, Brown M. Superior oblique tendon sheath syndrome of Brown. Am J Ophthalmol 1975;79:82–86.

Parks MM, Eustis HS. Simultaneous superior oblique tenotomy and inferior oblique recession in Brown's syndrome. Ophthalmology 1987;94:1043–1048.

Parks MM, Helveston EM. Direct visualization of the superior oblique tendon. Arch Ophthalmol 1970;84:491–494.

Parks MM. Surgery for Brown's Syndrome. In Symposium on Strabismus. Transactions of the New Orleans Academy of Ophthalmology. St. Louis: Mosby, 1978;157–177.

Sandford-Smith JH. Superior oblique tendon sheath syndrome and its relationship to stenosing tenosynovitis. Br J Ophthalmol 1973;57:859–865.

Smith E. Aetiology of apparent superior oblique tendon sheath syndrome. Trans Orthop Assoc Aust 1965;7:32.

Wang FM, Wertenbaker C, Behrens MM, Jacobs JC. Acquired Brown's syndrome in children with juvenile rheumatoid arthritis. Ophthalmology 1984;91:23–26.

Wilson ME, Eustis HS Jr, Parks MM. Brown's syndrome. Surv Ophthalmol 1989;34:153–172.

15

Divergent Vertical Deviation

ETIOLOGY

Stevens (1895) is credited with the discovery of divergent vertical deviation (DVD), but excellent descriptions and studies on the subject have been written by Bielschowsky (1940), Verhoeff (1941), Brown (1966), and Helveston (1980). Many terms have been used to describe DVD, including alternating supraduction, alternating hyperphoria (Crone, 1954), occlusion hypertropia, and double hypertropia. The term *divergent vertical deviation* has gained the widest acceptance and is used in this text.

The exact cause of DVD is unknown. White (1933) proposed that hyperfunction of the superior rectus muscles could be etiologic, and alternating eye depressor muscles could be paretic (Scobee, 1947). Aberrant impulses from a brain stem center, one that controls and allows vertical divergence, is another theory (Bielschowsky, 1938). Presumably, intermittent impulses to alternating sites could produce DVD. Crone (1954) suggested that deficient optomotor impulses from the inferonasal retina could account for DVD. Abnormalities of tone to the extraocular muscles could cause DVD, according to Posner (1944). The possibility that hypofunction of the superior oblique muscle could cause DVD seems to be contradicted by cases in which the superior oblique muscle overacts, ipsilateral to the eye with DVD (Helveston, 1969). The fact that DVD could be caused by a supranuclear disturbance has been discussed by Helveston (1991), who concluded that "divergent vertical deviation results from a neurologic oculomotor imbalance mediated by a presumed vertical vergence center or centers." This remains the best explanation for DVD, but the exact mechanism whereby DVD develops remains elusive.

DIAGNOSIS

Symptoms

DVD almost never causes symptoms. We have seen one child who experienced brow pain with DVD, but it was difficult to judge whether this was caused by DVD or some awareness that his eye was rotated up. Instead, DVD becomes apparent to friends and family of the patient as a wandering eye, most apparent at times of fatigue, lack of concentration, or illness.

Divergent Vertical Deviation and Hering's Law

DVD shows a number of clinical characteristics that help distinguish it from other vertical strabismus disorders. The hallmark of DVD is upward rotation of the eye, spontaneously or when occluded, associated with incyclotorsion. When the upwardly deviated eye returns to horizontal, the movement is not accompanied by a compensatory movement in the opposite direction by the fellow eye, as would be the case with a true vertical tropia. Thus, DVD does not obey Hering's law, which states that the yoke muscle (superior rectus muscle of the fellow eye) receives equal and simultaneous innervation.

Occasionally, DVD manifests as divergent exotropia. An occluded eye drifts out and returns to midline without any accompanying movement of the fellow eye (Wilson and McClatchey, 1991; Wilson et al., 1995).

Divergent Vertical Deviation Associations

Most patients with DVD have some other type of strabismus problem, too. Fifty to ninety percent of children with essential infantile esotropia (EIE) develop DVD (Lang, 1971; Manson and Parks, 1980), and in this setting DVD usually will become apparent by 3 years of age. Most children with DVD and EIE show nystagmus (Harcourt et al., 1980; Mein and Johnson, 1979). Binocular vision is virtually always impaired in patients with DVD (Harcourt et al., 1980; Helveston, 1980).

DVD occurs in a small percentage of patients with exotropia, as well. Helveston (1980) found the incidence to be 8.7%. There is also little question that DVD can occur as an isolated problem. We have examined a man with DVD in one eye and no other strabismus problem. His brother had congenital esotropia and DVD, suggesting that genetic factors could have been etiologic of his problem.

DVD also occasionally occurs with acquired (late-onset) strabismus, although the possibility that DVD was present all along cannot be excluded. Bielschowsky nystagmus, which is a slow, uniocular, vertical, pendular eye movement, may be nothing more (or less) than DVD. Bielschowsky's nystagmus occurs in the setting of dense amblyopia, at more advanced ages (typically adults) and is acquired

(Smith et al., 1982). If the cause of amblyopia is corrected, the nystagmus may resolve.

Bielschowsky's Phenomenon

Bielschowsky's phenomenon (1940) refers to the tendency for the elevated eye to fall when illumination in the fixing eye is reduced. This phenomenon occurs even when the falling eye is under cover. Conversely, increased illumination in an eye with DVD will cause it to drift vertically. This phenomenon is present in about 50% of patients with DVD.

Bielschowsky is also credited with the discovery of another interesting aspect of DVD. When a red lens is placed in front of either eye of a patient with DVD and a light source is visually fixated, a red image will always be seen below a white image. This finding helps distinguish DVD from vertical phorias or tropias, in which case the red image will be seen either above or below the white image, depending on whether the eye with the red lens is hypo- or hyperdeviated relative to the fellow eye.

Divergent Vertical Deviation and Head Tilt Testing

The head tilt test also yields an unpredicted result in DVD, causing the vertical deviation to worsen when the head is tilted away from the eye with DVD (Figure 15.1). In right DVD, for example, vertical deviation is often alleviated with right tilt and worsened with left tilt. Bilateral DVD may yield right hyperdeviation with left head tilt and left hyperdeviation with right tilt. The explanation for this phenomenon is unknown.

Incomitant Divergent Vertical Deviation

DVD may be worse in abduction or adduction. Inconcomitant DVD may be caused by superior oblique overaction (McCall and Rosenbaum, 1991). In this case, the amount of DVD is worse in abduction, moderate in primary gaze, and least in adduction. In some patients, the adducted eye with DVD may actually rest below the horizontal plane (Helveston, 1991). These patients usually also show some sort of horizontal ocular deviation and an **A** pattern, caused by superior oblique overaction.

Asymmetric Divergent Vertical Deviation

DVD may occur asymmetrically or may appear to be unilateral (Sprague et al., 1980; Braverman and Scott, 1977; Sargent, 1979; Knapp, 1978). A careful examination, including head tilt testing (see above) may elicit occult, bilateral DVD, although even very close examination may fail to disclose its presence (Helveston, 1980). DVD is usually worse in the nondominant (i.e., mildly amblyopic) eye (Magoon et al., 1982), or it may be worse in an eye with coexisting or preexisting hypertropia. Unfortunately, DVD in the fellow eye may become apparent only after unilateral surgery.

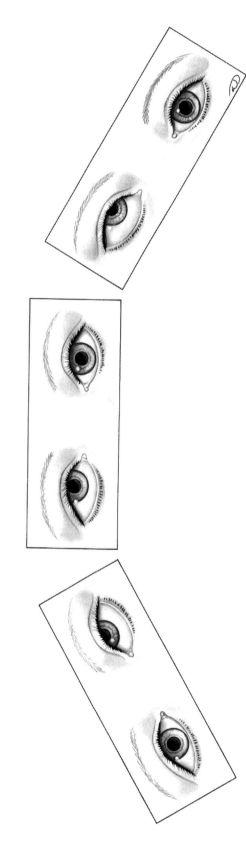

FIGURE 15.1 *In divergent vertical deviation (DVD), hypertropia may worsen on head tilt to the opposite side. Bilateral DVD would cause right hypertropia with left tilt and left hypertropia with right tilt.*

Measuring and Grading Divergent Vertical Deviation

Regrettably, the variability of DVD makes it hard to measure. Helveston (1980) indicated that measurements of DVD are less important than in other types of strabismus, since surgery is imprecise. Prolonged eye occlusion makes DVD worse, as does head tilt to the opposite side. Individual clinicians should develop a consistent approach to quantitating (and treating) DVD, and adhere to it.

Sargent (1979) categorized DVD in a given eye as small if it measured 0–9 prism diopters, moderate for 10–19 prism diopters, and large for 20 or more prism diopters. The manner in which the angle of DVD is measured is important. In some patients, a good estimate can be obtained by corneal light reflex testing. In others, accurate measurement requires simultaneous prism and cover testing. It is desirable to measure DVD on several occasions and prior to cover or alternate cover testing, because these examinations can affect the amount of DVD.

Divergent Vertical Deviation and Inferior Oblique Overaction:
Similarities and Differences

DVD must be distinguished from inferior oblique overaction (IOOA) to avoid inappropriate surgical management. Given the potential simultaneous occurrence of these conditions with EIE, the surgeon should be aware of the clinical characteristics of both. IOOA causes elevation of the eye in adduction, but when that same eye abducts, it will often depress due to IOOA of the other eye. DVD also causes elevation of the eye in adduction, but the same eye, when abducted, will elevate when the fellow eye fixates.

IOOA often causes a V-pattern deviation. No A or V pattern is seen with DVD. Torsion of the eye is an important aspect of DVD and is not seen in IOOA. The rate of elevation of the eye in DVD is slow. Elevation occurs quickly in IOOA. The vertical deviation in IOOA is usually uniform, but is variable in DVD (Figure 15.2).

Occasionally, cases are still ambiguous, in which case the eye with the vertical deviation can be patched for several hours. The patient is then returned to the examining room, and the patch is removed under cover. The patient fixes with the nonoccluded eye, and the alternating cover test is performed. The surgeon looks for development of hypotropia in the fixating eye when the cover is moved from the occluded to the previously fixating eye. Hypotropia indicates a true vertical tropia and a diagnosis of IOOA.

Forty percent of patients with DVD have some sort of simultaneous oblique overaction, usually inferior oblique (Helveston, 1980). The physical examination should search for the presence of a true vertical tropia even after DVD has been diagnosed. Wilson and colleagues

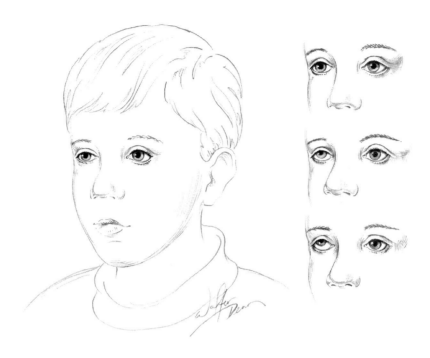

FIGURE 15.2 *Patients may have different amounts of divergent vertical deviation, depending on fatigue.*

(1989) have stated that in eyes in which both DVD and IOOA exist, opposing actions exist. The abducted eye, under cover, is under upward pressure from DVD and downward pressure from IOOA. Only when IOOA overcomes the DVD will a true hypertropia become manifest. On the other hand, the examiner should remember that the length of time that the eye is left under cover may influence the amount of DVD. Thus, an effort to elicit IOOA by detecting a hypertropia would best be accomplished by rapidly alternating the cover test.

Patients with DVD may tilt their heads. DVD is made worse on contralateral head tilt, the opposite finding of head tilt testing in superior oblique palsy. Inferior oblique palsy worsens on opposite head tilt. However, in inferior oblique palsy, the eye fails to elevate adequately on adduction; the opposite is found with DVD.

OPTICAL MANAGEMENT

Treatment of DVD is directed at the undesirable elevation of the involved eye. The surgeon should consider the possibility of optical correction as a first intervention. Any blurring of vision will exacerbate the DVD. Thus the best possible correction should be employed, after which the DVD can be reevaluated.

Conversely, deliberate blurring of one eye in cases of asymmetric DVD may be appropriate. For example, the fixating eye can be over-plussed, which will often stimulate fixation with the eye that previously demonstrated the manifest DVD. A technique for blurring has been described by Guyton (1988). The examination is performed with no cycloplegic agents. The fixating eye is given progressively stronger plus lenses until the fellow eye fixates. Glasses are then prescribed based on this examination—that is, the eye with DVD is given its best correction and the previously fixating eye is overplussed by the amount necessary to cause the other eye to fixate. Amblyopia in the eye with DVD may cause the new fixation pattern to be intolerable. According to Guyton, the deliberately blurred eye can be properly corrected after several years, and the patient may develop satisfactory alignment.

SURGICAL MANAGEMENT

The decision to operate for DVD is determined by the patient's appearance. The exact natural history of DVD is unknown, but there is some evidence that it may resolve with time in some patients (Good et al., 1993) or at least not worsen (Harcourt et al., 1980).

A number of surgical options are available. Faden sutures with or without superior rectus recession, inferior rectus resection with or without superior rectus recession, large superior rectus recessions, and anteriorization of the inferior oblique muscle have all been used, but very few trials have compared these techniques. Esswein and associates (1992) compared the effectiveness of 3- to 5-mm recessions of the superior rectus muscle, with or without Faden sutures, with large (7–9 mm) superior rectus recessions. The best long-term results were achieved with large superior rectus recessions. Lorenz and colleagues (1992) found the opposite to be true. Long-term effectiveness of superior rectus recession (3–5 mm) combined with Faden sutures exceeded large superior rectus recessions.

These mixed results are ever more difficult to interpret when one considers the fact that DVD is virtually never eliminated with any form of treatment. Surgery can cause improvement, and surgeons will base their approach to DVD on experience with given procedures.

Superior Rectus Recessions

Superior rectus recessions have been used in the treatment of DVD (Magoon et al., 1982). Using the hang-back technique, the superior rectus muscle is recessed as much as 14 mm. Surgery is usually performed bilaterally, even when DVD appears monocular, because unilateral surgery often unmasks DVD in the fellow eye. Bilateral surgery also helps to prevent the development of hypotropia in the operated eye.

Asymmetric DVD may be associated with hypertropia in the nonfixing eye. The etiology of the hypertropia may be underlying oblique dysfunction, but a long-standing DVD can eventually lead to true hypertropia if the superior rectus muscle tightens (Magoon et al., 1982). In the case of apparent monocular DVD, the examination should focus on the ability of the eye with DVD to take up fixation. If the eye never fixates, unilateral surgery may succeed in controlling the DVD. On the other hand, if that eye occasionally fixates, bilateral surgery is indicated.

Possible complications of larger superior rectus recessions include ptosis, palpebral fissure changes, eyelid retraction, and deficient elevation. When superior rectus recession is combined with ipsilateral inferior oblique weakening, elevation may be crippled more than would have been predicted.

Faden Operation

The Faden operation of Cuppers (1976) has been used in DVD, but use of the Faden procedure alone is usually ineffective. Sprague and associates (1980) combined the Faden operation on the superior rectus muscle with recession of that muscle. Success was achieved in the majority of cases. Complications included failure of surgery as follows: persistent DVD (evident immediately postoperatively), postoperative hypotropia in the nonfixing eye, and the need for a second operation (inferior rectus resection). Good results have also been obtained by other investigators using the Faden operation plus superior recession (von Noorden, 1978; Decker and Conrad, 1975).

Recess–Resect Surgery

Unilateral DVD can also be treated with a vertical recess–resect procedure; that is, the superior rectus muscle is recessed, usually 4–5 mm, and the inferior rectus muscle is resected, usually 6 mm (Knapp, 1976). Complications include narrowing of the palpebral fissure, caused by resection of the inferior rectus muscle, and complications, as listed above, with recession of the superior rectus muscle.

Superior Oblique Surgery

Superior oblique surgery has been used to treat DVD (Richard, 1987). Resection of the superior oblique tendon, combined with inferior oblique recessions, has been reported to be helpful. Kushner and Price (1988) advocate the use of the superior oblique tuck to manage DVD. The well-known complication of Brown's syndrome following this procedure has been temporary, in their experience, and hypotropia as a complication does not occur.

SPECIAL CONSIDERATIONS

Divergent Vertical Deviation and Ipsilateral Hypotropia

Sometimes patients present with DVD combined with hypotropia of the same eye. This problem is seen most commonly after a failed attempt to treat DVD and poses a complicated management problem. The goal is correction of an unacceptable DVD without worsening of the hypotropia. The involved eye can be treated with superior rectus recession plus the Faden operation. This usually must be counterbalanced to reduce any augmentation of the hypotropia. Options include ipsilateral inferior rectus recession and contralateral superior rectus recession (Kushner and Raab, 1988). In using the latter option, asymmetric recessions should be performed. For example, 12-mm recession of the involved eye could be balanced by an 8-mm recession of the uninvolved eye.

Incomitant Divergent Vertical Deviation

So-called incomitant DVD may require special surgical considerations. DVD combined with superior oblique overaction may lend itself to ipsilateral superior rectus recession combined with ipsilateral posterior tenotomy of the superior oblique muscle (McCall and Rosenbaum, 1991).

The simultaneous occurrence of DVD and IOOA may be an indication for anterior transposition of the inferior oblique muscle (Elliot and Nankin, 1981). This operation successfully eliminates the V pattern and helps reduce the amount of DVD. Anteriorization of the inferior oblique causes weakening of the muscle. Meanwhile, anteriorization also converts the inferior oblique muscle to a depressor, which accounts for hypotropia occasionally seen as a complication.

REFERENCES

Bielschowsky A. Lectures on motor anomalies. II. The theory of heterophoria. Am J Ophthalmol 1938;21:1129–1136.

Bielschowsky A. Lectures on Motor Anomalies. Hanover, NH: Dartmouth College Publications, 1940;33.

Braverman DE, Scott WE. Surgical correction of dissociated vertical deviations. J Pediatr Ophthalmol Strabismus 1977;14:337–342.

Brown HW. Dissociated Vertical Anomalies. In A Arugga (ed), International Strabismus Symposium. New York: S. Karger, 1966;175–179.

Crone RA. Alternating hyperphoria. Br J Ophthalmol 1954;38:591–604.

Cuppers C. The So-called Faden Operation. In P Fells (ed), The Second Congress of the International Strabismus Association. Marseilles, France: Lany, 1976;168.

Decker W, Conrad HG. Fadenoperation nach Cuppers bei komplizierten Augenmuskelstorungen und nichtakkommodativem Konvergenzexzess. Klin Monatsbl Augenheilkunde 1975;167:217–226.

Elliott RL, Nankin SJ. Anterior transposition of the inferior oblique. J Pediatr Ophthalmol Strabismus 1981;18:35–38.

Esswein MB, von Noorden GK, Coburn A. Comparison of surgical methods in the treatment of dissociated vertical deviation. Am J Ophthalmol 1992;113:287–290.

Good WV, da Sa LCF, Lyons CJ, Hoyt CS. Monocular visual outcome in untreated early onset esotropia. Br J Ophthalmol 1993;77:492–494.

Guyton DL. Correcting an ipsilateral manifest hypotropia and dissociated hypertropia (dissociated vertical deviation, DVD). Binoc Vis 1988;3:41–45.

Harcourt B, Mein J, Johnson F. Natural history and associations of dissociated vertical divergence. Trans Ophthalmol Soc UK 1980;100:495–497.

Helveston EM. A-exotropia, alternating sursumduction, and superior oblique overaction. Am J Ophthalmol 1969;67:377–380.

Helveston EM. Dissociated vertical deviation—a clinical and laboratory study. Trans Am Ophthalmol Soc 1980;78:734–779.

Helveston EM. Discussion of paper by LC McCall, AL Rosenbaum. Incomitant dissociated vertical deviation and superior oblique overaction. Ophthalmology 1991;98:911–918.

Knapp P. Dissociated Vertical Deviations. In P Fells (ed), The Second Congress of the International Strabismus Association. Marseilles, France: Lany, 1976;123.

Knapp P. Round Table Discussions. In Symposium on Strabismus: Transactions of the New Orleans Academy of Ophthalmology. St. Louis: Mosby, 1978:579–584.

Kushner BJ, Price RL. Correcting an ipsilateral manifest hypotropia and dissociated hypertropia (dissociated hypertropia, DVD). Binoc Vis 1988;3:41–45.

Kushner BJ, Raab E. Manifest hypotropia and dissociated hypertropia (dissociated vertical deviation, DVD). Binoc Vis 1988;3:41–45.

Lang J. Congenital convergent strabismus. Int Ophthalmol Clin 1971;11:88–92.

Lorenz B, Raab I, Boergen KP. Dissociated vertical deviation: what is the most effective surgical approach? J Pediatr Ophthalmol Strabismus 1992;29:21–29.

Magoon E, Cruciger M, Jampolsky A. Dissociated vertical deviation: an asymmetric condition treated with large bilateral superior rectus recession. J Pediatr Ophthalmol Strabismus 1982;19:152–156.

Manson R, Parks MM. Associated findings in congenital esotropia. Personal Communications in EM Helveston. Dissociated Vertical Deviation: A Clinical and Laboratory Study. Transactions of the American Ophthalmology Society 1980;78:734–779.

McCall LC, Rosenbaum AL. Incomitant dissociated vertical deviation and superior oblique overaction. Ophthalmology 1991;98:911–918.

Mein J, Johnson F. Dissociated Vertical Divergence and Its Association with Nystagmus. Transactions of the IV International Orthoptic Congress, Berne, Switzerland, 1979.

Posner A. Noncomitant heterophorias: considered as aberrations of the postural tonus of the muscular apparatus. Am J Ophthalmol 1994;27:1275–1279.

Richard JM. Combined superior oblique muscle tendon resection and inferior oblique recession for dissociated vertical deviation: a report of 25 cases. Binoc Vis Q 1987;2:137–150.

Sargent R. Dissociated hypertropia: surgical treatment. Transactions of the American Academy of Ophthalmology and Otolaryngology 1979;86:1428–1438.

Scobee RB. The Oculorotary Muscles. St. Louis: Mosby, 1947;143–145.

Smith JL, Flynn JT, Spiro JH. Monocular vertical oscillations of amblyopia: the Heimann-Bielschowsky phenomenon. J Clin Neuro-Ophthalmol 1982;2:85–91.

Sprague JB, Moore S, Eggers H, Knapp P. Dissociated vertical deviation: treatment with the Faden operation of Cuppers. Arch Ophthalmol 1980;98:465–468.

Stevens GT. Du strabisme vertical alternant et des déviations symmetriques moins pronounce que le strabisme. (On double vertical strabismus.) Ann Ocul 1895;113:225–232, 385–393.

Verhoeff FH. Occlusion hypertropia. Arch Ophthalmol 1941;25:780–795.

von Noorden G. Posterior Fixation Suture in Strabismus Surgery. In Symposium on Strabismus. Transactions of the New Orleans Academy of Ophthalmology. St. Louis: Mosby, 1978;307–320.

White JW. Paralysis of the superior rectus muscle. Trans Am Ophthalmol Soc 1933;3:551–584.

Wilson ME, Eustis HS Jr, Parks MM. Brown's syndrome. Surv Ophthalmol 1989;34:153–172.

Wilson ME, McClatchey SK. Dissociated horizontal deviation. J Pediatr Ophthalmol Strab 1991;28:90–95.

Wilson ME, Saunders RA, Berland JE. Dissociated horizontal deviation and accommodative esotropia: treatment options when an eso- and an exodeviation co-exist. J Pediatr Ophthalmol Strab 1995;32:228–230.

16

Inferior Oblique Palsy

THEORY AND ETIOLOGY

Isolated inferior oblique palsy is a rare disorder. The innervation to the inferior oblique muscle travels with the inferior division of the oculomotor nerve, which also supplies the inferior rectus muscle and pupil. Anything that damages the inferior division of the oculomotor nerve will therefore also affect these other muscles or functions. Indeed, even isolated involvement of the inferior division of the oculomotor nerve is rare (Cunningham and Good, 1994).

Isolated inferior oblique palsy secondary to central nervous system disease is even more rare (Castro et al., 1990). The oculomotor nucleus, however, is subdivided according to subnuclei, and there is one report of an inferior oblique palsy secondary to a midbrain lesion (Castro et al., 1990).

Inferior oblique palsy usually occurs with damage to the peripheral portion of the nerve (Scott and Nanken, 1977). Inferior oblique palsy has been reported following viral illnesses and orbital trauma. Dog bite injuries can cause inferior oblique palsy, and blepharoplasty surgery will occasionally traumatize the inferior oblique muscle. Such trauma usually also violates orbital fat, causing some degree of scarring and restrictive strabismus. In considering whether trauma is ever a cause of isolated palsy of the inferior oblique muscle, the reader should ask why deliberate destruction of the inferior oblique muscle (e.g., via myectomy) often does not cause it to underact.

DIAGNOSIS

Patients with inferior oblique palsy will complain of double vision. They show hypotropia in primary gaze when fixating with the normal fellow eye. Otherwise, hypertropia of the normal fellow eye may exist when the involved eye is used for visual fixation.

Assuming the usual circumstance of fixation with the uninvolved eye, the hypotropia worsens on adduction and improves on abduction. Limitation of elevation in the adducted position is also an important physical finding. Bielschowsky's head tilt test demonstrates worsening of the vertical deviation when the head is tilted toward the side of the uninvolved eye. Many patients, therefore, will demonstrate appropriate and helpful findings when the three-step test is applied diagnostically (Figure 16.1).

Patients with inferior oblique palsy may turn their head so that the involved eye is abducted. Some will elevate their chin so that they can avoid looking at objects in the most severely involved visual field— i.e., upgaze and adduction. The forced duction test is important and distinguishes inferior oblique palsy from other causes of hypotropia. The forced duction test should be free, indicating no restrictive disease (Figure 16.2).

DIFFERENTIAL DIAGNOSIS

Some authorities doubt the existence of an isolated inferior oblique palsy. In cases of presumed inferior oblique palsy, electromyographic studies demonstrate action potentials in the inferior oblique muscle (A Jampolsky, A Scott, personal communication). Most studies on inferior oblique palsy have failed to report results of forced duction testing. In trauma to the lower lid, a commonly reported cause of inferior oblique palsy, restriction of the globe secondary to fat adherence can account for physical findings simulating inferior oblique palsy (Jameson et al., 1992). Perhaps the most compelling argument against the existence of isolated inferior oblique palsy comes from results of weakening and denervation procedures performed on the inferior oblique muscle (Weakley and Stager, 1992). In our experience, even with an extirpation and denervation procedure of the inferior oblique muscle, that muscle may not underact, as it does in "isolated inferior oblique palsy."

Therefore, the strabismologist must look for conditions that can mimic inferior oblique palsy (Table 16.1). Signs of trauma should prompt an evaluation for the possibility of orbital floor injury. Entrapment of the inferior rectus muscle can cause restriction in elevation of the involved eye. Hypotropia can exist in primary gaze. In this situation, the forced duction test in the upward direction should be positive.

Occasionally, trauma in the area of the floor of the orbit (blowout fracture) can damage the nerve to the inferior rectus or infe-

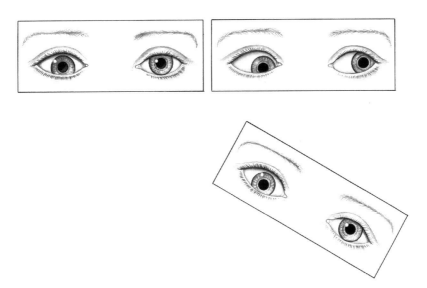

FIGURE 16.1   *Park's three-step test helps diagnose inferior oblique palsy. Right hypotropia is present in primary gaze and worse in left gaze and left head tilt. In this artist's drawing, the hypotropia is exaggerated intentionally. Seldom is the deviation more than 10 prism diopters.*

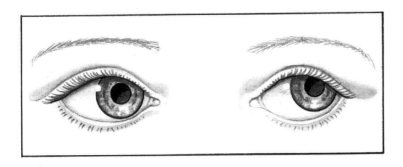

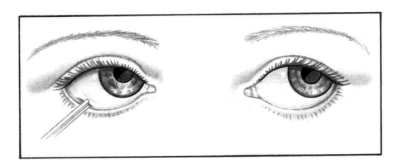

FIGURE 16.2   *In inferior oblique palsy, the involved eye underacts in elevation and adduction. The forced duction test is normal, distinguishing inferior oblique palsy from Brown's syndrome.*

TABLE 16.1   Conditions that mimic inferior oblique palsy

Blowout fracture
Fat adherence to the inferior rectus muscle
Palsy, inferior division of oculomotor nerve
Brown's syndrome
Double elevator palsy
Thyroid ophthalmopathy

rior oblique muscle, or both. In this case, the eye will not rotate down, but still could be hypotropic if the inferior extraocular muscles are trapped. When orbital fractures are suspected, a computed tomographic scan with coronal views should be obtained.

Injury to the lower lid, as can occur with a dog bite or blepharoplasty, is another reported cause of inferior oblique palsy or underaction (Harley et al., 1986). The strabismus surgeon is advised to carefully check forced duction testing in this situation, because restriction of the inferior rectus muscle or inferior globe, or both, can simulate inferior oblique palsy.

The differential diagnosis also includes conditions that can affect the inferior division of the oculomotor nerve. A careful examination for pupil findings (pupil will be dilated and weakly reactive or nonreactive in inferior division palsy) and for inferior rectus palsy should be performed. If inferior division palsy is suspected, the evaluation must include central nervous system imaging. Injury at any point in the course of the oculomotor nerve can lead to an isolated inferior division palsy.

Brown's syndrome is suspected from ortho- or hypotropia in primary gaze and from difficulty elevating the eye in adduction. It is distinguished from inferior oblique palsy on the basis of restriction in elevation and adduction, demonstrated in forced duction testing. In double elevator palsy, the affected eye does not rotate up completely in any field of gaze. Park's three-step test will usually not localize an affected muscle (Kushner, 1989).

Patients with Graves' disease similarly may show restriction of elevation on forced duction testing. However, the greater deficit of elevation is usually in the abducted position. Orbital imaging studies should demonstrate enlarged extraocular muscles.

MANAGEMENT

As usual, management is indicated when the patient has symptoms that interfere with normal living activities. Transient double vision (e.g., after blepharoplasty) may occur and last for several days (Rees and Wood-Smith, 1973). Spontaneous resolution of double vision can occur even weeks or months later (Neuhaus and Baylis, 1980). Therefore, surgery should be delayed until strabismus is stable.

Inferior oblique palsy will cause inconcomitant strabismus, but prisms may occasionally be useful for long-term management of this problem if the vertical deviation is small in primary gaze and relatively concomitant.

Surgery

Inferior Oblique Palsy with Superior Oblique Overaction

When superior oblique muscle overaction accompanies inferior oblique palsy, a weakening procedure of the superior oblique is a logical approach to the problem. This treatment should alleviate any hypotropia in primary gaze. The superior oblique overaction will also be cured with a weakening procedure. Problems with this intervention arise when the patient develops hypertropia in downgaze. This can be managed with a weakening procedure of the contralateral inferior rectus muscle (e.g., Faden operation).

Inferior Oblique Palsy with Hypotropia in Primary Gaze with No Superior Oblique Overaction

In this situation the surgeon should pay close attention to the results of the forced duction test. If positive (up and in), careful investigation for other causes is indicated (see Differential Diagnosis, above). When the forced duction test is negative, the surgeon has several choices. Surgery on the involved eye could be undertaken and would usually involve an inferior rectus recession. The rule of approximately 2.5 prism diopters of correction per millimeter of recession (for primary gaze deviation) should apply in this condition, again assuming there is no abnormality of the forced duction test.

Alternatively, the surgeon can attempt to match a defect in the involved eye with surgery in the uninvolved eye. For example, with certain symptoms in adduction and adduction in elevation, the surgeon could choose to perform a large superior rectus recession in the fellow eye. Ideally, these vertical rectus recessions should be done with adjustable sutures, depending on the age and status of the patient.

Inferior Oblique Palsy with Abnormal Forced Duction Test

The question of etiology of inferior oblique palsy can be argued, but the goal of treatment can usually be accomplished with the above-mentioned surgical procedures. To avoid inappropriate surgery, the surgeon is advised, once again, to carefully perform forced duction testing. In one case in which we believed the patient had suffered an isolated inferior oblique palsy, we were surprised to find restriction, albeit subtle, of the inferior rectus muscle and inferior globe (Jameson et al., 1992). The muscle involved with scarring should be operated on, if possible. A recession of the muscle can be performed. The results of surgery are less predictable than in cases where no scarring has occurred. Again, adjustable suture techniques are usually indicated.

If a restricted muscle cannot be operated on, the surgeon can still choose to operate on the fellow eye. In this circumstance, the goal would be to try to match a defect in elevation by performing a very large, contralateral superior rectus recession (e.g., 6–10 mm).

REFERENCES

Castro O, Johnson LN, Mamourian AC. Isolated inferior oblique paresis from brain-stem infarction: perspective on oculomotor fascicular organization in the ventral midbrain tegmentum. Arch Neurol 1990;47:235–237.

Cunningham E, Good WV. Inferior branch oculomotor nerve palsy. A case report. J Neuro-Ophthalmol 1994;14:21–23.

Harley RD, Nelson LB, Flanagan JC, Calhoun JH. Ocular motility disturbances following cosmetic blepharoplasty. Arch Ophthalmol 1986;104:542–544.

Jameson NA, Good WV, Hoyt CS. Inferior rectus restriction simulating inferior oblique palsy following blepharoplasty. Arch Ophthalmol 1992;110:1369.

Kushner BJ. Errors in the three-step test in the diagnosis of vertical strabismus. Ophthalmology 1989;96:127–132.

Neuhaus RW, Baylis HI. Complications of Lower Eyelid Blepharoplasty. In AM Putterman (ed), Cosmetic Oculoplastic Surgery. New York: Grune & Stratton, 1982;275–306.

Rees TD, Wood-Smith D. Cosmetic Facial Surgery. Philadelphia: Saunders, 1973;52.

Scott WE, Nankin SJ. Isolated inferior oblique paresis. Arch Ophthalmol 1977;95:1586–1593.

Weakley DR Jr, Stager DR. A new surgical procedure: nasal myectomy of the inferior oblique muscle combined with anterior transposition of the insertion; results in ten cases. Binoc Vis Eye Muscle Surg 1992;7:215–218.

17

Inferior Rectus Palsy

Michael C. Brodsky

ETIOLOGY

Inferior rectus muscle dysfunction is seen most commonly as a component of a third cranial nerve palsy. Isolated inferior rectus palsy, once thought to be rare, is now a well-recognized condition that reflects a limited number of underlying conditions (Pusateri et al., 1987; Roper-Hall and Burde, 1975; Spoor and Shippman, 1979) (Table 17.1). The diagnostic evaluation of the patient with inferior rectus palsy is guided by the clinical history as well as associated neuro-ophthalmic findings.

The infrequent occurrence of isolated inferior rectus palsy reflects the complex neuroanatomy of the oculomotor nerve (Roper-Hall and Burde, 1975; Warren et al., 1982; Van Dalen and van Mourik-Noordenbos, 1984). Most compressive, ischemic, or inflammatory third nerve lesions affect the nerve's fascicular portion, located between the oculomotor nucleus in the dorsal midbrain and the nerve's bifurcation into superior and inferior divisions in the anterior cavernous sinus. Here, axons destined to innervate the extraocular muscles are in close apposition. Such injuries almost invariably affect innervation to multiple extraocular muscles, not just the inferior rectus muscle.

Neuroanatomically, there are two sites where a third nerve injury could produce an isolated paresis of the inferior rectus muscle (Spoor and Shippman, 1979; Van Dalen and van Mourk-Noordenbos, 1984). One site is the oculomotor nucleus, where cell bodies of neurons that are destined for each target muscle are segregated into a distinct subnucleus. A focal vascular demyelinating or metastatic lesion involving the inferior rectus subnucleus can result in isolated inferior rectus

TABLE 17.1 Diagnostic categories of inferior rectus palsy

Unilateral
    Myasthenia gravis
    Nuclear third nerve palsy (metastatic, ischemic, demyelinative)
    Orbital disease (blowout fracture, orbital tumor, dysthyroid
       orbitopathy with superior rectus restriction)
    Basilar artery aneurysm
    Iatrogenic (following inferior oblique myectomy, lower lid ble-
       pharoplasty, retrobulbar injection)
    Congenital
    Idiopathic
Bilateral (alternating skew deviation)
    Structural abnormalities involving the craniocervical junction
       (Arnold-Chiari malformation, platybasia, syringomyelia, Klippel-
       Feil anomaly, high cervical meningioma)
    Drug induced (lithium, alcohol)
    Spinocerebellar degenerations
    Multiple sclerosis
    Vascular infarction
    Idiopathic

palsy. The orbit is the second site where an injury or disease process involving the portion of the inferior division of the third nerve destined for the inferior rectus muscle, the myoneural junction, or the muscle itself could produce an isolated inferior rectus palsy (Spoor and Shippman, 1979). The organization of the oculomotor nerve is such that a lesion anywhere along its course could produce an isolated inferior rectus palsy. A basilar artery aneurysm can do this, for example (Kardon et al., 1991), although it is likely to affect several aspects of nerve function.

DIAGNOSIS

The patient with an inferior rectus palsy complains of vertical diplopia that increases on downgaze. On examination, the patient manifests incomitant hypertropia that increases on downgaze and abduction (Figure 17.1).

A comparison of forced duction testing between the two eyes shows decreased rotation of the involved eye into downgaze and abduction when the fellow eye is covered. von Noorden has stressed that the three-step test cannot be relied on to confirm the diagnosis of

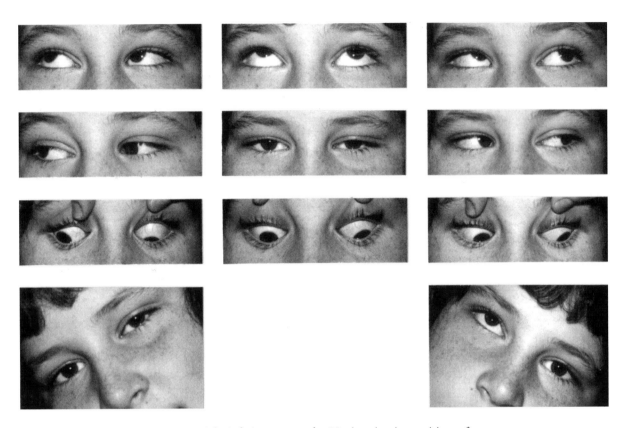

FIGURE 17.1   *Right inferior rectus palsy. Versions in nine positions of gaze show right hypertropia that is worse in downgaze and abduction and with left head tilt. These findings correspond to the diagnosis of right inferior rectus palsy on Park's three-step test. There is an **A** pattern corresponding to loss of secondary adduction from the paretic inferior rectus muscle.*

inferior rectus palsy (von Noorden and Hansell, 1991). Similarly, the position of compensatory face turn may be opposite that expected in an inferior rectus palsy, presumably reflecting the patient's attempt to maximally separate the double images and minimize the annoyance caused by the unwanted image (von Noorden and Hansell, 1991). Double Maddox rod testing often shows incyclotropia of the involved eye, but may also show paradoxical incyclotropia of the fellow eye (von Noorden and Hansell, 1991). Patients with congenital inferior rectus palsy may have complete absence of cyclotropia (von Noorden and Hansell, 1991).

DIFFERENTIAL DIAGNOSIS

A methodologic approach to the evaluation of a patient with inferior rectus palsy relies on a careful history and physical examination, in addition to a limited panel of diagnostic tests. A history of variability or remissions is highly suggestive of myasthenia gravis (Cleary, 1973; Spoor and Shippmann, 1979). In this setting, a careful history and neurologic examination to elicit other myasthenic symptoms and an edrophonium chloride (Tensilon) test are crucial to establish the diagnosis.

A history of previous orbital trauma suggests an orbital blowout fracture (Kushner, 1982). Close examination may reveal limited supraduction and enophthalmos. A forced duction test can be performed in the office to confirm the presence of orbital restriction. It may be difficult to rotate the eye up passively. Passive rotation downward may be normal (indicating paralysis of the inferior rectus) or abnormal if the ipsilateral superior rectus has tightened. Orbital computed tomographic scanning with direct axial and coronal views definitively establishes the diagnosis.

Patients with Graves' ophthalmopathy may have ocular motility findings of inferior rectus palsy secondary to a tight superior rectus muscle (Buckley and Meekins, 1988). Careful inspection may reveal orbital signs of Graves' orbitopathy (proptosis, lid retraction, chemosis, injection over the extraocular muscle sites). If these signs are present, a positive forced duction test (rotating the eye up) followed by a high-resolution orbital computed tomographic scan usually confirms the diagnosis.

The patient who develops an acute inferior rectus palsy following strabismus surgery, lower lid blepharoplasty, or retrobulbar injection usually has an iatrogenic injury to the inferior rectus muscle (Brodsky et al., 1992; De Faber and von Noorden, 1991). Iatrogenic inferior rectus palsy is a presumptive diagnosis that is supported by normal neuroimaging studies and a negative Tensilon test.

Bilateral inferior rectus palsies have been described as "alternating skew deviation" and "alternating abducting hypertropia" (Moster et al., 1988). This well-defined neurologic condition is often seen in association with downbeating nystagmus. The finding of bilateral inferior rectus palsies in a patient with a history of intermittent neurologic symptoms (headache, oscillopsia, unsteadiness, imbalance, weakness, dysphagia) suggests the possibility of an Arnold-Chiari malformation or other structural anomalies at the cervicomedullary junction. Sagittal magnetic resonance imaging is the best noninvasive neuroimaging modality to depict structural abnormalities of the craniocervical junction. Less commonly, bilateral inferior rectus palsies are associated with other conditions (see Table 17.1). A clinical algorithm to facilitate diagnostic evaluation of a patient with inferior rectus palsy is provided in Figure 17.2.

TREATMENT

Patients with inferior rectus palsy secondary to myasthenia gravis are treated with pyridostigmine bromide (Mestinon), often in combination with prednisone. When inferior rectus palsy is attributable to other causes, the patient should be observed for 6 months to confirm that the ocular motility findings are stable. During this period, vertical prisms will rarely eliminate diplopia, but they are usually ineffective because of the horizontal incomitance that is associated with inferior rectus palsy. If the deviation remains unchanged after 6 months, strabismus surgery is the definitive treatment. Inferior rectus palsy responds well to surgical treatment because these patients generally retain excellent fusional potential (von Noorden and Hansell, 1991). The use of adjustable suture surgery is preferable in adults to adjust ocular alignment postoperatively. von Noorden and Hansell (1991) noted that of 21 patients treated surgically for inferior rectus palsy, 14 were cured, 6 improved, and 1 was unchanged.

Mild Inferior Rectus Palsy

Small deviations that are limited to the field of action of the inferior rectus muscle (i.e., downgaze) are successfully managed by a 3- to 4-mm resection of the paretic inferior rectus muscle (von Noorden and Hansell, 1991).

Moderate to Severe Inferior Rectus Palsy

An inferior rectus resection of more than 4 mm for large deviations carries the risk of restricted ocular elevation postoperatively (iatrogenic double elevator palsy). Large deviations (i.e., those that affect primary gaze) require resection of the inferior rectus muscle (4 mm) combined with recession of the ipsilateral superior rectus muscle (5–7 mm).

Inferior Rectus Palsy in Orbital Blowout Fracture

Patients who have vertical diplopia in downgaze from an orbital blowout fracture may fail to improve following blowout fracture repair partly due to paresis of the inferior rectus muscle (i.e., nerve injury) and partly due to scarring and contracture or residual entrapment of

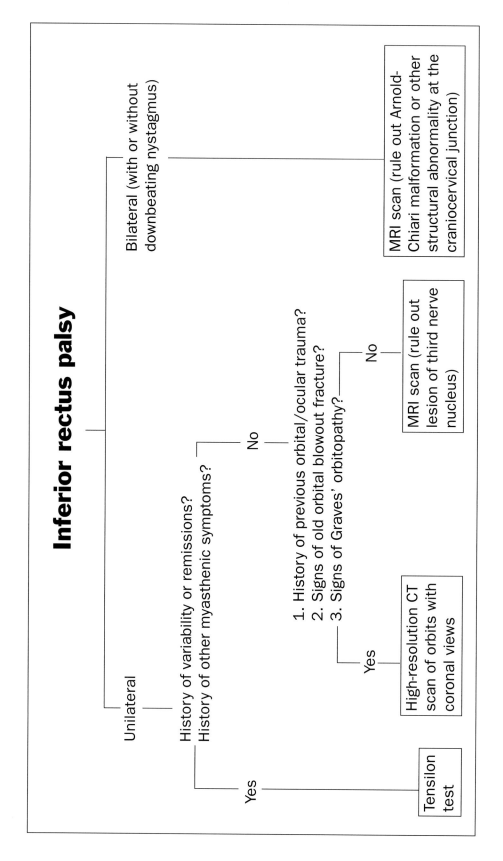

FIGURE 17.2 *Diagnostic evaluation of inferior rectus palsy.*

the injured inferior rectus muscle. Orbital blowout fractures can produce two distinct ocular motility disturbances which may be present before or after fracture repair.

First is vertical diplopia limited to downgaze associated with decreased infraduction, normal ocular alignment in primary gaze, and normal supraduction. For this situation, Saunders (1984) and Buckley and Meekins (1988) have advocated performing a posterior fixation suture on the contralateral inferior rectus muscle to produce a contralateral infraduction lag that will "match the defect." They have also used this surgical approach successfully in patients with dysthyroid orbitopathy who have unilaterally decreased infraduction secondary to a tight superior rectus muscle. The inferior rectus posterior fixation suture is placed 13 mm posterior to the muscle insertion (just anterior to the location of the vortex vein). This operation is reserved for patients with normal ocular alignment in primary gaze and diplopia limited to downgaze. Although this operation may not completely eliminate the diplopia in extreme downgaze, it significantly expands the window of single binocular vision and often restores single vision in the normal reading position (approximately 9 degrees of downgaze).

Second is vertical diplopia in upgaze and downgaze associated with decreased infraduction, decreased supraduction, and normal ocular alignment in primary gaze. This motility pattern results from inferior rectus dysfunction brought on by a variety of causes (e.g., palsy, muscle injury, residual entrapment, scarring, contracture), producing impaired infraduction together with restricted supraduction. Kushner (1982) recommended performing an inferior rectus recession (6 mm) with an ipsilateral superior rectus recession (6 mm). This procedure improves both infraduction and supraduction and thereby expands the field of single binocular vision without disrupting primary gaze. This procedure can be modified slightly or performed with adjustable sutures if the patient also has vertical heterotropia in primary gaze. Blowout fractures are discussed in Chapter 20.

REFERENCES

Brodsky MC, Fritz KJ, Carney SH. Iatrogenic inferior rectus palsy. J Pediatr Ophthalmol Strabismus 1992;29:113–115.

Buckley EG, Meekins BB. Faden operation for the management of complicated incomitant vertical strabismus. Am J Ophthalmol 1988;105:304–312.

Cleary PE. Ocular manifestations of myasthenia gravis. Br Orthop J 1973;30–51.

De Faber JT, von Noorden GK. Inferior rectus muscle palsy following retrobulbar anesthesia [letter]. Am J Ophthalmol 1991;112:209–211.

Kardon RH, Traynelis VC, Biller J. Inferior division paresis of the oculomotor nerve caused by basilar artery aneurysm. Cerebrovasc Dis 1991;1:171–176.

Kushner BJ. Paresis and restriction of the inferior rectus muscle after orbital floor fracture. Am J Ophthalmol 1982;94:81–86.

Moster ML, Schatz NJ, Savino PF et al. Alternating skew on lateral gaze (bilateral abducting hypertropia). Ann Neurol 1988;23:190–192.

Pusateri TJ, Sedwick LA, Margo CE. Isolated inferior rectus muscle palsy from a solitary metastasis to the oculomotor nucleus. Arch Ophthalmol 1987;105:675–677.

Roper-Hall G, Burde RM. Inferior rectus palsies as a manifestation of atypical third cranial nerve disease. Am Orthop J 1975;25:122–130.

Saunders RA. Incomitant vertical strabismus treatment with posterior fixation of the inferior rectus muscle. Arch Ophthalmol 1984;102:1174–1177.

Smith JL. The "nuclear third" question. J Clin Neuro-Ophthalmol 1982;2:61–63.

Spoor TC, Shippman S. Myasthenia gravis presenting as an isolated inferior rectus paresis. Ophthalmology 1979;86:2158–2160.

Van Dalen JTW, van Mourik-Noordenbos AM. Isolated inferior rectus paresis: a report of six cases. Neuro-Ophthalmol 1984;4:89–94.

von Noorden GK, Hansell R. Clinical characteristics and treatment of isolated inferior rectus paralysis. Ophthalmology 1991;98:253–257.

Warren W, Burde RM, Klingele TG et al. Atypical oculomotor paresis. J Clin Neuro-Ophthalmol 1982;2:13–18.

V

Restrictive Eye Muscle Disease

18

Congenital Fibrosis Syndromes

David S. I. Taylor and Richard Gregson

OCULAR FIBROSIS AND RESTRICTIVE STRABISMUS

The hallmark of a restrictive strabismus is reduced movement of the eye away from the direction of action of the affected muscle. This can be confirmed by a positive forced duction test. Thus, if there is fibrosis of the inferior rectus muscle, the eye cannot be fully elevated; if there is fibrosis of the medial rectus muscle, the eye cannot be fully abducted; and if there is generalized fibrosis of the extraocular muscles, all movements of the eye are reduced. Extraocular muscle fibrosis can be congenital or acquired. The congenital form may be due to primary fibrosis of the extraocular muscles, or the fibrosis may be secondary to abnormal innervation of the muscles.

HEREDITARY EXTRAOCULAR FIBROSIS

In 1889, Gast described a case of congenital external ophthalmoplegia and was probably referring to the condition of hereditary extraocular fibrosis. However, the condition and its hereditary nature were first accurately described by Bradbourne in 1912, when he reported on a large pedigree of obviously autosomal dominantly inherited extraocular muscle fibrosis with ptosis. The syndrome is rare, but since then there have been several other descriptions of similarly affected families (Apt and Axelrod, 1978; Brown, 1950; Harley et al., 1978; Laughlin, 1956; Bell et al., 1990). The clinical picture is characteristic (Figure 18.1).

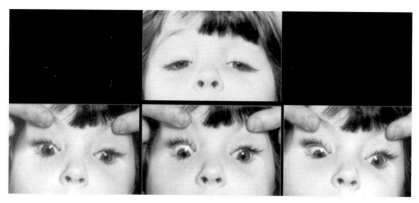

FIGURE 18.1   *A child with congenital fibrosis and characteristic head posture, which is caused by an inability to elevate the eyes.*

Affected family members have a chin-up posture with ptosis and eyes that are fixed in a downgazing esotropic position. Most ocular movements are impossible, although there may be some horizontal twitch of the eyes on attempted upgaze. There is no single binocular vision, and amblyopia is common. Management consists of attempting to prevent amblyopia by patching and through surgery, if indicated, to move the dominant eye into a better functional position (Fells et al., 1984). During surgery, fibrosis of all the extraocular muscles is found, as well as fibrosis of Tenon's capsule and adhesions between the muscles (Harley et al., 1978). There is an inelasticity and fragility of the conjunctiva. The cause of this syndrome is unknown, although it may be due to an abnormality of innervation, with the fibrotic changes being secondary to this. Reported associations include musculoskeletal abnormalities (Kishore and Kumar, 1991), Prader-Willi syndrome (Kalpakian et al., 1986), and Joubert's syndrome (Appleton et al., 1989).

SURGICAL MANAGEMENT

Although surgery can do nothing to improve ocular motility, it is possible to relieve the abnormal head posture somewhat. The dominant eye should be moved horizontally into the midline by recession of the tightest horizontal muscle (e.g., the medial rectus muscle in a case of fixed esodeviation). Usually the recessions have to be very large, and "hang-back" sutures may be used. Having released the muscle from the globe during the recession procedure, the forced duction test should be repeated to make sure that the eye can now be moved. Occasionally a fibrotic band is found attached to the globe behind the medial rectus muscle in these patients, and this too needs to be cut before the eye can be passively abducted.

The optimal vertical position of the eye depends on a number of factors, including the likely final height of the patient—a very tall person requires more downgaze than a very short one. Usually the inferior rectus muscle is more fibrotic than the superior muscle, and so the eye can be elevated slightly by means of an inferior rectus recession. It is wise to leave the eye in a slight degree of downgaze to avoid the risks of corneal exposure after ptosis surgery.

If correction of the ptosis is required, this cannot be achieved by surgery to the fibrotic levator palpebrae superioris muscle, which generally has only minimal function in this condition; bilateral brow suspension is needed (Collin, 1968).

SURGICAL COMPLICATIONS

Wong and Jampolsky (1974) have noticed that the anterior ciliary circulation to the eye may be aberrant in some children with congenital fibrosis. Operating on even one muscle may be problematic (i.e., ischemia) if no other muscles are present. Therefore, an examination of other muscles may be advisable before detaching any muscle.

DOUBLE ELEVATOR PALSY

Double elevator palsy is also considered in Chapter 13 but is discussed again here because in most cases double elevator palsy is a form of congenital restrictive disease.

The term *double elevator palsy* was coined by White in 1942, who described monocular paralysis of the inferior oblique and superior rectus muscles presenting as a failure of upgaze. The term is now generally reserved for the congenital form of the condition, which is unusual (Rosner, 1963).

Differential Diagnosis

Acquired cases of restriction of upgaze are more common and are usually caused by a condition producing fibrosis and contracture of a rectus muscle, such as dysthyroid eye disease, cellulitis, orbital blowout fracture, third nerve palsy, traumatic or postsurgical rectus muscle disinsertion, or various other conditions producing rectus muscle rigidity (Barsoum-Homsy, 1983; Bell et al., 1990; Metz, 1981). In congenital double elevator palsy there is a limitation of upgaze in adduction, primary position, and abduction (Figure 18.2).

The presence of some elevation on abduction should raise the suspicion of congenital Brown's syndrome. If the clinical examination cannot exclude this condition, forced duction testing under

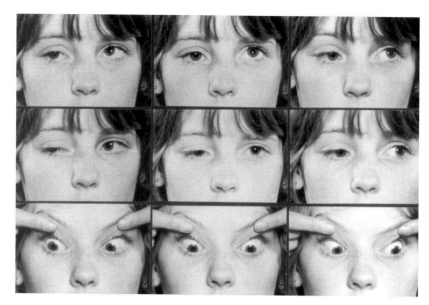

FIGURE 18.2   *A child with double elevator palsy (right eye), which causes a monocular elevation deficit in adduction and abduction.*

anesthesia may be used, especially if the surgeon makes sure to perform the forced duction test with the eye in a position of protrusion, thus tightening the rectus muscles, and also in a position of retraction, which more specifically tightens the superior and inferior oblique muscles. Double elevator palsy due to supranuclear disease presents as a unilateral failure of upgaze, often with an associated ptosis and sometimes with Marcus-Gunn jaw-winking (Metz, 1981). Bell's phenomenon may be absent or may be normal, demonstrating that this is a supranuclear unilateral failure of upgaze (Jampel and Fells, 1968). If the affected eye can be elevated to the primary position, amblyopia may not be present, but more commonly the eye is hypotropic with little active elevation possible, and amblyopia is profound. The fellow eye is usually normal, although bilateral cases have been described (Metz, 1981).

If a forced duction test is performed early enough, little passive resistance is encountered on elevation of the affected eye, but in later life the traction tests often become positive due to inferior rectus fibrosis (von Noorden, 1970). This is probably a secondary phenomenon, although McNeer and Jampolsky (1965) described one case in which an anomalous insertion of an extra band of the inferior rectus muscle produced the clinical picture of a double elevator palsy. Some patients, however, do not have a restriction of passive upgaze, as the presence of Bell's phenomenon demonstrates.

Etiology

The etiologic mechanism of double elevator palsy due to supranuclear disease is obscure, especially if one accepts that the nerve fibers to the superior rectus muscle from the oculomotor nucleus are crossed, whereas those nerve fibers to the inferior oblique muscle are not (Warwick, 1953). Jampel and Fells (1968), from a series of eight patients, suggested that the condition was due to a discrete lesion in the pretectum in the midbrain. Lessel (1975) reported on a patient who developed a double elevator palsy in his left eye and was found at autopsy to have a metastatic tumor in the right side of the pretectum. The condition may have a supranuclear origin, with the fibrotic changes being secondary.

Management

The management of double elevator palsy is essentially conservative. Amblyopia is the major problem, and cosmesis is a secondary problem that may best be approached when the child is older. In some cases, there is no deviation in the primary position, so surgery for double elevator palsy is contraindicated because any surgery is likely to compromise the patient's otherwise excellent chances of developing single binocular vision. More often, there is hypodeviation in the primary position, with or without an associated ptosis. In these cases, surgery is definitely indicated because the affected eye will become deeply amblyopic without surgery.

Surgical Management

The presence of Bell's phenomenon and a normal forced duction test indicate the absence of inferior rectus fibrosis, and in this situation a Knapp procedure (1969) is the treatment of choice. The medial and lateral recti are disinserted and brought around to the insertion of the superior rectus muscle. Depending on how close their insertions are brought to that of the superior rectus muscle, 20–35 prism diopters of hypotropia may be corrected this way. Levator resection may be required to correct a ptosis sufficient to occlude the pupil, but if the ptosis does not occlude the pupil, ptosis surgery is better left until later in childhood. The ptosis is most frequently a pseudoptosis, and therefore treatment should be delayed until the eye position is optimized. Following successful surgical elevation of the eye, vigorous patching of the fellow eye may permit the development of useful vision, but the prognosis should be guarded (von Noorden, 1970).

SURGICAL MANAGEMENT OF UNIOCULAR INFERIOR RECTUS FIBROSIS

Acquired isolated fibrosis of the inferior rectus muscle appears to be more common than fibrosis of any other rectus muscle in isolation. It can also be congenital and may represent fibrotic changes secondary to a double elevator palsy, or it may be primarily caused by an inability to elevate the eye. Inferior rectus fibrosis produces a hypodeviation in the primary position and restricts upgaze. Management consists of confirming the diagnosis by a forced duction test and a large recession of the inferior rectus muscle. Once the inferior rectus muscle has been isolated and detached from the globe, the forced duction test should be repeated to ensure that the globe is now free to move into elevation. The large recession of the inferior rectus muscle may result in a recession of the lower lid, requiring more surgery later on. Lower lid retraction may be avoided by dissection of the lower lid retractors from the inferior rectus muscle and their reattachment to the site of the original insertion of the inferior rectus muscle.

OTHER ACQUIRED FIBROSIS SYNDROMES

Extraocular muscle fibrosis may be acquired as a result of inflammation (e.g., dysthyroid ophthalmopathy), infiltration (e.g., amyloidosis affecting the medial recti [Sharma et al., 1991]), denervation (e.g., in very long-standing third nerve palsies), or trauma (e.g., blowout fractures of the orbit), or it may be idiopathic (e.g., progressive esotropia of high myopia). The general principles of surgical management are the same throughout: Large recessions are usually required, using an adjustable suture technique wherever possible, and resections should be avoided in all cases where the extraocular muscles are abnormally tight.

REFERENCES

Appleton RE, Chitayat D, Jan JE et al. Joubert's syndrome associated with congenital ocular fibrosis and histidinemia. Arch Neurol 1989;46:579–582.

Apt L, Axelrod RN. Generalized fibrosis of the extraocular muscles. Am J Ophthalmol 1978;85:822–829.

Barsoum-Homsy M. Congenital double elevator palsy. J Pediatr Ophthalmol Strabismus 1983;20:185–191.

Bell JA, Fielder AR, Viney S. Congenital double elevator palsy in identical twins. J Clin Neuro-Ophthalmol 1990;10:32–34.

Bradbourne AA. Hereditary ophthalmoplegia in five generations. Trans Ophthalmol Soc UK 1912;32:142–153.

Brown HW. Congenital Muscle Anomalies. In JH Allen (ed), Strabismus Ophthalmic Symposium. St. Louis: Mosby, 1950;229–233.

Collin JRO. A Manual of Systematic Eyelid Surgery. London: Butterworth, 1968.

Fells P, Waddell E, Alvarez M. Progressive Exaggerated A-Pattern Strabismus with Presumed Fibrosis of Extraocular Muscles. In RD Reiniecke (ed), Strabismus II: Proceedings of the Fourth Meeting of the Strabismological Association. Orlando: Grune & Stratton 1984;355–343.

Gast R. Ein fall von ophthalmoplegia bilateralis exterior congenita. Klin Monatsbl Augenheilkd 1889;27:214–217.

Harley RD, Rodrigues MM, Crawford JS. Congenital fibrosis of the extraocular muscles. J Pediatr Ophthalmol Strabismus 1978;15:346–358.

Jampel RS, Fells P. Monocular elevation paresis caused by a central nervous system lesion. Arch Ophthalmol 1968;80:45–47.

Kalpakian B, Bateman JB, Sparkes RS, Wood GK. Congenital ocular fibrosis syndrome associated with the Prader-Willi syndrome. J Pediatr Ophthalmol Strabismus 1986;23:170–173.

Kishore K, Kumar H. Congenital ocular fibrosis with musculoskeletal abnormality: a new association. J Pediatr Ophthalmol Strabismus 1991;28:283–286.

Knapp P. Surgical treatment of double elevator paralysis. Trans Am Ophthalmol Soc 1969;67:304–323.

Laughlin RC. Congenital fibrosis of the extraocular muscles: a report of six cases. Am J Ophthalmol 1956;41:432–438.

Lessell S. Supranuclear paralysis of monocular elevation. Neurology 1975;25:1134–1136.

McNeer KW, Jampolsky A. Double elevator palsy caused by anomalous insertion of the inferior rectus. Am J Ophthalmol 1965;59:317–319.

Metz HS. Double elevator palsy. J Pediatr Ophthalmol Strabismus 1981;18:31–35.

Rosner RS. Double elevator paralysis. Am J Ophthalmol 1963;55:87–93.

Sharma P, Gupta NK, Arora R et al. Strabismus fixus convergens secondary to amyloidosis. J Pediatr Ophthalmol Strabismus 1991;28:236–237.

von Noorden GK. Congenital hereditary ptosis with inferior rectus fibrosis. Arch Ophthalmol 1970;83:378–380.

Warwick R. Representation of the extraocular muscles in the oculomotor nuclei of the monkey. J Comp Neurol 1953;98:449–504.

White JW. Paralysis of the superior rectus and inferior oblique muscle of the same eye. Arch Ophthalmol 1942;27:366–371.

Wong GY, Jampolsky A. Agenesis of three horizontal rectus muscles. Ann Ophthalmol 1974;6:909–915.

19

Thyroid Eye Disease

ETIOLOGY

Graves' disease is a systemic illness that consists of thyroid abnormalities (hypothyroidism, diffused goiter, elevated thyroid levels), pretibial myxedema, and ophthalmopathy. The most common cause of acquired double vision in adults is thyroid myopathy. Unilateral and bilateral proptosis is usually caused by thyroid ophthalmopathy, although the differential diagnosis includes other orbital disease processes.

The etiology of thyroid myopathy is unknown. Ophthalmopathy is less frequent in Asians (Tellez et al., 1992), but gender and age are not risk factors (Utiger, 1992). Human leukocyte antigen (HLA) typing cannot distinguish patients at risk for ophthalmopathy.

Hyperthyroidism could have a role in aggravating ophthalmopathy. Tallstedt and colleagues (1992) showed that thyroid ophthalmopathy is more likely to occur in patients treated with iodine 131, perhaps because this treatment elevates serum levels of triiodothyronine. Obviously this hormone is now implicated in the etiology of Graves' disease. This finding corroborates clinical data, which show that ophthalmopathy starts at the same time or after the onset of symptoms of hyperthyroidism in most cases (Marcocci et al., 1989). However, thyroid ophthalmopathy could also be an immunologic disorder in which T cells react against thyroid and extraocular muscles (Volpe, 1978; Wall et al., 1981; Sergott and Glaser, 1981). Yet another theory holds that thyroglobulin binds to antigens that are shared by the thyroid gland and extraocular muscles, and that this incites an immunologic reaction (Kriss et al., 1975). Smoking also apparently increases the risk of severe ophthalmopathy in patients with Graves' disease (Hagg and Asplund, 1987).

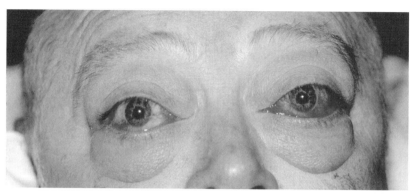

A

FIGURE 19.1   *Soft-tissue signs in thyroid ophthalmopathy include chemosis, lid edema, and injection. Note lid edema (A), injection over extraocular muscles (B, C), and more generalized injection (D). (Courtesy of Stuart R. Seiff, M.D.)*

DIAGNOSIS

It is important to remember that thyroid myopathy is part of a spectrum of orbital and ocular abnormalities that can occur in patients with Graves' disease. Most classification schemes for thyroid ophthalmopathy include four categories of abnormalities: soft-tissue involvement, exophthalmos, extraocular involvement, and optic neuropathy (Solem et al., 1979; Werner, 1969). Patients do not necessarily progress from one aspect of eye involvement to another. For example, soft-tissue signs may precede or be followed by extraocular muscle involvement. Sight-threatening involvement can also occur early in the course of thyroid ophthalmopathy.

The soft-tissue signs of thyroid ophthalmopathy include conjunctival chemosis, eyelid edema, and redness of the bulbar conjunctiva (Figure 19.1). Initial symptoms include mild ocular discomfort, photophobia, and even a sensation of deep orbital pressure (Bahn et al., 1990; Bahn and Heufelder, 1993).

Proptosis in thyroid ophthalmopathy is the result of enlargement of the extraocular muscles (Figure 19.2). Proptosis may be mild or severe and is responsible for another external disease abnormality, that of keratopathy caused by exposure of the cornea and inability of the eyelids to protect the cornea.

Vision loss in thyroid ophthalmopathy is presumably due to enlargement of extraocular muscles, causing compromise of optic nerve function. Undoubtedly, different patients show different vulnerabilities to this enlargement, accounting for the fact that some patients develop optic neuropathy even with mild degrees of enlargement of extraocular muscles.

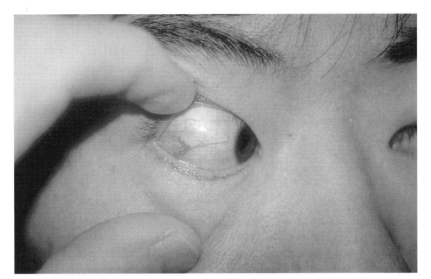

B

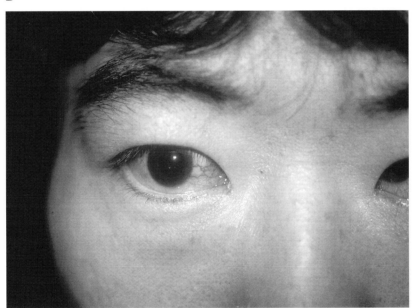

C

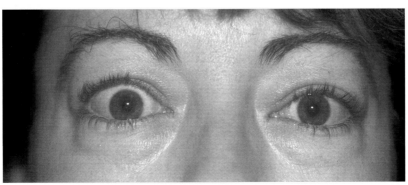

D

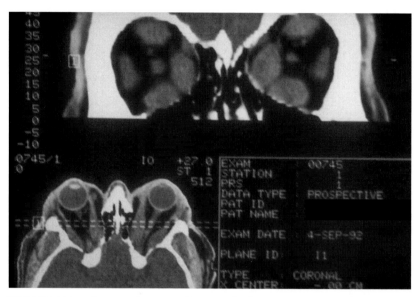

FIGURE 19.2 *Computed tomographic scan of orbits in a patient with thyroid myopathy. Note the enlarged extraocular muscles. (Courtesy of Stuart R. Seiff, M.D.)*

LABORATORY INVESTIGATION

Laboratory investigations can also help to support a diagnosis of thyroid myopathy. There is a strong link between thyroid myopathy and systemic hyperthyroidism (Amino et al., 1980). Eighty-five percent of patients who present with Graves' ophthalmopathy will develop hyperthyroidism within 18 months (Marcocci et al., 1989). Even though 10% of patients with thyroid ophthalmopathy are not hyperthyroid, most of these patients have laboratory evidence for thyroid autoimmune disease (Salvi et al., 1990). The HLA-DR3 is associated with thyroid ophthalmopathy (Frecker et al., 1986), but its relevance to predictive risk of ophthalmopathy is debated (Utiger, 1992).

Eye findings can occur before or after thyroid disease (Pequegnat et al., 1967). Occasionally patients remain euthyroid throughout the course of their thyroid ophthalmopathy condition.

STRABISMUS IN THYROID OPHTHALMOPATHY

Patients with Graves' disease virtually always suffer enlargement of extraocular muscles (Coleman et al., 1972; Forrester et al., 1977) but only some will develop diplopia. Thyroid myopathy should be suspected in patients with acute onset of diplopia, particularly when restrictive eye muscle disease can be diagnosed.

Therefore, the diagnosis of thyroid myopathy is based partly on the presence of abnormal forced duction tests. The inferior rectus muscle is most commonly involved, followed in frequency of involvement by medial, superior, and lateral rectus muscles. The patient's attempts to elevate the eyes may cause diplopia due to asymmetric restriction of the inferior rectus muscles. When the eyes are passively rotated up (for inferior rectus involvement) or out (for medial rectus involvement), positive forced duction findings indicate restrictive disease.

Involvement of extraocular muscles can be diagnosed by ultrasonography, even when there are minimal signs of Graves' disease (Skalka, 1980; Hodes and Stern, 1975). Nearly every patient with Graves' disease can be diagnosed in this fashion.

The most common strabismus abnormality is vertical restriction due to inferior rectus involvement (Figure 19.3). The involvement may be symmetric or asymmetric. Because the inferior rectus muscle plays a secondary role in adduction (Jampolsky, 1978), tightness of this muscle or muscles can cause esotropia as well.

Restriction of upward movement of the eyes caused by inferior rectus muscle disease is responsible for the physical finding of intraocular pressure increases when patients look up. An increase in intraocular pressure of 4 mm Hg correlates with restriction of the inferior rectus muscle (Char, 1990). Increased intraocular pressure may occur even in primary gaze, again, due to the tethering effect of involved extraocular muscles (Gamblin et al., 1983; Allen et al., 1985).

DIFFERENTIAL DIAGNOSIS

Conditions that can mimic thyroid ophthalmopathy should be investigated. Double elevator palsy usually manifests in childhood. It is not accompanied by other signs of thyroid ophthalmopathy. Restriction in elevation occurs on abduction and adduction, in contrast to thyroid ophthalmopathy, in which a restriction in elevation is usually more marked in the abducted position.

Brown's syndrome causes restriction of elevation of the eye in the adducted position. Forced duction testing in Brown's syndrome is abnormal when the eye is elevated and adducted.

Orbital blowout fractures can cause restriction of the inferior rectus muscle. Computed tomographic scans usually show the fracture, and the condition may be accompanied by enophthalmos. In thyroid ophthalmopathy, exophthalmos is the rule.

A number of conditions can cause enlargement of the extraocular muscle or muscles. Tumor metastases to extraocular muscles are rare but can cause restriction of eye movement. A carotid cavernous fistula can also cause enlargement of one or more extraocular muscles, presumably due to increased blood flow through the muscle. Idiopathic myositis causes enlargement of extraocular muscles. The

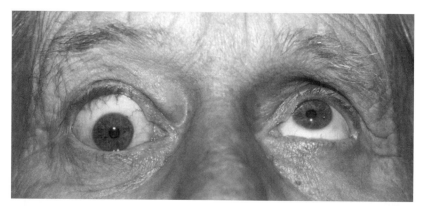

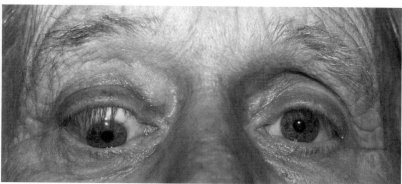

FIGURE 19.3   *This patient with thyroid myopathy had restriction of upgaze due to restrictive disease of his right inferior rectus muscle.*

muscle enlargement includes the tendon; in thyroid myopathy, the tendon is usually spared.

Finally, the clinician must always remember that myasthenia gravis accompanies Graves' disease in up to 5% of patients. Because ocular findings in myasthenia gravis can mimic almost any strabismic condition, the clinician should perform serial examinations on patients and investigate for myasthenia gravis in cases that do not conform to the usual conditions of strabismus seen in thyroid ophthalmopathy (Verde, 1990). Exotropia in Graves' ophthalmopathy is particularly uncommon and should suggest a diagnosis of Graves' disease and myasthenia gravis (Vargas et al., 1993).

MANAGEMENT

Medical Management of Thyroid Myopathy

Extraocular muscles involved in thyroid myopathy progress from an acute inflammatory stage where lymphocytes are found in the extracellular matrix to a fibrotic stage. Before the fibrotic stage is reached, strabismus abnormalities may be transient or variable, or both. Patients with newly diagnosed hyperthyroidism with acute symptoms of double vision can be treated with systemic steroids. Up to 20% of patients may improve either spontaneously or with systemic steroids (Sterk et al., 1985). On the other hand, *chronic* diplopia is seldom managed effectively with any form of medical treatment.

Other treatment modalities for acute thyroid ophthalmopathy and myopathy include cyclosporine A and radiation. When retrobulbar radiation is compared to oral prednisone, both are equally effective in controlling moderately severe Graves' ophthalmopathy (Prummel et al., 1993). No form of immunosuppression is effective in the management of chronic (fibrotic) Graves' myopathy.

Optical Management

A reasonable goal in managing diplopia associated with Graves' myopathy is achievement of single vision in primary gaze and in the reading gaze position. To this effect, the use of prisms can be helpful. Fusional amplitudes in newly acquired vertical strabismus of any variety are not large. Therefore, small amounts of prism to manage small angles of vertical deviation may be extremely helpful. Regrettably, thyroid myopathy often causes incomitant strabismus, limiting the usefulness of prisms. Still, with deviations of as much as 15 prism diopters, prisms may provide a permanent, satisfactory solution.

The patient's refraction may change either as a result of the thyroid myopathy or of surgery. Large changes in astigmatic correction are known to occur. Therefore, one of the mainstays of treating thyroid eye disease is a careful refraction performed at various stages of the disease.

Botulinum Toxin Treatment

Botulinum toxin has been used to manage diplopia associated with thyroid myopathy in the first 6 months of the disease (Dunn et al., 1986). Evidently, some patients develop lateral rectus palsy if they receive botulinum toxin and have previously undergone an orbital decompression (Char, 1990). Botulinum toxin is probably of no or limited value once the myopathy has reached the fibrotic stage.

Surgery

Timing of Strabismus Surgery

A logical approach to the surgical management of thyroid ophthalmopathy has been presented by Shorr and Seiff (1986). If an orbital decompression is necessary, this should be performed prior to strabismus surgery, since almost 80% of patients who undergo decompression experience postoperative double vision (Rosenbaum, 1982; Fells, 1987). The reason for postoperative diplopia has to do with reposition of the eyes in the orbits and the potential for the extraocular muscles to fall into the surgically induced bony defects. Many patients also undoubtedly have diplopia before decompression surgery.

Another reason for performing orbital decompression before strabismus surgery has to do with the risk of exposure keratitis. Any recession of extraocular muscles augments proptosis and can further aggravate exposure keratitis. In our experience, conventional recessions of two muscles in the same eye can induce as much as 3–4 mm of proptosis in patients with Graves' myopathy.

On the other hand, due to the tendency for vertical muscle surgery to move the position of the eyelids, any procedure to change lid position should probably be performed after a strabismus operation. The stare that thyroid patients may show is partially induced by efforts to elevate the eyes. A simple inferior rectus recession can alleviate upper eyelid retraction and result in a considerable cosmetic improvement. Similarly, hypotropia may be associated with a pseudoptosis. Again, once the eye is elevated with an inferior rectus recession, the ptosis may be considerably improved.

The decision to correct strabismus with surgery should await stabilization of the eye movement problem (strabismus). Eye movement problems can improve with control of systemic hyperthyroidism (Sterk et al., 1985; Hamilton et al., 1960). Most surgeons would prefer to wait 4–6 months and to document a stable strabismus examination before undertaking a surgical procedure.

Vertical Deviation
Vertical strabismus is the most common type of misalignment caused by thyroid myopathy. One or both inferior rectus muscles undergo fibrotic changes, resulting in hypotropia (Scott and Thalacker, 1981). When prisms have failed to provide satisfactory alignment, surgery is a reasonable option.

Forced duction tests should be positive, indicating restricted upgaze. Even though a large unilateral hypotropia may be present, forced duction tests in the fellow eye should be observed, since lesser amounts of inferior rectus fibrosis may be present in the contralateral eye.

Treatment usually consists of an inferior rectus recession. In cases of hypotropia where both eyes elevate above the midline easily, an ipsilateral inferior rectus recession can be performed. The expected effect of 2.5 prism diopters per millimeter of recession of the inferior rectus muscle does not hold as well for thyroid myopathy. For that reason, the use of an adjustable suture on the operated muscle may be especially helpful.

With marked restriction of both inferior rectus muscles, or with asymmetric movement of the inferior rectus muscles, bilateral inferior rectus recessions can be performed. The amount of recession should be greater on the more involved side. Both muscles can be operated on with adjustable sutures, allowing considerable flexibility in postoperative adjustments.

An important risk in recessing one or both inferior rectus muscles is that of overcorrection. The patient may achieve orthotropia in primary gaze but suffer hypertropia in downgaze due to overcorrection of the involved and operated muscle. Lesser amounts of recession in the fellow eye may help reduce the risk of this complication, but the surgeon should also pay attention to ipsilateral superior rectus contracture. Long-standing hypotropia results in a considerable effort to elevate both eyes. The result is that the superior rectus muscle can become tightened and may hold the eye up in the upward position, inhibiting its ability to rotate down with efforts toward downgaze, especially after recession. Forced duction testing in the downward direction at the time of surgery may indicate tightness of the superior rectus muscle. In this case, the surgeon should consider the apparently paradoxical maneuver of performing an ipsilateral superior rectus recession (also on an adjustable suture) in conjunction with recession of the inferior rectus muscle (Jampolsky, personal communication).

A slowly progressive overcorrection is also known to occur, perhaps due to the same mechanisms as discussed above. Occasionally, the hypotropia is caused by such marked inferior rectus fibrosis that the eye cannot be rotated above the horizontal plane. The surgeon may be surprised to find that in severe cases the eye cannot even be rotated to the horizontal or midline position with forced duction testing at the time of surgery, and with the inferior rectus muscle detached from the globe. In this case, unconventional amounts of recession of the inferior rectus muscle in the involved eye may be necessary to achieve satisfactory eye alignment. Recession of as much as 12–16 mm may be necessary. On occasion we have had to suture the inferior rectus muscle to posterior Tenon's, accompanied by a large recession of the fascia to provide the patient with the ability to elevate the eye above the midline.

With recessions of more than 6 mm, the lower eyelid position in relation to the globe often changes. A careful dissection of the connections between the inferior rectus muscle and lower eyelid may partially help to prevent this complication. Nevertheless, patients should be forewarned that lower eyelid ptosis can occur and may require subsequent eyelid surgery.

Vertical Strabismus Associated with Esotropia
Some patients show esotropia associated with hypotropia. Deficient abduction can occur as a result of tightening of the inferior rectus muscle. Jampolsky (1978) advocated recessing the inferior rectus muscle or muscles as an approach to managing both horizontal and vertical strabismus.

The inferior rectus muscle can be recessed and placed on adjustable sutures. At the same time, forced duction tests are performed on the medial rectus muscles (into abduction). If tightness exists, the surgeon can consider performing a simultaneous unilateral or bilateral medial rectus recession. Again, the use of adjustable sutures is advised.

The risk of performing simultaneous inferior and medial rectus recessions is that of overcorrection, which causes certain problems in downgaze (i.e., the patient develops exotropia and has double vision in the reading position).

Esotropia

Some patients may demonstrate a reasonably pure and concomitant esotropia. Abduction is deficient in one or both eyes. In this case, medial rectus recessions can be performed. Approximately 3 prism diopters of shift occur per millimeter of recession, but this depends to some extent on surgical technique, and adjustable sutures remain advisable, since the effect is somewhat unpredictable.

A Patterns

Some patients may show a preoperative, significant A-pattern esotropia. This may be combined with various amounts of vertical strabismus, as well. Inferior rectus recessions can be used to manage the vertical strabismus. They may also reduce the esotropia in primary gaze but contribute to worsening of the A pattern. In this setting, weakening of the superior oblique muscles can be entertained. A "posterior seven-eighths" procedure can be performed in which the posterior seven-eighths or so of the superior oblique tendon is isolated and cut. The effect of this procedure is to reduce the abducting effect of the superior oblique muscles in downgaze without changing the vertical or torsional orientation of the eye. *Bilateral* superior oblique surgery is advisable.

Torsional Problems

Patients with thyroid myopathy seldom complain of cyclotorsion of one eye or both, even though torsion can be measured in nearly 50% of them (Trobe, 1984; Caygill, 1972). The majority of patients show excyclotorsion, but incyclotorsion, when it occurs, is highly specific for thyroid myopathy (Trobe, 1984). The inferior rectus muscles induce excyclotorsion as they become fibrotic. Presumably, restriction of other muscles (e.g., superior rectus) is responsible for incyclotorsion.

Recession of the inferior rectus muscle or muscles alleviates excyclotorsion. However, patients adjust to the excyclotorsion and may experience torsional symptoms as a result of recession of the inferior rectus muscles. The best treatment for this postoperative problem is a period of observation. Most people will grow accustomed to the realignment of their eyes and cease complaining after 3–6 months. Surgical management of torsion is discussed in Chapter 14.

Surgical Complications

There are several complications specifically related to the surgical management of thyroid myopathy. Scleritis and sector ischemia of the anterior segment of the eye are more common when two adjacent muscles are operated on simultaneously. Signs of this problem include increased redness and discomfort. Fortunately, the problem usually resolves after a period of several months. Treatment can include ocular lubricants or topical steroids, or no treatment at all.

Fibrotic muscles, once recessed, may continue to slip. The surgeon may wish to aim for a slight undercorrection when recessing an inferior rectus muscle. The tendency will be for that muscle to continue to weaken somewhat. An accurate alignment on the first postoperative day may result in an overcorrection noted 3–6 months later. In our experience, undercorrection is more common, especially in severe cases. Usually, the surgeon fails to recess a muscle far enough even though forced duction testing indicates that more aggressive surgery is indicated. With adjustable suture techniques, the surgeon should feel less inhibited about performing a large recession, since the operated muscle can be repositioned postoperatively.

REFERENCES

Allen C, Stetz D, Roman SH et al. Prevalence and clinical associations of intraocular pressure changes in Graves' disease. J Clin Endocrinol Metab 1985;61:183–187.

Amino N, Yuasa T, Yabu Y et al. Exophthalmos in autoimmune thyroid disease. J Clin Endocrinol Metab 1980;51:1232–1234.

Bahn RS, Garrity JA, Gorman CA. Diagnosis and management of Graves' ophthalmopathy. J Clin Endocrinol Metab 1990;71:559–563.

Bahn RS, Heufelder AE. Pathogenesis of Graves' ophthalmopathy. N Engl J Med 1993;329:1468–1475.

Caygill WM. Excyclotropia in dysthyroid ophthalmopathy. Am J Ophthalmol 1972;73:437–441.

Char D. Thyroid Eye Disease. New York: Churchill Livingstone, 1990.

Coleman DJ, Jack RL, Franzen LA, Werner SC. High resolution B-scan ultrasonography of the orbit. V. Eye changes of Graves' disease. Arch Ophthalmol 1972;88:465–471.

Dunn WJ, Arnold AC, O'Connor PS. Botulinum toxin for the treatment of dysthyroid ocular myopathy. Ophthalmology 1986;93:470–475.

Fells P. Orbital decompression for severe dysthyroid eye disease. Br J Ophthalmol 1987;71:107–111.

Forrester JV, Sutherland GR, McDougall IR. Dysthyroid ophthalmopathy: orbital evaluation with B-scan ultrasonography. J Clin Endocrinol Metab 1977;45:221–224.

Frecker M, Stenszky V, Balazs C et al. Genetic factors in Graves' ophthalmopathy. Clin Endocrinol 1986;25:479–485.

Gamblin GT, Harper DG, Galentine P et al. Prevalence of increased intraocular pressure in Graves' disease—evidence of frequent subclinical ophthalmopathy. N Engl J Med 1983;308:420–424.

Hagg E, Asplund K. Is endocrine ophthalmopathy related to smoking? Br Med J Clin Res Ed 1987;295:634–635.

Hamilton HE, Schultz RO, DeGowin EL. The endocrine eye lesion in hyperthyroidism. Arch Intern Med 1960;105:575–585.

Hodes BL, Stern G. Contact B-scan echographic diagnosis of ophthalmopathic Graves' disease. J Clin Ultrasound 1975;3:255–261.

Jampolsky A. Surgical Leashes in Strabismus Surgical Management. In Symposium on Strabismus. Transactions of the New Orleans Academy of Ophthalmology. St. Louis: Mosby, 1978;244–268.

Kriss JP, Konishi J, Herman M. Studies on the pathogenesis of Graves' ophthalmopathy (with some related observations regarding therapy). Recent Prog Horm Res 1975;31:533–566.

Marcocci C, Bartalena L, Bogazzi F et al. Studies on the occurrence of ophthalmopathy in Graves' disease. Acta Endocrinol 1989;120:473–478.

Pequegnat EP, Mayberry WE, McConahey WM, Wyse EP. Large doses of radioiodide in Graves' disease: effect on ophthalmopathy and long-acting thyroid stimulator. Mayo Clin Proc 1967;42:802–811.

Prummel MF, Mourits MP, Blank L et al. Randomized double-blind trial of prednisone versus radiotherapy in Graves' ophthalmopathy. Lancet 1993;342:949–954.

Rosenbaum AL. Discussion. Ophthalmology 1982;89:327–328.

Salvi M, Zhang Z-G, Haegert D et al. Patients with endocrine ophthalmopathy not associated with overt thyroid disease have multiple thyroid immunological abnormalities. J Clin Endocrinol Metab 1990;70:89–94.

Scott WE, Thalacker JA. Diagnosis and treatment of thyroid myopathy. Ophthalmology 1981;88:493–498.

Sergott RC, Glaser JS. Graves' ophthalmopathy. A clinical and immunologic review. Surv Ophthalmol 1981;26:1–21.

Shorr N, Seiff SR. The four stages of surgical rehabilitation of the patient with dysthyroid ophthalmopathy. Ophthalmology 1986;93:476–483.

Skalka HW. The use of ultrasonography in the diagnosis of endocrine orbitopathy. Neuro-Ophthalmol 1980;1:109–261.

Solem JH, Segaard E, Ytteborg J. The course of endocrine ophthalmopathy during anti-thyroid therapy in a prospective study. Acta Med Scand 1979;205:111–114.

Sterk CC, Bierlaagh JJ, de Keizer RJ. Motility disorders in endocrine ophthalmopathy. Doc Ophthalmol 1985;59:71–75.

Tallstedt L, Lundell G, Torring O et al. Occurrence of ophthalmopathy after treatment for Graves' hyperthyroidism.The Thyroid Study Group. N Engl J Med 1992;326:1733–1738.

Tellez M, Cooper J, Edmonds C. Graves' ophthalmopathy in relation to cigarette smoking and ethnic origin. Clin Endocrinol 1992;36:291–294.

Trobe JD. Cyclodeviation in acquired vertical strabismus. Arch Ophthalmol 1984;102:717–720.

Utiger RD. Pathogenesis of Graves' ophthalmopathy. N Engl J Med 1992;326:1772–1773.

Vargas ME, Warren FA, Kupersmith MJ. Exotropia as a sign of myasthenia gravis in dysthyroid ophthalmopathy. Br J Ophthalmol 1993;77:822–823.

Verde RM. Graves' ophthalmopathy and the special problem of concomitant ocular myasthenia gravis. Am Orthop J 1990;40:37–50.

Volpe R. The pathogenesis of Graves' disease: an overview. Clin Endocrinol Metab 1978;7:3–29.

Wall JR, Henderson J, Strakosch CR, Joyner DM. Graves' ophthalmopathy. Can Med Assoc J 1981;124:855–866.

Werner SC. Classification of the eye changes of Graves' disease. J Clin Endocrinol Metab 1969;29:982–984.

20

Orbital Fractures and Strabismus

ETIOLOGY

Lang (1889) recognized that blunt trauma to the eye and orbit can cause an orbital bone fracture, but Smith and Regan (1957) were the first to use the term *blowout fracture*. The work of Smith and Regan confirmed the theory that pressure on the globe is transmitted to the orbital floor, resulting in its buckling (Figure 20.1).

This so-called hydraulic theory probably accounts for the majority of orbital fractures and has been confirmed by investigations in animals (Green et al., 1990). However, some orbital floor fractures are caused by the transmission of forces posteriorly from below to the orbital rim (Fujino and Sato, 1987). When the orbital floor is fractured, the orbital contents may shift inferiorly. Because the inferior rectus muscle is closest to the fracture site, its injury or entrapment is most likely. Most floor fractures occur in the posteromedial region (Whyte, 1968). This region is apposed to the equator of the globe. The location of the fracture, particularly whether it is anterior or posterior, can determine the strabismus pattern.

The medial wall of the orbit can also be fractured (Figure 20.2). Medial wall injury usually accompanies an injury to the orbital floor (Converse et al., 1967), but occasionally, isolated medial wall fractures are encountered. Damage to the medial wall of the orbit is most likely to injure or entrap the medial rectus muscle, in which case horizontal strabismus would be expected.

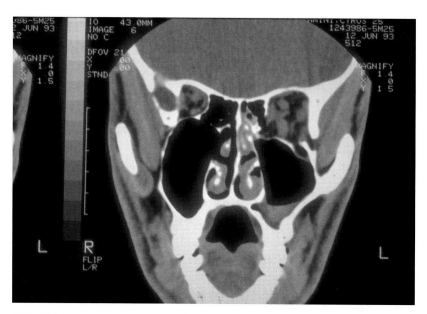

FIGURE 20.1 *Coronal computed tomographic scan shows a defect in the left orbital floor. Note the air–fluid level in the left maxillary sinus, a frequent finding in blowout fracture.*

The mechanism of strabismus in fractures of the orbital roof differs from that of fractures of the orbital floor. A sort of "blow-in" fracture can occur in which trauma to the frontal bone causes transmission of forces inferiorly, resulting in encroachment of the orbit by the fracture fragments (Baker and Epstein, 1991). Damage to the superior rectus muscle is most likely in this type of fracture. Paralysis of the superior rectus muscle or its entrapment can result.

Because the lateral wall of the orbit is so solid, its isolated damage is extremely rare. Usually, the patient with lateral orbital fracture also suffers massive facial damage and requires extensive maxillofacial surgical intervention.

DIAGNOSIS

The blowout or blow-in fracture should be suspected on the basis of the patient's history and physical findings. A history of blunt trauma to the eye or inferior orbital rim should lead to a careful physical examination. Blunt trauma to the forehead can also cause fractures of the orbital roof. Blunt trauma to the nose can cause fractures of the medial wall of the orbit. Signs and symptoms related to fractures in these areas should be sought.

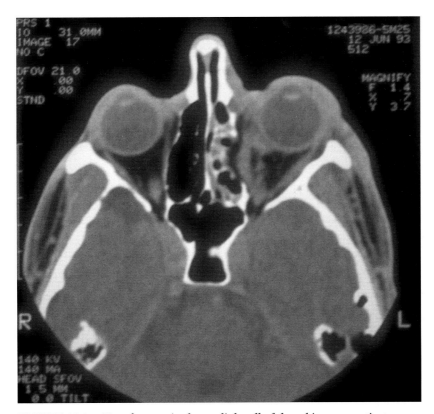

FIGURE 20.2 *Note fracture in the medial wall of the orbit, same patient.*

Enophthalmos occurs when a floor fracture allows the orbital contents to collapse inferiorly and posteriorly. Occasionally, a fracture can be palpated on the bony orbital rim in any location.

Strabismus is usually vertical. When the inferior rectus muscle is entrapped, the patient may show difficulty elevating the involved eye. Hypotropia may be present in primary gaze and in downgaze as well.

Paradoxically, a posterior entrapment of the inferior rectus muscle can lead to hypertropia of the involved eye (Cole and Smith, 1963). This occurs because the muscle can tether the eye and actually cause the back part of the globe to rotate inferiorly (and the anterior globe to rotate superiorly), or, perhaps, because the inferior rectus becomes paralyzed (Metz et al., 1974). Paralysis of the inferior rectus muscle can occur as an isolated finding or can accompany either of the types of entrapment previously mentioned (anterior or posterior floor entrapment). A paralyzed inferior rectus muscle leads to a large-angle hypertropia on the affected side (Figure 20.3). The eye would only rotate to approximately the horizontal level in attempted downgaze. The vertical deviation is worse in abduction than in adduction.

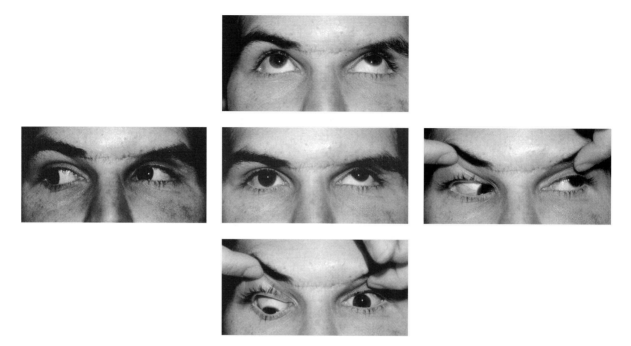

FIGURE 20.3   *This man suffered a blowout fracture in an automobile accident. He has a large hypertropia in primary gaze and deficient left infraduction. Forced duction tests were normal.*

Brown's syndrome has been reported both with floor (Zipf and Trokel, 1973) and roof fractures of the orbit (Baldwin and Baker, 1988; Jackson et al., 1979; Baker and Conklin, 1987). Therefore, physical findings of Brown's syndrome do not necessarily localize the site of the fracture. In most cases (when orbital fractures are involved), Brown's syndrome is caused by posttraumatic inflammation of the superior oblique tendon or trochlea, but Baldwin and Baker (1988) reported a case in which Brown's syndrome was caused by actual entrapment of the superior oblique tendon within a superior orbital fracture (Figure 20.4).

Fractures of the medial wall of the orbit can produce a retraction syndrome (Miller and Glaser, 1966; Edwards and Ridley, 1968; Mirsky and Saunders, 1979). Mirsky and Saunders (1979) noted that minor trauma may produce a medial orbital wall blowout fracture. In this syndrome, adduction may be limited, and abduction is deficient and associated with retraction of the globe. The presumed mechanism of globe retraction is that the medial rectus muscle tethers the eye and fails to allow it to abduct. The tethering action supports the eye and causes it to retract during abduction. Gittinger and colleagues (1986) noted an association between this so-called acquired retraction syn-

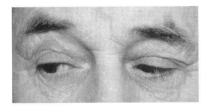
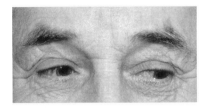
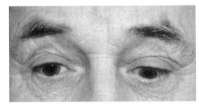
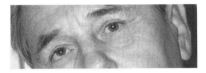
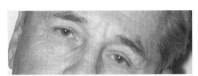
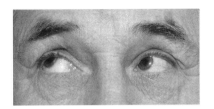
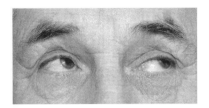
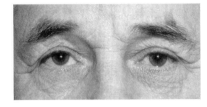

FIGURE 20.4 *This man fell off his motorcycle in 1968, fracturing the floor and roof of his left orbit. He has left Brown's syndrome with deficient elevation on adduction. Gradually he developed a head tilt to the left to maintain sensory fusion. Note that right tilt causes a large right hypertropia. At the time of surgery, a tight right superior rectus muscle was diagnosed.*

drome and African-American patients. They hypothesized that this population may be at greater risk for this type of injury.

Because retraction syndrome mimics Duane's syndrome (Duane et al., 1976), a careful history of eye trauma is important in this setting.

Fractures of the orbital roof can produce symptoms of eye movement abnormalities, enophthalmos, ptosis, and central nervous system abnormalities (McClurg and Swanson, 1976; McLachlan et al., 1982; Smith and Regan, 1957; Greenwald et al., 1987). Pulsating exophthalmos has been reported (Baker and Epstein, 1991; Smith and Blount, 1971). We have seen a child with a cerebrospinal fluid leak that caused recurrent upper eyelid edema. The edema resolved after neurosurgical patching of the dura and superior orbital fracture.

Eye movement abnormalities associated with orbital roof fractures usually consist of vertical gaze problems. In one case, superior rectus underaction was noted in a patient with a subperiosteal hemorrhage (Ohtsuka and Nakaoka, 1987). Brown's syndrome caused by damage to the superior oblique trochlea can occur (Al-Qurainy et al., 1988; Baldwin and Baker, 1988). Difficulty in elevating the involved eye can also occur as a result of damage to the superior rectus muscle, caused by bone fragments from the orbital roof (McLachlan et al., 1982; Milauskas and Fueger, 1966).

Forced duction testing has an important role in the diagnosis of motility problems associated with orbital fractures. With entrapped muscles, the forced duction test is positive, attempting to move the eye away from the field of action of that muscle. For example, a trapped inferior rectus muscle results in a positive forced duction test when the eye is rotated superiorly. The forced duction test may be positive with medial wall blowout fractures. Attempts to rotate the eye laterally meet with resistance. The forced duction test is usually normal with orbital roof fractures since the cause of the motility disturbance is underaction of the superior rectus muscle.

Forced generation testing may also be useful. An underacting or paralyzed muscle will fail to generate normal eye movement against resistance. This examination requires a cooperative patient and an experienced physician to judge whether the eye movement force is normal or less than normal.

DIFFERENTIAL DIAGNOSIS

The differential diagnosis for orbital fractures associated with motility disturbances falls into two broad categories. First, vertical strabismus problems may mimic the strabismus associated with blowout fractures. Second, a variety of ocular motor disturbances caused by trauma may occur but do not involve a mechanism of orbital bone fracture.

Any vertical strabismus problem may mimic strabismus associated with a blowout fracture. Fourth nerve palsies cause hypertropia that worsens on ipsilateral head tilt and on adduction of the involved eye. However, in an orbital floor fracture (i.e., with an entrapped inferior rectus muscle), contralateral hypertropia may exist, which worsens on elevation. Forced duction testing will reveal that the inferior rectus muscle is trapped in the blowout fracture (Figure 20.5). Forced duction testing in superior oblique palsy is usually normal. Fourth nerve palsies can occur with head trauma, and this can confuse the examiner if he or she is not looking out for it.

A tight inferior rectus muscle occurs with congenital fibrosis syndrome, double elevator palsy, and thyroid myopathy. The first two conditions are usually congenital. Thyroid myopathy is acquired, usually in adulthood, and is associated with other signs of Graves'

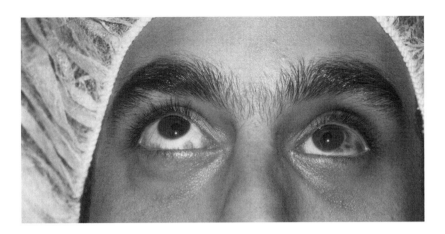

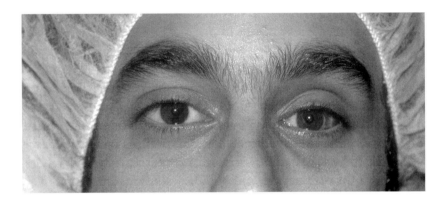

FIGURE 20.5 *This patient had a trapped inferior rectus muscle as a result of a blowout fracture. He is nearly orthotropic in primary gaze but has restricted upgaze of his left eye.*

disease and/or enlargement of the extraocular muscles. The important test to perform to distinguish these conditions is an orbital computed tomographic scan. A fracture would be noted in the case of orbital bone damage. Enlargement of the extraocular muscle or muscles occurs with thyroid myopathy.

Trauma in the absence of blowout fracture can cause a variety of ocular motor abnormalities (Baker and Epstein, 1991). The third, fourth, and sixth cranial nerves can be damaged with head trauma (Miller, 1977; Rush and Younge, 1981). The diagnosis and management of these cranial neuropathies are discussed in Chapters 14, 25, and 26. A combination of cranial neuropathies may occur with trauma that damages the supero-orbital fissure or cavernous sinus.

Miller (1985) has described this as the sphenocavernous syndrome. In this situation, a nearly total ophthalmoplegia (external and internal) may occur.

Internuclear ophthalmoplegia has been reported following trauma and may mimic lateral rectus entrapment (Turazzi and Bricolo, 1977; Doslak et al., 1980). An ipsilateral adduction deficit is associated with a contralateral abducting nystagmus. The patient may demonstrate exotropia in primary gaze. If the pontine paramedian reticular formation is involved, an ipsilateral gaze palsy affecting both eyes will occur (Klingele et al., 1980; Daroff and Troost, 1987). Forced duction testing in gaze palsies is normal. Most traumatic cases improve, unlike when vascular disease is implicated (Daroff and Hoyt, 1971).

Vertical gaze problems can also occur as a result of central nervous system trauma. Paralysis of downgaze and upgaze has been reported to occur as a result of presumed traumatic lesions in the dorsal midbrain of a child (Cogan, 1974). Baker and Epstein (1991) noted that upgaze paresis is usually associated with other signs of dorsal midbrain damage, and these should be sought very carefully during physical examination. These physical findings fall under the general category of Parinaud's syndrome. Physical findings include paralysis of upgaze (bilateral), eyelid retraction, a convergence type of nystagmus associated with upgaze, and pupillary abnormalities. Pupil findings consist of failure of the pupils to react to light but preserved pupillary reactions to accommodation.

Skew deviation also can occur in association with dorsal midbrain lesions. This deviation is usually concomitant and consists of a vertical misalignment of the eyes. Hypertropia exists and is caused by supranuclear disorder of input to the vertical ocular motor system. Traumatic skew deviation has been studied carefully by Keane (1975). In his review of 100 patients, he noted that in traumatic cases the lesion was usually in the pons. In skew deviation, the forced duction test is normal. Concomitancy as a physical finding is most helpful in distinguishing skew from entrapped extraocular muscles or fourth nerve palsy.

MANAGEMENT

The notion that blowout fractures spare the eye and adnexae from concurrent injury is wrong. Leibshon and associates (1976) have shown a very high incidence of concurrent eye injury. Their series demonstrated that the eye itself can suffer virtually any type of traumatic injury. Traumatic iridoplegia was most common. Optic nerve damage occurred in 28 of 119 injured orbits. We have seen many patients with associated hyphema or eye wall laceration (see also Walker et al., 1990). Injuries to orbital bones may accompany other serious systemic and neurologic injuries. Orbital roof fractures are commonly associated with neurologic damage (McLachlan et al., 1982). Motor vehicle accidents may be the most common cause of fractures of the orbital roof (Leibsohn et al., 1976).

Therefore, the initial management of the patient with a blowout fracture should consist of very careful physical, neurologic, and ocular examinations (Milauskas and Fueger, 1966). Patients should be evaluated for symptoms of injuries to other parts of their body. Mental status and neurologic examinations are critical. The eye examination should very carefully document associated ocular injuries.

Timing of Intervention

The incidence of diplopia following a blowout fracture is high. Leibsohn and colleagues (1976) noted an incidence of 36%, but Converse and associates (1967) and Helveston (1977) suggested that the incidence may be nearly 100% if diplopia is tested for in extremes of gaze.

However, when orbital fractures are repaired early (within the first week), the incidence of the diplopia does not appear to be altered. Emery and colleagues (1970) demonstrated that patients operated on within 1 week of injury suffered the same rate of diplopia as those operated on later. These authors also noted that a substantial number of patients have spontaneous resolution of diplopia within 2 weeks of injury. These studies were corroborated by Putterman and associates (1974), leading to the current clinical trend to recommend orbital repair for diplopia after waiting 2–4 weeks (Dulley and Fells, 1975; Wilkins and Havins, 1982).

On the other hand, large fractures or fractures associated with other facial or neurologic injuries should potentially be operated on earlier. Many surgeons prefer to allow edema and hemorrhage to resorb and to operate on large fractures after 1 week. Enophthalmos secondary to orbital fractures often cannot be adequately evaluated until the edematous phase has resolved.

Strabismus Management by Repairing Orbit Fractures

Is there any evidence that repair of the orbital fracture itself cures diplopia? Metz and colleagues (1974) attempted to identify patients at risk for permanent diplopia after blowout fracture. These investigators studied saccadic velocity in downward movement of the involved eye and compared it to upward movement of the same eye. Their study showed that if the speed of downward movement was no more than 30% less than the speed of upward movement, diplopia would resolve spontaneously. On the other hand, if downward movement was 51% slower, diplopia would persist. This study suggests that muscle fiber impairment and nerve damage to the muscle, rather than entrapment of the muscle in a bony defect, may often be responsible for diplopia. The fact that so many patients experience spontaneous resolution of diplopia also suggests that soft-tissue swelling and/or nerve damage to the muscle is often responsible for diplopia, rather than involvement of the muscle in a bony defect.

Nevertheless, there are patients in whom repair of an orbital fracture may be helpful in curing diplopia. The problem is identifying which patients should be managed for their orbital fracture and which should be managed purely for their strabismus. Metz and associates (1974) demonstrated that forced duction testing does not necessarily indicate an entrapped muscle. Soft-tissue swelling and hemorrhage can cause the forced duction test to be positive. A posterior fracture causing hypertropia of the affected eye may indicate entrapment of the inferior rectus muscle, well behind its arc of contact with the globe. In this situation, repair of the fracture may ameliorate the strabismus (Seiff, 1992). Otherwise, there simply are no adequate guidelines to determine whether a patient's diplopia will improve with repair of the fracture, or whether an operation on extraocular muscles will be required.

Nonsurgical Management of Strabismus in Blowout Fracture

Some patients with small amounts of relatively concomitant strabismus can be managed by the use of prisms. Because diplopia secondary to a blowout fracture is often inconcomitant, prisms may fail to provide satisfactory improvement of symptoms. As usual, a very careful refraction is advisable, since good sensory input is important for fusion.

Surgical Management of Strabismus

Entrapment of the Inferior Rectus with Hypotropia

Whether or not the patient has undergone repair of the blowout fracture, hypotropia of the involved eye with a positive forced duction test can be managed with recession of the involved inferior rectus muscle (Harley, 1975). The amount of recession that is necessary to manage the deviation is difficult to determine because a restricted muscle will behave differently than one that is not entrapped or restricted. Therefore, the use of adjustable sutures is advised.

Paresis of the Inferior Rectus Muscle

The management of paresis of the inferior rectus muscle depends on the strabismus status in primary gaze. If hypotropia of the involved eye accompanies a deficiency of depression of that eye, then a recession of the involved inferior rectus muscle is indicated. A rough rule would be a calculation of 2.5 prism diopters of shift per millimeter of recession of the muscle. Of course, the actual amount of effect may vary due to possible tightening of the muscle; therefore, adjustable sutures are advisable.

Recession of the inferior rectus muscle may still leave the patient hypertropic in downgaze. At least two options exist for managing this problem. First, a Faden suture applied to the contralateral (normal) inferior rectus muscle can be used (Saunders, 1984). The purpose of this suture is to prevent the eye from rotating inferiorly, without compromising its position in primary (neutral) gaze. In effect, this suture matches the defect in the involved eye, so the patient still has a reduced ability to look down. A second operation, designed to increase inferior binocular visual fields, is the inverse Knapp procedure (Lipton et al., 1990). Horizontal muscles are transposed inferiorly and sutured on either side of the inferior rectus muscle (Dunlap, 1971). This procedure improves inferior binocular visual fields and apparently has the unexpected effect of improving superior visual fields, as well (Lipton et al., 1990).

Hypertropia of the involved eye with downgaze deficiency can occur. This can be managed with a superior rectus recession of the involved eye with or without resection of the inferior rectus muscle of the involved eye. The primary position of the eye is improved but the eye still does not rotate down because the inferior rectus muscle is paralyzed (Lipton, 1990).

A recession of the superior rectus muscle can be large, up to 15 mm. This has the effect of producing a deficiency of elevation of the eye but does not usually pose any great deficit in *function*. The disadvantage to resecting the inferior rectus muscle is that it may draw the lower lid superiorly if great care is not taken to dissect the connections between the inferior rectus muscle and the lower lid retractors.

Surgery of the vertical rectus muscle probably should be accompanied by either a large recession of the contralateral inferior rectus muscle or a Faden suture in this muscle, or both, to try to match the downgaze deficit in the involved eye. A contralateral inferior rectus recession will affect the position of that eye in neutral position, so the surgeon should be careful to avoid overcorrection.

Medial Rectus Entrapment

Management of medial rectus entrapment usually begins with an attempt to repair the medial orbital wall and free the medial rectus muscle (Rumelt and Ernest, 1972). The strabismus problem is usually etiologically tied to entrapment of the medial rectus muscle. Therefore, its release from bony entrapment may be useful.

Strabismus surgery should also attempt to free the medial rectus muscle if it is trapped. This can be done by performing a conjunctival peritomy on the muscle (Mirsky and Saunders, 1979). Success in freeing the medial rectus muscle can be judged by changes in the forced duction test. If the medial rectus muscle is trapped, its freedom will result in improvement in the ability to passively abduct the eye.

Delayed Management of Ocular Motility Problems Associated with Orbital Fractures

Helveston (1977) discussed the problems associated with delayed management of ocular motility problems caused by orbital fractures. Scarring with adhesions, paresis of muscles, and hematoma can all hinder successful surgical ocular realignment. The surgeon, therefore, must employ surgical techniques such as traction sutures and muscle transposition procedures. For example, a patient with complete paralysis of an inferior rectus muscle will have hypertropia in all directions of downgaze. A recession of the superior rectus muscle and resection of the inferior rectus muscle may alleviate the problem but may not provide the patient with single vision in reading position. It may not be desirable to entirely cripple the contralateral inferior rectus muscle, thus preventing it from rotating down. Therefore, a vertical transposition procedure—moving the medial and lateral rectus muscle down to the inferior rectus muscle of the involved eye—may be helpful. Similarly, a strong silk traction suture can be used to place the eye on traction in downgaze for several days. This is painful for the patient and may be poorly tolerated, however.

REFERENCES

Al-Qurainy IA, Dutton GN, Moos KF et al. Orbital injury complicated by entrapment of the superior oblique tendon: a case report. Br J Oral Maxillofac Surg 1988;26:336–340.

Baker RS, Conklin JD Jr. Acquired Brown's syndrome from blunt orbital trauma. J Pediatr Ophthalmol Strabismus 1987;24:17–21.

Baker RS, Epstein AD. Ocular motor abnormalities from head trauma. Surv Ophthalmol 1991;35:245–267.

Baldwin L, Baker RS. Acquired Brown's syndrome in a patient with an orbital roof fracture. J Clin Neuro-Ophthalmol 1988;8:127–130.

Cogan D. Paralysis of down-gaze. Arch Ophthalmol 1974;92:192–199.

Cole HG, Smith B. Eye muscle imbalance complicating orbital floor fractures. Am J Ophthalmol 1963;55:930–935.

Converse JN, Smith B, Obear MF et al. Orbital blow-out fractures: a ten year survey. Plast Reconstr Surg 1967;39:20–36.

Daroff RB, Hoyt WF. Supranuclear Disorders of Ocular Control Systems in Man. In P Bach-y-Rita, CC Collins, JE Hyde (eds), Control of Eye Movements. New York: Academic Press, 1971;175–235.

Daroff RB, Troost BT. Supranuclear Disorders of Eye Movements. In TD Duane, EA Jager (eds), Clinical Ophthalmology. Vol. 2. New York; Harper & Row, 1987;10.

Doslak MJ, Kline LB, Dell-Osso LF, Daroff RB. Internuclear ophthalmoplegia: recovery and plasticity. Invest Ophthalmol Vis Sci 1980;19:1506–1511.

Duane TD, Schatz NJ, Caputo AR. Pseudo-Duane's retraction syndrome. Trans Am Ophthalmol Soc 1976;74:122–132.

Dulley B, Fells P. Long-term follow-up of orbital blow-out fractures with and without surgery. Mod Probl Ophthalmol 1975;14:467–470.

Dunlap EA. Vertical Displacement of Horizontal Rectus. In Symposium on Strabismus. Transactions of the New Orleans Academy of Ophthalmology. St. Louis: Mosby, 1971;307–329.

Edwards WC, Ridley RW. Blowout fracture of medial orbital wall. Am J Ophthalmol 1968;65:248–249.

Emery JM, von Noorden GK, Schlernitzauer DA. Orbital floor fractures: long-term follow-up of cases with and without surgical repair. Trans Am Acad Ophthalmol Otolaryngol 1971;75:802–812.

Fujino T, Sato TB. Mechanism of orbital blow-out fracture. Experimental study by three-dimensional eye model. Orbit 1987;6:237–246.

Gittinger JW, Hughes JP, Suran EL. Medial orbital wall blow-out fracture producing an acquired retraction syndrome. J Clin Neuro-Ophthalmol 1986;6:153–156.

Green RP, Peters DR, Shore JW et al. Force necessary to fracture the orbital floor. Ophthal Plast Reconstr Surg 1990;6:211–217.

Greenwald MJ, Lissner GS, Tomita T, Naidich TP. Isolated orbital roof fracture with traumatic encephalocele. J Ped Ophthalmol Strabismus 1987;24:141–144.

Harley RD. Surgical management of persistent diplopia in blowout fractures of the orbit. Ann Ophthalmol 1975;7:1621–1626.

Helveston EM. The relationship of extraocular muscle problems to orbital floor fractures: early and late management. Trans Am Acad Ophthalmol Otolaryngol 1977;83:660–662.

Jackson OB Jr, Nankin SJ, Scott WE. Traumatic simulated Brown's syndrome: a case report. J Pediatr Ophthalmol Strabismus 1979;16:160–162.

Keane JR. Ocular skew deviation. Analysis of 100 cases. Arch Neurol 1975;32:185–190.

Klingele TG, Schultz R, Murphy MG. Pontine gaze paresis due to traumatic craniocervical hyperextension. A report of two cases. J Neurosurg 1980;53:249–251.

Lang W. Traumatic enophthalmos with retention of perfect acuity of vision. Trans Ophthalmol Soc UK 1889;9:41–45.

Leibsohn J, Burton TC, Scott WE. Orbital floor fractures: a retrospective study. Ann Ophthalmol 1976;8:1057–1062.

Lipton JR, Page AB, Lee JP. Management of diplopia on down-gaze following orbital trauma. Eye 1990;4:535–537.

McClurg FL Jr, Swanson PJ. An orbital roof fracture causing diplopia. Arch Otolaryngol 1976;102:497–498.

McLachlan DL, Flanagan JC, Shannon GM. Complications of orbital roof fractures. Ophthalmology 1982;89:1274–1278.

Metz H, Scott WE, Madson E, Scott AB. Saccadic velocity and active force studies in blow-out fractures of the orbit. Am J Ophthalmol 1974;78:665–670.

Milauskas AT, Fueger GF. Serious ocular complications associated with blowout fractures of the orbit. Am J Ophthalmol 1966;62:670–672.

Miller GR, Glaser JS. The retraction syndrome and trauma. Arch Ophthalmol 1966;76:662–663.

Miller NR. Solitary oculomotor nerve palsy in childhood. Am J Ophthalmol 1977;83:106–111.

Miller NR. Walsh and Hoyt's Clinical Neuro-Ophthalmology (4th ed). Vol 2. Baltimore: Williams & Wilkins, 1985;454–456, 528–544, 672–674, 707–732.

Mirsky RG, Saunders RA. A case of isolated medial wall fracture with medial rectus entrapment following seemingly trivial trauma. J Ped Ophthalmol Strabismus 1979;16:287–290.

Ohtsuka H, Nakaoka H. Impaired upward gaze due to subperiosteal hemorrhage of the orbital roof. Ann Plast Surg 1987;18:547–549.

Putterman AM, Stevens T, Urist MJ. Nonsurgical management of blow-out fractures of the orbital floor. Am J Ophthalmol 1974;77:232–239.

Rumelt MB, Ernest JT. Isolated blowout fracture of the medial orbital wall with medial rectus muscle entrapment. Am J Ophthalmol 1972;73:451–453.

Rush JA, Younge BR. Paralysis of cranial nerves III, IV and VI: cause and prognosis in 1,000 cases. Arch Ophthalmol 1981;99:76–79.

Saunders RA. Incomitant vertical strabismus. Treatment with posterior fixation of the inferior rectus muscle. Arch Ophthalmol 1984;102:1174–1177.

Seiff SR. Hypertropia and the Posterior Blowout Fracture. Presented at the American Society of Ophthalmic Plastic and Reconstructive Surgery, Dallas, Texas, 1992.

Smith B, Regan WF. Blow-out fracture of the orbit. Mechanism and correction of internal orbital fracture. Am J Ophthalmol 1957;44:733–739.

Smith RR, Blount RL. Blowout fracture of the orbital roof with pulsating exophthalmos, blepharoptosis and superior gaze paresis. Am J Ophthalmol 1971;71:1052–1054.

Trobe JD. Cyclodeviation in acquired vertical strabismus. Arch Ophthalmol 1984;102:717–720.

Trokel SL, Potter GD. Radiographic diagnosis of fracture of the medial wall of the orbit. Am J Ophthalmol 1969;67:772–773.

Turazzi S, Bricolo A. Acute pontine syndromes following head injury. Lancet 1977;2:62–64.

Walker J, Davidorf FH, Kelly DR, Doyle WJ. Laceration of the globe due to a blow-out fracture. Arch Ophthalmol 1990;108:1522–1523.

Whyte DK. Blowout fractures of the orbit. Br J Ophthalmol 1968;52:721–728.

Wilkins RB, Havins WE. Current treatment of blow-out fractures. Ophthalmology 1982;89:464–466.

Zipf RG, Trokel SL. Simulated superior oblique tendon sheath syndrome following orbital floor fracture. Am J Ophthalmol 1973;75:700–705.

VI

Postoperative Strabismus

21

Strabismus After Cataract Surgery

ETIOLOGY

An understanding of the various causes of diplopia after cataract surgery allows a systematic approach to management (Hamed, 1991). "Binocular" diplopia may be caused by preexisting disorders of eye movements or refractive errors, by the effect of prolonged occlusion from the cataract predating the surgery, by surgical trauma to the rectus muscles and soft tissue during cataract surgery, and by optical problems related to aphakia, pseudophakia, or anisometropia after surgery (Hamed, 1991). Monocular diplopia is caused by monocular eye disease.

TRANSIENT DIPLOPIA AFTER CATARACT SURGERY

Occasionally, patients experience transient diplopia after cataract surgery. This is presumed to be secondary to prolongation of the effect of the local anesthetic agent (Burns and Seigel, 1988). Prolonged occlusion of an eye, as might occur with postoperative patching for persistent corneal epithelial defect, can cause a vertical tropia. This tropia should resolve swiftly once the patch is removed. Similarly, a preexisting phoria can be turned into a tropia with prolonged occlusion (e.g., dense cataract) in one eye. Up to 40% of patients with cataracts show heterotropia when examined preoperatively (Brent, 1986), and the risk for developing heterotropia increases as vision decreases.

OPTICAL CAUSES OF DIPLOPIA
AFTER CATARACT SURGERY

Cataract surgery can lead to monocular diplopia for many reasons. A corneal opacification (preexisting or the result of endothelial damage during surgery) can cause the perception of double images. The mechanism may involve a prismatic effect induced by corneal edema or light scatter from the opacity.

When an intraocular lens decenters, diplopia can occur. Tilting of the lens, as occurs when one haptic is fixated in the sulcus and one in the capsule, must be extreme to cause substantial astigmatism. The axis of astigmatism (plus axis) is the same as the imaginary line along which the lens tilts (Rubin, 1974). Decentration of the lens implant could position a lens edge in the visual axis and render the eye partially (optically) aphakic, possibly causing diplopia.

Problems with anisometropia or high amounts of astigmatism secondary to the surgical procedure can cause diplopia. An inadvertently poor choice of intraocular lens power can cause substantial anisometropia. This is most likely to occur with very small or very large eyes, because the lens implant calculation formulas are unreliable with less "normal" eyes. Diplopia may be binocular and is caused by anisokeinia. Problems with spectacles can cause monocular or binocular double vision. Dense lenses have a prismatic effect; anisometropia results from the need to place a different power "prism" in front of each eye. With well-centered and -framed lenses, primary gaze should be unaffected. However, inadvertent decentration of one lens induces a prismatic effect and is a potential cause of diplopia. Image jump can also pose a problem for patients wearing bifocals. The bifocal add has a prismatic effect. If corrective lenses differ (as in anisometropia), vertical strabismus can be caused by the bifocals.

Recent emphasis on astigmatism control in cataract surgery will undoubtedly reduce the incidence of monocular double vision. However, a radical change in the amount of astigmatism, even if toward a more normal direction (e.g., attempting to match astigmatism with the fellow eye), can pose problems insofar as patient adaptation. In patients with monocular defects, high amounts of astigmatism are usually well tolerated, but the presence of asymmetric and altered astigmatism poses a potential problem for patients and may lead to lengthy periods of adaptation (American Academy of Ophthalmology, 1988).

PREEXISTING EYE MOVEMENT ABNORMALITIES

Previously unsuspected abnormalities of eye movements may be revealed by cataract surgery, as may be the case for thyroid eye disease presenting after cataract surgery (Hamed and Lingua, 1990). Some patients demonstrate laboratory and ocular motility findings characteristic of Graves' myopathy, including enlarged extraocular muscles, following cataract surgery. Diplopia may have been masked by occlusion of vision caused by the cataract, or surgical trauma and manipulation of the eye could aggravate thyroid ophthalmopathy.

A previously undiagnosed superior oblique palsy can be discovered during cataract surgery (Hamed et al., 1987). Results of Park's three-step test are usually, but not always, diagnostic in this case (Kushner, 1989). At least two reasons exist for symptoms after, but not before, cataract surgery: either the patient did not experience double vision because one eye was occluded by the cataract, or a period of reduced vision in the eye postoperatively caused reduction in the vertical fusional amplitudes that had been used to control the vertical deviation in the first place.

INTRACTABLE DIPLOPIA AFTER CATARACT SURGERY: LOSS OF FUSIONAL ABILITY

Several investigators have demonstrated that some patients lose the ability to use their eyes together for sensory fusion after prolonged occlusion from a unilateral cataract (Kushner, 1986; Pratt-Johnson and Tillson, 1989). In the study by Pratt-Johnson and Tilson, patients ranged in age from 6 to 39 years. All had suffered unilateral traumatic cataracts of a prolonged interval (longer than 2½ years) between cataract formation and surgical correction. All patients showed a secondary strabismus after developing cataracts. The strabismus was assumed to be an indicator of the possibility of intractable diplopia after cataract surgery. In these authors' patients, correction of strabismus was of no value in treating the diplopia, which was experienced as a sort of oscillation of the second image.

We have seen this so-called central fusion disruption on occasion. However, the majority of patients who have strabismus in association with a long-standing dense cataract are able to fuse after cataract surgery or, if strabismus is also present, after cataract surgery and strabismus surgery.

INFERIOR RECTUS MUSCLE INJURY DURING CATARACT SURGERY

The inferior rectus muscle may be damaged, or its effect on eye movements altered, as a result of cataract surgery (Hamed and Mancuso, 1991; Kushner, 1988). The mechanism of alteration in function is debated. One hypothesis holds that anesthetic agents are myotoxic (Rainin and Carlson, 1985; Rao and Kawatra, 1988). Local anesthetic agents used in rats caused substantial muscle fiber degeneration. However, when the effect of bupivacaine on extraocular muscles was studied in cynomolgus monkeys, the muscles showed only mild structural changes (Porter et al., 1988).

A second theory is that Volkmann's ischemic contracture of the inferior rectus muscle is created by the administration of the anesthetic agent (Hamed, 1991). Volkmann's ischemic contracture is a fibrotic change in peripheral skeletal muscle caused by increased pressure within the muscles' fascial compartment (Volkmann, 1881; Mubarak and Carroll, 1979). Vascular compromise of the inferior rectus muscle could be the result of trauma to the ciliary artery or compression of the artery by a hematoma or bolus of anesthetic agent.

Subconjunctival injections can also cause fibrosis of rectus muscles (Kushner, 1988). An inflammatory reaction could cause progressive restriction and enlargement of the involved muscle. The motility examination would then be expected to show either a stable or progressive tropia.

STRABISMUS CAUSED BY ALTERATIONS IN THE SUPERIOR RECTUS MUSCLE

It is surprising that diplopia occurs so seldom when a superior rectus bridle suture is used for traction of the globe. Most surgeons pass the suture blindly underneath the superior rectus muscle, often catching some of the muscle and even some of the episclera beneath it. An adhesion can be created between the muscle and the globe, creating a Faden-like effect (Hamed et al., 1987); that is, the globe fails to rotate superiorly. Alternatively, the superior rectus muscle can be damaged during needle placement, resulting in deficient elevation of the operated eye and hypotropia that worsens in gaze toward the involved side (Catalano et al., 1987). Damage to the superior rectus muscle could also cause fibrotic changes, resulting in restriction of upward eye movement (Catalano et al., 1987). Motility findings would consist of hypertropia in primary gaze, worsening in gaze toward the involved side.

Superior rectus overaction could result from transient paralysis of the ipsilateral inferior rectus muscle (Grimmett and Lambert, 1992). Presumably, a short period of time during which the superior rectus muscle is unopposed allows it to strengthen. Motility findings consist of hypertropia in primary gaze that increases in upgaze and improves in downgaze.

CONTRALATERAL OPHTHALMOPLEGIA AFTER RETROBULBAR INJECTION

A retrobulbar injection can inadvertently penetrate the subarachnoid space around the optic nerve. An anesthetic agent can diffuse to the brain stem and other cranial nerves, resulting in an important constellation of findings: contralateral vision loss, drowsiness, slowing of vital signs, especially respirations, and contralateral as well as ipsilateral ophthalmoparesis (Friedberg and Kline, 1986; Ahn and Stanley, 1987).

DIAGNOSIS

It is worth reiterating that a careful and complete ophthalmology examination is crucial to the appropriate diagnosis of diplopia after cataract surgery. In our experience, the possibility of significant astigmatism or refractive error after cataract surgery is often overlooked. Many patients can be managed satisfactorily with refraction and appropriate optical correction.

Despite the wide variety of potential causes of diplopia after cataract surgery, a few physical findings occur with regularity. Damage to the inferior rectus muscle from subconjunctival injections may cause a small-angle hypotropia (Figure 21.1). The hypotropia worsens on abduction, and there may be some restriction of elevation. The forced duction test is helpful (and positive), since inferior rectus injury can mimic underaction of the superior rectus muscle, as occurs with the Faden effect from a bridle suture (Figure 21.2). Damage to, or contracture of, the superior rectus muscle causes an ipsilateral hypertropia that worsens on abduction (Figure 21.3).

The importance of diagnosing fusional disruption prior to cataract surgery cannot be overemphasized. An absence of fusion will lead to intractable diplopia after surgery. Although most patients with dense unilateral cataracts will have greatly reduced vision, limiting preoperative sensory tests, a corneal light reflex test can demonstrate the presence of strabismus. Many patients can then answer questions as to whether they see one light or two when a single light source is shined on the eyes. Then the surgeon should attempt to establish that the patient can use the eyes together by neutralizing the ocular deviation with prisms.

MANAGEMENT

Postoperative Optical Problems

Ideally, postoperative astigmatism is recognized within a few weeks of surgery and can be managed with suture adjustment. Astigmatism

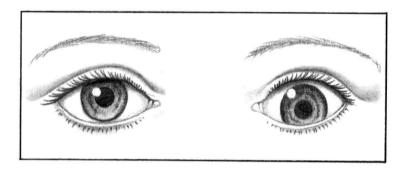

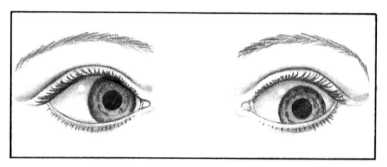

FIGURE 21.1 *With left inferior rectus muscle restriction, hypotropia in primary gaze worsens in left gaze. The forced head tilt test may not be helpful in diagnosing cases of restrictive disease (Kushner, 1989), but the forced duction test should be positive, rotating the eye up.*

with plus axis in the vertical meridian can be reduced by cutting one or more sutures. On the other hand, astigmatism at 180 degrees cannot be managed in this fashion. The surgeon must attempt to determine whether the astigmatism will be tolerated by the patient once it is neutralized with glasses. If the patient will have trouble tolerating the astigmatism, then readjustment of the cataract wound with additional tight sutures may be advisable.

At a certain point after surgery, manipulation of the wound becomes less effective in increasing or reducing astigmatism. At this point, usually 6–8 weeks postoperatively, a number of options are available to help the patient. First, a waiting period may be advisable. Many patients will be able to adjust and adapt to the astigmatism, given enough time. A contact lens can be used to manage astigmatism. The surgeon as well as the patient may feel defeated in this regard, since an intraocular lens has usually been placed inside the eye to avoid the necessity of using a contact lens. Lastly, corneal refractive surgery is also an option for controlling astigmatism.

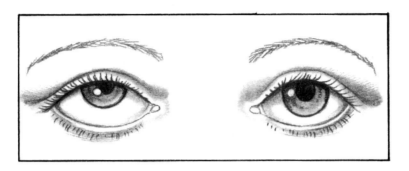

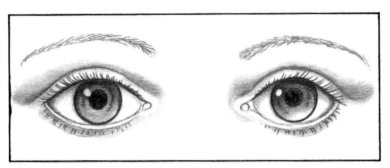

FIGURE 21.2 *When the cause of strabismus after cataract surgery is the Faden effect of bridle suture placement in the superior rectus muscle, the eyes are usually orthotopic in primary gaze. The involved eye fails to rotate up, causing hypotropia in upgaze.*

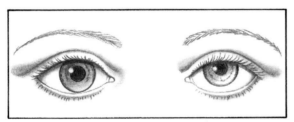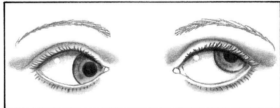

FIGURE 21.3 *With left superior rectus restriction, hypertropia in primary gaze worsens on abduction. The forced duction test should be positive, rotating the eye down.*

Problems arise with significant postoperative anisometropia. Bifocals may create problems for the patient when he or she attempts to look down through the segment. A prismatic effect is created by the bifocal, causing double vision in the reading position. This problem can be managed with the slab-off technique for grinding bifocals, or simply by providing the patient with a separate pair of reading glasses. When anisometropia causes double vision in primary gaze, and there is no demonstrable strabismus, the cause can be assumed to be anisokeinia.

One option for treating this problem is to provide the patient with monovision; that is, one eye is refracted for distance vision, the other for reading. Many, but not all, patients can tolerate spectacles designed thus.

The closer a lens is placed to the eye, the less it causes image size alteration. Therefore, a second option is to treat the patient with a contact lens to correct the refractive error in one or both eyes. If this also proves unsuccessful, then blurring the vision in one eye may be effective. Surgical options also exist, including intraocular lens exchanges to reduce or minimize the amount of anisometropia.

Disrupted Fusion

The most important aspect in the management of fusional disruption is its recognition. Ideally, the problem will be recognized before cataract surgery is undertaken. However, if fusional disruption is recognized after cataract surgery, it may be advisable to avoid strabismus surgery, since double images that are far apart are better tolerated than double images that are close together. Further management interventions can include blurring one eye or occluding one eye (e.g., with Scotch tape or opaque lens in glasses) to eliminate the diplopia.

Faden Effect from Bridle Suture

Three options exist for the management of a Faden effect created by the superior rectus bridle suture. First, the eyes should be left alone, or prism glasses should be used if a small deviation exists in primary gaze. A second option is to match the defect in the eye with the Faden effect, with a Faden suture in the superior rectus muscle of the fellow eye. Faden sutures are most effective when positioned posteriorly in the rectus muscle. If double vision occurs promptly on attempted elevation, the Faden effect in the eye with the cataract surgery is probably posteriorly located in the superior rectus muscle. The surgeon would therefore match this problem by placing a fixation suture more posteriorly in the superior rectus muscle of the fellow eye. A third option is to dissect the involved superior rectus muscle and remove its adhesion to the globe. This may prove effective in the short term, but the scarring response persists after surgery and could recreate the Faden effect.

Inferior Rectus Muscle Injury After Cataract Surgery

The best method for managing inferior rectus muscle injury is to avoid it. Subconjunctival antibiotics might best be given in quadrants rather than directly over a rectus muscle. Local anesthetic agents require administration in the region of the inferior rectus muscle, but an inferotemporal approach with the retrobulbar needle minimizes the chance of damaging this muscle.

For hypotropia in the eye with cataract surgery, prisms can be tried. If prisms fail, the inferior rectus muscle can be recessed. The usual guideline for the amount of shift in prism diopters per millimeter of recession do not hold as well after a muscle has been injured. Nevertheless, a rough guideline of 2.5 prism diopters of shift in primary gaze per millimeter of recession can be used.

Deviations of up to 15 prism diopters can be managed with an inferior rectus recession up to 5 mm (Burns and Seigel, 1988). Recessions of as little as 2 mm may be adequate for small amounts of deviation. For deviations greater than 15 prism diopters, an inferior rectus recession and ipsilateral superior rectus resection can be undertaken. This has the possible disadvantage of causing an overcorrection in downgaze (Pachtman, 1988). An ipsilateral inferior rectus recession and contralateral superior rectus recession may help to avoid this problem. We recommend the use of an adjustable suture. This provides the surgeon with the flexibility of changing the position of the muscle in an office procedure after surgery.

REFERENCES

Ahn JC, Stanley JA. Subarachnoid injection as a complication of retrobulbar anesthesia. Am J Ophthalmol 1987;103:225–230.

American Academy of Ophthalmology. Optics, Refraction and Contact Lenses. San Francisco: American Academy of Ophthalmology, 1988–1989; 120–128.

Brent P. Cataract patients. Preoperative assessment for fusion potential. Am Orthopt J 1986;36:135–138.

Burns CL, Seigel LA. Inferior rectus recession for vertical tropia after cataract surgery. Ophthalmology 1988;95:1120–1124.

Catalano RA, Nelson LB, Calhoun JH et al. Persistent strabismus presenting after cataract surgery. Ophthalmology 1987;94:491–494.

Friedberg HL, Kline OR Jr. Contralateral amaurosis after retrobulbar injection. Am J Ophthalmol 1986;101:688–690.

Grimmett MR, Lambert SR. Superior rectus muscle overaction after cataract extraction. Am J Ophthalmol 1992;114:72–80.

Hamed LM, Helveston EM, Ellis FD. Persistent binocular diplopia after cataract surgery. Am J Ophthalmol 1987;103:741–744.

Hamed LM, Lingua RW. Thyroid eye disease presenting after cataract surgery. J Pediatr Ophthalmol Strabismus 1990;27:10–15.

Hamed LM. Strabismus presenting after cataract surgery. Ophthalmology 1991;98:247–252.

Hamed LM, Mancuso A. Inferior rectus muscle contracture syndrome after retrobulbar anesthesia. Ophthalmology 1991;98:1506–1512.

Kushner BJ. Abnormal sensory findings secondary to monocular cataracts in children and strabismic adults. Am J Ophthalmol 1986;102:349–352.

Kushner BJ. Case report. Ocular muscle fibrosis following cataract extraction. Arch Ophthalmol 1988;106:18–19.

Kushner BJ. Errors in the three-step test in the diagnosis of vertical strabismus. Ophthalmology 1989;96:127–132.

Mubarak SJ, Carroll NC. Volkmann's contracture in children: aetiology and prevention. J Bone Joint Surg [Br] 1979;61:285–293.

Pachtman M. Personal communication. Cited in CL Burns, LA Seigel. Inferior rectus recession for vertical tropia after cataract surgery. Ophthalmology 1988;95:1120–1124.

Porter JD, Edney DP, McMahon EJ, Burns LA. Extraocular myotoxicity in the retrobulbar anesthetic bupivacaine hydrochloride. Invest Ophthalmol Vis Sci 1988;29:163–174.

Pratt-Johnson JA, Tillson G. Intractable diplopia after vision restoration in unilateral cataract. Am J Ophthalmol 1989;107:23–26.

Rainin EA, Carlson BM. Postoperative diplopia and ptosis: a clinical hypothesis based on the myotoxicity of local anesthetics. Arch Ophthalmol 1985;103:1337–1339.

Rao VA, Kawatra UK. Ocular myotoxic effects of local anesthetics. Can J Ophthalmol 1988;23:171–173.

Rubin M. Optics for Clinicians. Gainesville, FL: Triad Publishing, 1974;308–310.

Volkmann R. Die ischaemischen Muskellähmungen und-Kontrakturen. Centralb Chir 1881;8:801–803.

22

Strabismus After Retinal Detachment Surgery and Glaucoma Surgery

Diplopia after retinal detachment surgery occurs in more than 50% of cases. Most cases resolve within 6 months, leaving perhaps 10–20% of patients with some form of permanent diplopia requiring intervention (Sewell et al., 1974). In defining an appropriate treatment plan, it is important to understand the many causes of diplopia in the setting of retinal detachment surgery.

RISK FACTORS FOR STRABISMUS AFTER RETINAL DETACHMENT SURGERY

Diplopia following retinal detachment surgery is more likely to occur with the use of encircling elements than with radial exoplants (Kutschera and Antlanger, 1979). Pneumatic retinopexy, which does not involve the use of an exoplant, does not cause strabismus. On the other hand, many cases that could be treated with pneumatic retinopexy can also be treated by radial scleral buckle, which carries a low risk for postoperative strabismus (Smiddy et al., 1989). Preexisting heterophoria increases the risk of diplopia. Poor postoperative visual acuity and delay in recovery of vision are also risk factors for diplopia. Encircling elements and exoplants can create myopia and astigmatism, both of which may be responsible for diplopia or asthenopic symptoms (Sewell et al., 1974). Increased size of the exoplant may also make strabismus more likely (Table 22.1).

TABLE 22.1   Risk factors for strabismus following retinal detachment surgery

Encircling element
Preexisting heterophoria
Poor or slow return of vision postoperatively
Multiple operations
Large exoplant size
Change in refraction

Silicone Oil and Diplopia

Silicone oil used for complicated retinal detachment surgery induces a large amount of astigmatism in the axis of the meniscus of the oil. Astigmatism with an axis of plus cylinder at 90 degrees occurs when the patient is in the upright position. The axis shifts when the patient's head position changes. Fortunately, silicone is not a permanent intervention, and in many cases the patient's acuity is too poor for silicone-induced optical aberrations to be a problem.

Almost 33% of patients treated with silicone oil develop diplopia (Eckardt et al., 1990). However, except as noted previously, the oil itself probably does not cause diplopia. The use of silicone oil is a marker for other strabismus risk factors after retinal detachment surgery, because its use usually indicates multiple previous surgical procedures.

ETIOLOGY OF VERTICAL STRABISMUS

Vertical strabismus is more common than horizontal strabismus after retinal detachment surgery, for many reasons (Muñoz and Rosenbaum, 1987). Smaller vertical (vs. horizontal) fusional amplitudes undoubtedly contribute to this fact. Problems in the management of the superior oblique tendon in positioning the exoplant could also contribute. The tendon's entrapment causes torsional and vertical diplopia (see below). Violation of Tenon's capsule may be more likely to occur with surgery around the superior and inferior rectus muscles than around the horizontal muscles.

FAT ADHERENCE AFTER RETINAL DETACHMENT SURGERY

The fact that surgical manipulation of Tenon's capsule may be a factor in causing diplopia is suggested by the observation that transconjunctival cryotherapy (vs. bare sclera therapy), used to close retinal holes, does not cause strabismus. Adhesions may form after manipulation of Tenon's capsule. These adhesions and fat extrusion have a role in the development of strabismus after retinal detachment surgery (Wright, 1986). Fat adherence occurs at the muscle sleeve; that is, the anatomic point where the rectus muscle penetrates Tenon's capsule and is surrounded by orbital fat (Figure 22.1). This location is commonly traumatized by retinal surgeons who strip the muscle of fascial attachments with a cotton tip or blunt object.

REVERSE LEASH PHENOMENON

A type of reverse leash effect can result from retinal detachment surgery. Adhesions between bulbar fascia and reflected fascia can occur and lead to a positive forced duction in the field of gaze of the position of the leash (Jampolsky, 1978). For example, adhesions in the nasal region would cause a restriction of gaze nasally and a forced duction that becomes positive only after the eye has been rotated a considerable distance nasally.

EXOPLANT AS A CAUSE OF STRABISMUS

In some cases, the scleral exoplant itself may cause a type of restrictive strabismus. Research by Wright (1986) and by Price and Pederzolli (1982) suggests that this is seldom the case, and that fat adhesions and scarring usually account for strabismus that is restrictive in nature. Nevertheless, there are cases in which restriction will exist in the field of action of a muscle juxtaposed by a retinal sponge. In some of these cases, removal of the sponge cures the strabismus, a fact which at least circumstantially supports the role of the exoplant in causing the strabismus.

ETIOLOGY OF TORSIONAL DIPLOPIA AFTER RETINAL DETACHMENT SURGERY

Torsional diplopia related to surgical trauma to the superior oblique tendon is an uncommon cause of diplopia after retinal detachment surgery (Metz and Norris, 1987). Torsional changes in the position of the eye may occur more commonly, but the ability to tolerate as much as 5 degrees of torsion without symptoms prevents the patient from experiencing torsional diplopia. The mechanism of torsional diplopia could be related to movement of the superior oblique tendon anteriorly, particularly with a posteriorly displaced encircling element. In this case, hyperdeviation, esodeviation, and excyclotorsion have been

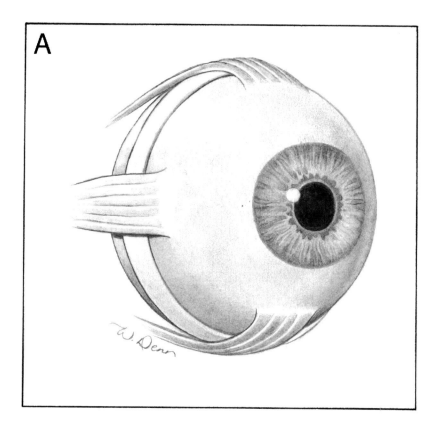

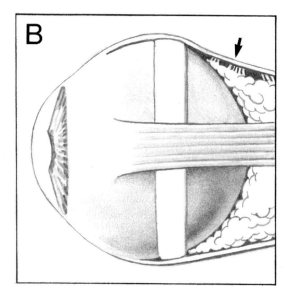

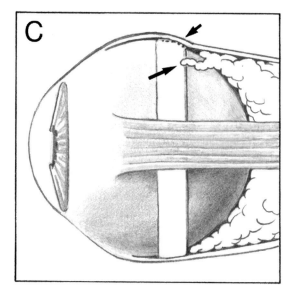

FIGURE 22.1   *A. Violation of extraconal fat can lead to the so-called fat adherence syndrome. Fat and scarring (B and C) (arrows) restrict eye movement away from the muscle involved and may pull the eye toward the scarring.*

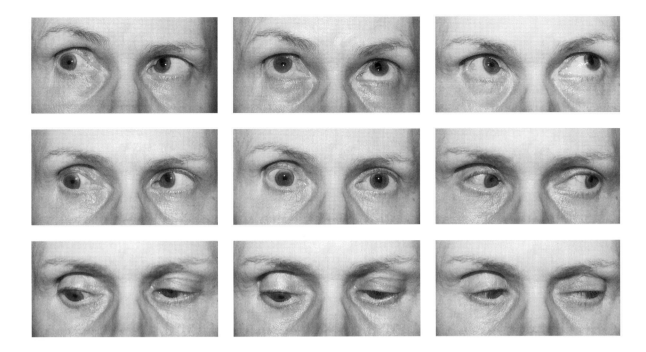

FIGURE 22.1   D. *Multiple operations for retinal detachment, left eye, resulted in a left hypertropia and fat adherence and scarring in this patient. Forced duction testing was positive, rotating the left eye down.*

noted. In another case, incyclotorsion was noted and was partially relieved by strabismus surgery (Metz and Norris, 1987).

If the superior oblique tendon inadvertently is elevated with the muscle hook, allowing the encircling band to pass underneath, the tendon could be anchored to the globe farther nasally, where the band might actually rest on top of the tendon (Price and Pederzolli, 1982). This could potentially prevent the tendon from passing through the trochlea, leading to Brown's syndrome.

THE ROLE OF PREEXISTING PHORIAS

Preexisting phorias undoubtedly can be aggravated by retinal detachment surgery. They represent another cause of diplopia in this setting (Kutschera and Antlanger, 1979). Decompensation of phorias occurs in the setting of decreased vision in one eye, a common finding in retinal detachment.

REFRACTIVE ERRORS INDUCED BY RETINAL DETACHMENT SURGERY

Placement of buckles and sponges around the globe causes a change in the refraction of the eye. A segmental sponge could cause plus astigmatism in the axis of the sponge, but segmental exoplants and encircling elements are equally likely to cause astigmatism (Smiddy et al., 1989). Induced astigmatism is likely to be transient (Fiore and Newton, 1970). Risk factors for alterations in refractive error are height of the buckle (Goel et al., 1983), anterior location of the buckle (Rubin, 1975), and medial rectus disinsertion. Irregular astigmatism can also occur in the setting of any type of scleral buckle (Burton, 1973).

An encircling band may cause elongation of the globe and relative myopia. In a prospective study on refractive changes after scleral buckling surgery, Smiddy and colleagues (1989) found that an average increased axial length of 0.99 mm correlated to 2.75 D of myopia. Any of these various refractive changes can cause monocular diplopia.

THE EXOPLANT AS POSTERIOR FIXATION SUTURE

In some cases, the exoplant or surgical adhesions may function like a posterior fixation suture (Muñoz and Rosenbaum, 1987). We have seen cases in which an encircling element eroded through the muscle and put pressure on the muscle, effectively altering the functional attachment of the muscle to the globe. Adhesions between muscle and globe could produce the same effect.

LOST MUSCLES IN SURGERY

Rectus muscles are occasionally detached from the globe, either deliberately or unintentionally. Loss of a muscle or the faulty repositioning of a muscle represents another cause of diplopia after retinal detachment surgery.

ECTOPIC MACULA

One of the most formidable causes of diplopia in the setting of retinal surgery is surgically induced displacement of the fovea. Retinal laser surgery will occasionally cause traction of the fovea, drawing it superiorly or inferiorly (Figure 22.2). Macular gliosis (epiretinal membrane formation), a complication of retinal detachment surgery, can also cause macular ectopia. The patient has preserved peripheral binocular fields with central diplopia.

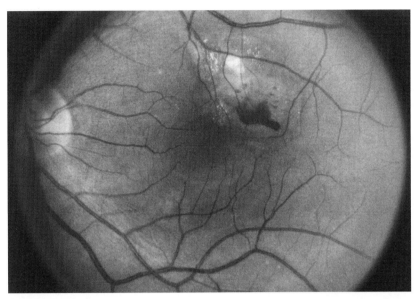

A

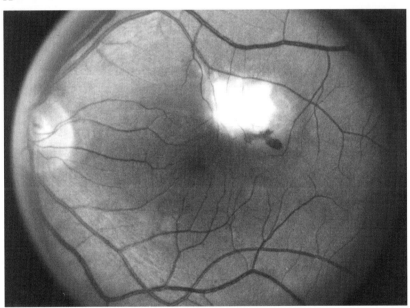

B

FIGURE 22.2   *An ectopic fovea can occur after laser treatment and cause diplopia. This patient had subretinal neovascularization due to histoplasmosis (A). Laser treatment was applied (B) and led to scarring and displacement of the fovea (C). Note the change in position of the fovea. (Courtesy of Howard Schatz, M.D.)*

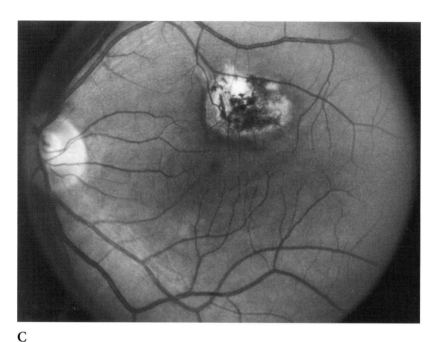

C

FIGURE 22.2 *(continued)*

Burian (1939, 1941) showed that peripheral retinal fields are more important for fusion than are central, macular fields. With macular ectopia, peripheral fields are preserved and continue to override central stimuli. The patient experiences central confusion—that is, he or she perceives objects at two different loci in space.

DIAGNOSIS

Seldom is there any difficulty in discerning a problem after retinal detachment surgery. Patients with diplopia will describe the problem in detail. The surgeon should remember, though, that patients with retinal detachment may be unhappy about low vision or morbidity, and may focus on the symptom, diplopia, for secondary gain. Strabismus could have predated retinal surgery. The evaluation should begin with a careful history, exploring preexisting symptoms such as diplopia, asthenopia, fatigue with prolonged reading, the use of preoperative prisms, and previous ophthalmologic examinations.

The diagnosis of fat adherence syndrome is suggested by restriction of ductions in the operated eye and by positive forced duction in the field of action of the restriction. For example, fat adherence around the inferior rectus muscle would cause restriction in upgaze. The diagnosis of adhesions would be supported by difficulty in passively elevating the eye with forceps. The diagnosis is ultimately confirmed if and when the patient is operated on, at which time the adhesions can be found. Once the adhesions are dissected, the positive forced duction should be eliminated. Regrettably, fat adherence syndrome often returns after surgery, for once Tenon's capsule is violated, a scarring mechanism is established that is difficult to control.

In diagnosing fat adherence syndrome, the surgeon should always consider the possibility that a preexisting condition is responsible for restrictive strabismus. One series showed that 40% of patients scheduled for retinal detachment surgery had not had a motility examination (Roth and Sypnicki, 1975). Preexisting trochlear nerve palsy and Graves' disease are examples of conditions that may be overlooked by the surgeon in his or her haste to deal with the retinal detachment.

MANAGEMENT

The best management for strabismus after retinal detachment surgery is prevention. Exposure of extraconal fat and disruption of Tenon's capsule during surgery for retinal detachment cause the majority of cases of restrictive strabismus in this setting.

A Waiting Period

Because most cases of strabismus following retinal detachment surgery resolve spontaneously, no surgical intervention is advised for 4–6 months. This recommendation is bolstered by the knowledge that early manipulation of the exoplant carries the risk of redetachment of the retina (Hilton and Wallyn, 1978). Phoria adaptation accounts for a large percentage of spontaneous cures. Retinal surgery causes a shift in ocular motor balance, which is then compensated by a shift in range of fusion.

Regrettably, a considerable number of patients with retinal detachment are left with subnormal vision, even following successful surgery. Up to 30% of patients adapt by learning to suppress vision from one eye (Arruga, 1973, 1977). However, the presence of low vision after retinal detachment, or even of preexisting amblyopia, does not preclude the development of strabismus and diplopia (von Noorden, 1985a).

Refraction

Management should begin with a careful refraction and comparison to refraction prior to treatment. Simply correcting a refractive error is useful, even with binocular diplopia. Cases of monocular diplopia will benefit from optical correction.

Prism Treatment

In cases of concomitant strabismus, prisms often will be useful. When the deviation in primary gaze is large, or there is incomitant strabismus, prisms are unlikely to be beneficial. Prisms should be used as a temporizing treatment while waiting for maturation of the retinal detachment surgery. Overall, prisms will provide successful treatment in approximately 40% of cases (Fison and Chignell, 1987).

After 4 months, the surgeon has the option of removing the retinal exoplant. Removal of the prosthesis is most likely to be of benefit when the prosthesis itself is responsible for strabismus. This would be most obvious in the case of a sectoral or radial exoplant and strabismus accentuated toward or directly away from the location of the exoplant. Our experience with removal of exoplants has been disappointing. Most cases of diplopia persist after exoplant removal, presumably because fat adherence syndrome is the etiology.

Botulinum Neurotoxin

Use of botulinum neurotoxin to manage strabismus after retinal detachment surgery has been evaluated by Scott (1990) and Petitto and Buckley (1991), who reported encouraging results. Restoration of fusion was possible in 60% and 85% of Scott's and Pettito and Buckley's cases, respectively. Success may depend, in part, on visual acuity and the number of previous retinal reattachment procedures (Lee et al., 1991). Nevertheless, treatment with botulinum toxin has potential advantages over surgery.

Botulinum neurotoxin injection is an office procedure. In skilled hands and with electromyographic control, the risk of ocular perforation is remote. There is no risk of anterior segment ischemia, as might occur with strabismus surgery in the setting of an exoplant, and the surgeon avoids the technical problems involved in operating in the area of previous retinal detachment surgery. The risk of redetachment of the retina is nill. The comfort level of the patient is considerably improved. Injections may have to be repeated. Inadvertent effects such as ptosis or worsening of diplopia can occur, but are transient.

Surgery

Progressive strabismus during the first 4 months after retinal detachment surgery indicates that the strabismus will not resolve spontaneously. The surgeon and patient then have the option of surgery to correct the deviation. If the exoplant is present, it need not be removed unless it contributes markedly to the strabismus.

Dissection of adhesions to relieve the restrictive components of strabismus involves meticulous identification of the muscle and removal of scar. The surgeon should avoid further disruption of the fat cone. Removal of adhesions is not adequate to cure the strabismus, since rectus muscles will have "taken up slack," showing an altered relationship to the globe. Thus, removal of adhesions usually needs to be complemented by rectus muscle surgery. For example, inferior adhesions causing a restriction in upgaze would be removed at surgery, and a recession of the inferior rectus muscle would be performed.

The amount of surgery to the adhesions should be guided by the results of intraoperative forced duction tests. Similarly, rectus muscle recession amounts are also guided by forced duction testing. Usual rules for the amount of recession per prism diopter of deviation are difficult to apply in cases of restrictive disease, but, in general, more effect is created per millimeter of recession than in nonrestrictive strabismus, in our experience.

A technique for adjustable sutures with retinal detachment surgery has been described by Mallette et al. (1988). The rectus muscle is identified, dissected, and sutured with a double-armed 5-0 or 6-0 Vicryl suture near its insertion. The muscle is then disinserted and "hung back," allowing the Vicryl sutures to pass over the exoplant. The sutures are attached to the globe anterior to the exoplant. Muñoz and Rosenbaum (1987) have noted success using adjustable sutures in 80% of operated cases. Their definition of success was single binocular vision in primary gaze, however. The surgeon's success will be modified by the preoperative degree of incomitancy of strabismus.

The uncertainty of how much surgery to perform in restrictive cases makes adjustable suturing a valuable technique. The surgeon biases the amount of surgery to permit pulling the suture at the time of adjustment. It is far more difficult to recess the muscle farther than to pull it forward with the adjustable technique.

Incomitancy

A Faden suture may be useful in the management of some incomitant cases of strabismus after retinal detachment surgery. The most important goal is to achieve single binocular vision in primary gaze and downgaze, if possible. To this effect, a Faden, or posterior fixation, suture can restrict eye movement in the field of gaze of the sutured muscle. Efforts to correct diplopia surgically in eccentric fields of gaze by other means, when the patient has single vision in primary gaze, should be avoided, lest the patient suffer diplopia in primary gaze.

Ectopic Fovea

The management of ectopic fovea is problematic. Prisms may be partially beneficial (Burgess et al., 1980). Occlusion of the central visual field with tape placed on the spectacles may also be useful. Occasionally, a patient will improve spontaneously. Surgery is probably of no benefit, since peripheral and central fusions are not synchronous.

STRABISMUS AFTER GLAUCOMA EXOPLANT SURGERY

Etiology

Exoplants for drainage of aqueous for glaucoma management are now used regularly in cases where conventional surgery has failed. A variety of strabismus problems has been reported, all of which can also occur with retinal detachment surgery.

The surface area of the exoplant establishes the amount of aqueous drainage and, therefore, the intraocular pressure. Unfortunately, the drainage plates assume an entire quadrant between the extraocular muscles. Two plates usually are required for adequate drainage.

Many surgeons prefer to place the drainage plates in the superior quadrant(s) of the eye. Brown's syndrome can occur if the plate(s) are positioned on the superior oblique tendon (Ball et al., 1992) (Figure 22.3).

FAT ADHERENCE SYNDROME AND RESTRICTIVE STRABISMUS

Similar to the situation with placement of retinal detachment exoplants, glaucoma exoplants can violate Tenon's capsule and create a restrictive strabismus. The sheer bulk of glaucoma exoplants probably restricts ductions (to some degree) in nearly all cases (Figure 22.4). Patients may remain asymptomatic if vision is poor or if diplopia occurs only in extremes of gaze. Vertical strabismus has been reported with superiorly positioned devices (Muñoz and Parrish, 1992) and with inferiorly located plates (Wilson-Holt et al., 1990).

Diagnosis

Diagnostic features are similar to those in retinal detachment surgery, with the possible exception that forced duction testing is often positive (abnormal) in all fields of gaze.

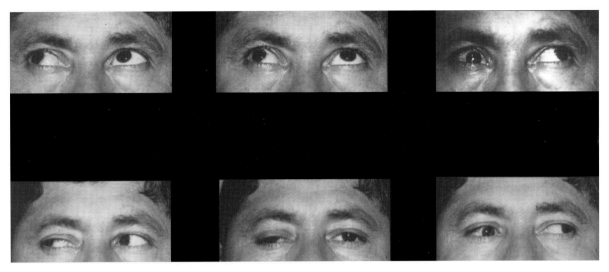

FIGURE 22.3 *This patient developed Brown's syndrome after placement of a Molteno valve exoplant in two superior quadrants. Note that he is not able to elevate his right eye in the adducted position.*

Management

Brown's syndrome can be managed by repositioning a superonasal plate. The plate can be moved to another quadrant (Ball et al., 1992), or, if this is not possible, an attempt can be made to weaken the superior oblique tendon.

Restriction caused by glaucoma exoplants is difficult to manage. Botulinum toxin may be useful, but the incomitancy of the strabismus may limit its effectiveness. Removal of the exoplant affects glaucoma control and may not affect the strabismus. Recession of rectus muscles to allow orthotropia in primary gaze may be helpful.

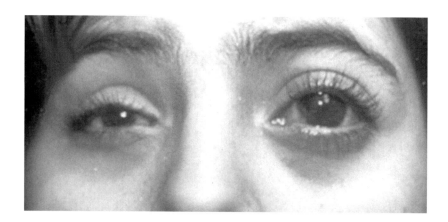

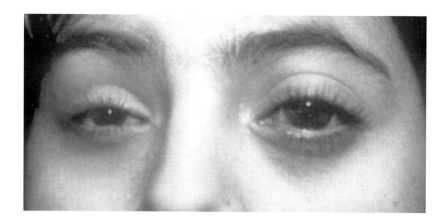

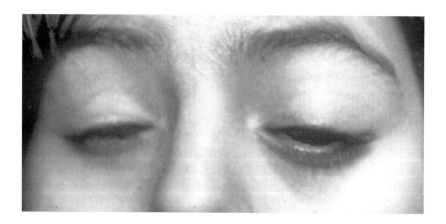

FIGURE 22.4   *This monocular patient was asymptomatic after Molteno valve surgery for left eye glaucoma, but note restriction of eye movement in all vertical fields of gaze.*

REFERENCES

Arruga A. Binocularity after retinal detachment surgery. Doc Ophthalmol 1973;34:41–45.

Arruga A. Motility disturbances induced by operations for retinal detachment. Mod Probl in Ophthalmol 1977;18:408–414.

Ball SF, Ellis GS Jr, Herrington RG, Liang K. Brown's superior oblique tendon syndrome after Baerveldt glaucoma implant [letter]. Arch Ophthalmol 1992;110:1368.

Burgess D, Roper-Hall G, Burde RM. Binocular diplopia associated with subretinal neovascular membranes. Arch Ophthalmol 1980;98:311–317.

Burian HM. Fusional movements: role of peripheral retinal stimuli. Arch Ophthalmol 1939;21:486–491.

Burian HM. Fusional movements in permanent strabismus: a study of the role of central and peripheral retinal regions in the act of binocular vision in squint. Arch Ophthalmol 1941;26:626–652.

Burton TC. Irregular astigmatism following episcleral buckling procedure with the use of silicone rubber sponges. Arch Ophthalmol 1973;90:447–448.

Eckardt C, Zwick A, de Decker W. Visual acuity and binocular vision following surgery of extreme retinal detachment. Fortschr Ophthalmol 1990;87:274–278.

Fiore JV Jr, Newton JC. Anterior segment changes following the scleral buckling procedure. Arch Ophthalmol 1970;84:284–287.

Fison PN, Chignell AH. Diplopia after retinal detachment surgery. Br J Ophthalmol 1987;71:521–525.

Goel R, Crewdson J, Chignell AH. Astigmatism following retinal detachment surgery. Br J Ophthalmol 1983;67:327–329.

Hilton GF, Wallyn RH. The removal of scleral buckles. Arch Ophthalmol 1978;96:2061–2063.

Jampolsky A. Surgical leashes and reverse leashes in strabismus surgical management. Transactions of the New Orleans Academy of Ophthalmology. St. Louis: Mosby, 1978;244–268.

Kutschera E, Antlanger H. Influence of retinal detachment surgery on eye motility and binocularity. Mod Probl Ophthalmol 1979;20:354–358.

Lee J, Page B, Lipton J. Treatment of strabismus after retinal detachment surgery with botulinum neurotoxin A. Eye 1991;5:451–455.

Mallette RA, Kwon JY, Guyton DL. A technique for repairing strabismus after scleral buckling surgery. Am J Ophthalmol 1988;906:364–365.

Metz HS, Norris A. Cyclotorsional diplopia following retinal detachment surgery. J Pediatr Ophthalmol Strabismus 1987;24:287–290.

Muñoz J, Rosenbaum AL. Long-term strabismus complications following retinal detachment surgery. J Pediatr Ophthalmol Strabismus 1987;24:309–314.

Muñoz M, Parrish R. Hypertropia after implantation of a Molteno drainage device [letter]. Am J Ophthalmol 1992;113:98–100.

Petitto VB, Buckley EG. Use of botulinum toxin in strabismus after retinal detachment surgery. Ophthalmology 1991;98:509–512.

Price RL, Pederzolli A. Strabismus following retinal detachment surgery. Am Orthop J 1982;32:9–17.

Roth AM, Sypnicki BA. Motility dysfunction following surgery for retinal detachment. Am Orthop J 1975;25:118–121.

Rubin ML. The induction of refractive errors by retinal detachment surgery. Trans Am Ophthalmol Soc 1975;73:452–490.

Scott AB. Botulinum treatment of strabismus following retinal detachment surgery. Arch Ophthalmol 1990;108:509–510.

Sewell JJ, Knobloch WH, Eifrig DE. Extraocular muscle imbalance after surgical treatment for retinal detachment. Am J Ophthalmol 1974;78:321–323.

Smiddy WE, Loupe D, Michels RG et al. Extraocular muscle imbalance after scleral buckling surgery. Ophthalmology 1989;96:1485–1490.

von Noorden GK. Amblyopia: a multidisciplinary approach. Proctor lecture. Invest Ophthalmol Vis Sci 1985a;26:1704–1716.

von Noorden GK. Idiopathic amblyopia. Am J Ophthalmol 1985b;100:214–217.

Wilson-Holt N, Franks W, Noureddin B et al. Hypertropia following inferiorly sited double plated Molteno tubes. Ophthalmology 1990;97(Suppl):143.

Wright KW. The fat adherence syndrome and strabismus after retina surgery. Ophthalmology 1986;93:411–415.

VII

Paralytic Strabismus

23

Sixth Nerve Palsy

J. Raymond Buncic

The sixth cranial nerve, with its long, tortuous course, is the ocular motor cranial nerve most commonly involved in paralytic strabismus. The resultant horizontal diplopia, compensatory face turn, secondary amblyopia in susceptible children, and psychosocial aspects of the esotropia pose challenges that can be solved in the majority of cases.

ANATOMY

The clinical picture resulting from interruptions of sixth cranial nerve function is governed by the pattern of adjacent anatomic structures as the nerve fibers pass from their origin in the nucleus of the sixth nerve in the pons to the lateral rectus muscle in the orbit, which the fibers eventually innervate. The sixth (abducens) nucleus is found in the more caudal part of the paramedian pontine tegmentum, just underneath the floor of the fourth ventricle. In the tightly packed neural structures of the pons, the sixth nerve nucleus and fascicle are in close proximity to cranial nerves V, VII, and VIII. Brain stem lesions in this area produce dysfunctions of these adjacent nerves.

The facial nerve fibers, as they loop intimately around the sixth nerve nucleus before leaving the brain stem at the cerebellar pontine angle, are easily damaged, along with the sixth nerve. The sixth nerve brain stem syndrome is the first of the "six syndromes of the sixth nerve" (VI[1]), as classified by Bajandas (1980).

After leaving the lower pons, approximately 1 cm lateral to the midline, the nerve rises along the pons, is crossed by the anteroinferior cerebellar artery, and then projects anteriorly to pierce the dura of the clivus. It passes beneath the petroclinoid ligament of Gruber and then enters the cavernous sinus. It is in this area (i.e., extra-axial) that elevated intracranial pressure of hydrocephalus, resulting in downward displacement of the brain stem, can result in stretching of the sixth nerve in this tethered position, producing paresis (elevated intracranial pressure syndrome, or VI[2]) (Bajandas, 1980). The close contact of the sixth cranial nerve with the tip of the petrus pyramid within Dorello's canal creates a susceptibility to inflammations in this area (i.e., Gradenigo's syndrome, or sixth nerve palsy with hearing loss) and pain following otitis media (VI[3]) (Bajandas, 1980).

The nerve emerges into the cavernous sinus from beneath the petroclinoid ligament, where it lies free and thereafter passes through the annular segment of the superior orbital fissure to eventually innervate the lateral rectus muscle. Within the cavernous sinus, lesions of the sixth nerve may also involve cranial nerves III, IV, and V, as well as the ocular sympathetic plexus (i.e., cavernous sinus syndrome [VI[4]]). In its most anterior position, the sixth nerve may be involved with other signs of orbital involvement (i.e., orbital syndrome [VI[5]]), or it may be an isolated sixth nerve paresis (VI[6]).

DIAGNOSIS

The resultant clinical picture of sixth nerve palsy is governed partially by the degree of loss of abduction ability, the amount of esotropia, and the ocular fixation pattern. In mild cases, the patient may complain of intermittent diplopia with only an esophoria that is incomitant, becoming exaggerated on side gaze and breaking down after prolonged alternate cover testing. The patient is able to fuse distance images as long as the image or deviation falls within the range of the patient's amplitude for fusion during distance fixation. In mild unilateral cases, binocularity may be maintained easily with a small head turn. As the esotropia becomes more marked, however, the compensatory face turn becomes too large to be maintained for practical purposes. When the better eye of an amblyope is paretic and used for fixation, the resultant esotropia is larger (secondary deviation) and the compensatory face turn is usually not evoked, since binocularity serves less as a stimulus. Typically, the esotropia measures greater during fixation than at near, and greater in the direction of the paretic muscle. In bilateral cases, however, the distance measurement may be fairly symmetric in all positions of gaze.

"Burying the white" indicates no visible sclera on the nasal side of the normal (fellow) eye when gaze is directed toward the paretic muscle.

It is not a reliable sign of the degree of paresis in mild cases of sixth cranial nerve paresis. Some healthy individuals with prominent globes never bury the white in full lateral position. Muscle paretic nystagmus in abduction, inadequate maintenance of the eye in the abducted position, and decreased saccadic velocities of abduction are useful observations in mild cases. In terms of prism therapy for diplopia and judgments made for surgery later on, esotropia measurement with the prism and cover test is still the ultimate measurement. The clinical course of paralytic strabismus can be followed by sequential prism measurement, Lee or Hess screen, and the plotting of binocular single visual fields using the Goldmann perimeter. Loss of abduction power can be graded clinically on a scale of 0 to –4, with 0 being full abduction and –4 representing total loss of abduction (i.e., the eye cannot move beyond a primary position). Esotropia can be documented photographically to capture all positions of gaze, including primary gaze for comparative reasons.

CAUSES OF SIXTH NERVE PALSY

In children, isolated sixth nerve palsies, most often unilateral without associated neurologic or other signs, will often resolve spontaneously (Glaser, 1990). Many are associated with a viral-like illness. In Knox and colleagues' experience (1967), children developed a transiently isolated abducens palsy 1 to 3 weeks after a nonspecific febrile or respiratory illness. The palsy recovered generally within 10 weeks; patients ranged in age from 18 months to the early teens. Similarly, transient sixth nerve palsies were seen following other specific viral illness such as varicella or following immunization. In the newborn, transient sixth nerve paresis weakness has been recorded with spontaneous resolution by 6 weeks. In the case of so-called benign sixth nerve palsies of childhood, there can be recurrences with spontaneous remissions, and with no other general neurologic implications.

Interestingly, in Robertson and associates' series (1970) of 122 children reported from the Mayo Clinic, approximately one half of "isolated" sixth nerve palsies were due to trauma and neoplasm in nearly equal distribution. It is noted, however, that in their series, papilledema was an additional finding in one third of the children with neoplasms, and nystagmus was found in one half of those at the initial examination. Moreover, other additional neurologic signs became apparent within several months. Similarly, in Harley's series (1985) of sixth nerve palsies as an overall group, trauma was responsible for one third and tumors for one fourth. In our in-patient population at The Hospital for Sick Children in Toronto, hydrocephalus was a significant cause of sixth nerve palsy, bilateral or unilateral.

TABLE 23.1   Differential diagnosis of abducens palsy

Graves' myopathy
Myasthenia gravis
Pseudotumor
Medial wall blowout fracture
Congenital fibrosis
Duane's syndrome
Convergence spasm
Essential infantile esotropia
Möbius' syndrome

In general, the causes of sixth nerve palsy in children tend to reflect the nature of pediatric diseases. As one considers the older age groups, ischemia and aneurysms have a larger role in the mechanism producing sixth nerve palsies. In the adult populations, microvascular causes (hypertension, diabetes) are more important (Glaser, 1990). Although trauma and neoplasm remain important causes, aneurysms do cause a significant number of sixth nerve pareses. Causes that are undetermined constitute approximately 20–25% of these studies. Multiple sclerosis is an uncommon cause.

DIFFERENTIAL DIAGNOSIS

In reaching a diagnosis of isolated sixth nerve palsy, other causes of abduction deficit must be considered (Glaser, 1990) (Table 23.1). Graves' orbitopathy with muscle involvement, specifically a tight medial rectus muscle, can be verified by a traction test and neuroimaging or ultrasonographic modalities to demonstrate the enlarged extraocular muscles.

Myasthenic involvement of the muscles is suggested by the presence of variable ptosis and variable strabismus. The diagnosis can be corroborated by a Tensilon test, if necessary. The amount of ptosis and diplopia can be quantified during the Tensilon test to determine its effect on the eye movement problem.

External evidence of inflammation involving the orbit, the globe itself, and the other extraocular muscles with signs of congestion and tenderness characterizes an inflammatory orbital process such as inflammatory pseudotumor.

A history of orbital trauma with resultant horizontal diplopia and abduction difficulty would suggest medial rectus entrapment, which can be verified with forced duction testing of the medial rectus muscle. Neuroimaging of the orbit may demonstrate physical entrapment of the medial rectus muscle in the adjacent orbital wall. In fibro-

TABLE 23.2 Features that distinguish Duane's syndrome from abducens palsy

Feature	Abducens Palsy	Duane's Syndrome
Angle of deviation in primary gaze	Usually >30 prism diopters	Usually <30 prism diopters
Lid fissure	No change on adduction	Narrows on adduction
Medial rectus function	Normal or overacts	May underact
Oblique function	Normal	May overact
A or V pattern	V pattern often	None usually

sis syndromes (e.g., medial rectus muscle), the degree of abduction loss in the affected eye is severe or complete. The forced duction test is positive. Sometimes the diagnosis can only be determined at the time of surgery, when a fibrotic extraocular muscle is found.

In Duane's syndrome (Table 23.2), there is usually no diplopia present. Patients maintain good binocular vision and stereopsis in the areas of binocular single vision. The narrowing of the palpebral fissure is an important sign in Duane's syndrome during attempted adduction, especially in bilateral cases. In unilateral or bilateral Duane's syndrome, the angle of esotropia is small (<30 prism diopters), compared to the dramatic loss of abduction present in both eyes. In addition, there is more often a history of recent discovery of the problem by an examiner or the patient rather than any other history to suggest sixth nerve palsy due to medical reasons. Corroborating the diagnosis of Duane's syndrome would be long-term follow-up during which the ocular findings would remain completely unchanged.

Spasm of convergence may occur in children who are neurologically impaired with cerebral palsy or other developmental disorders. These cases tend to be intermittent and quite variable during an examination, with full abduction sometimes demonstrated when the child performs oculocephalic maneuvers. Similarly, the convergence spasm intermittently seen as part of convergence retraction nystagmus in people with a dorsal midbrain syndrome secondary to midbrain involvement (e.g., pinealoma) can result in transient deficits of abduction in association with momentary diplopia (pseudoabducens palsy). These spasms are very short in duration. Here, again, abduction can be shown to be full with prolonged observation of the patient in extremes of gaze and also by vestibulo-ocular testing. In addition, the other stigmata of the dorsal midbrain syndrome, i.e., vertical gaze paresis of some degree and light near dissociation of the pupils, will be apparent. The longer lasting (i.e., seconds to minutes) convergence of spasm seen in cases of malingering, and sometimes following head trauma, is associated with variable and intermittent miosis during the spasm phase and can be shown to have full abduction during the ocular cephalic maneuver. This sign is usually present without neurologic signs, while simple testing of versions with both eyes open will usually not result in demonstration of full amplitude of eye movements. Monocular testing using the oculocephalic maneuver, however, will usually demonstrate full abduction ability. Repetitive testing may be necessary.

Congenital esotropia may mimic bilateral sixth nerve palsies, especially in children with neurologic disease. The presence of dissociated vertical deviation, latent nystagmus, or overaction of the inferior oblique muscles would support the infantile type of esotropia rather than sixth nerve paresis. I find the most useful method for demonstrating abduction in such cases is to turn the child's head quickly back and forth with one eye covered. Rotation of the infant will also often demonstrate the presence of abducting saccades in the lateral rectus muscle in question, but demonstration of full amplitudes of movement of the lateral rectus is most helpful.

One must always be alert to the possibility of a patient with known childhood esotropia developing an increasing degree of strabismus. An increasing or new face turn with or without diplopia may represent the additional problem of sixth nerve paresis. Once alerted to this possibility, the clinical identifications of increased abduction difficulty, decreased saccadic ability of abduction, and greater measurements for distance fixation will point to a sixth nerve paresis that is new.

Confusion of sixth nerve palsies with Möbius' syndrome is only a problem in the most mild of Möbius cases. In a classic case of Möbius' syndrome, there exists a facial diplegia of variable degree, with paralysis of lateral gaze (and often an esotropia). This is present from birth and is nonprogressive. There is usually no complaint of diplopia. The children often substitute convergence movements to allow them to cross-fixate in their strategy to fixate to the side. In addition, the clinician will find signs of congenital abnormality, including tongue hemiatrophy, deformities of the head and extremities, as well as difficulty with hearing, speech, and swallowing. Vertical gaze and the convergence mechanism are most often preserved. (See Chapter 7 on Möbius' syndrome.)

MANAGEMENT

The neurogenic nature of paralytic esotropia should be established. That is, when possible, other myopathic or local problems should be ruled out with a forced duction test and an intravenous Tensilon test, if appropriate. If the child has acute sixth nerve palsy and no other abnormal neurologic findings, the child should be followed for several months. If the situation does not improve by 2 months, neuroimaging of the head and orbits should be done.

The possibility of microvascular disease (diabetes mellitus, hypertension, cranial arteritis) should be considered in adults. With no other neuroabnormalities, observing the patient without scanning is appropriate. If the sixth nerve palsy persists (>6 weeks) a scan is indicated.

In cases of painful ophthalmoplegia secondary to inflammatory pseudotumor of the orbit, a trial course of oral corticosteroids should result in a dramatic relief of pain and symptoms, although, because of the possibility of neoplasm, these cases should be followed on a regular basis and restudied, as necessary.

Whenever an isolated sixth nerve palsy lingers without improvement for 6 weeks, neuroimaging investigation should be pursued, often with the help of a neurologist.

Ophthalmologic Management

In all cases, it is important to advise the patient or parent of the nature of the paralytic esotropia and its visual consequences and outline realistically the long-term goals of treatment and the nature of both conservative and more invasive treatments (e.g., botulinum injection, surgery).

In both unilateral and bilateral acute sixth nerve palsies or pareses, the aim of treatment is to alleviate symptoms of diplopia and problematic anomalous head position or face turn; maintain binocular single vision in some useful field of gaze, if possible; and prevent amblyopia in susceptible children. If the horizontal face turn is small and allows binocular or single vision in a reasonable area of gaze, the patient may be advised simply to maintain a small face turn to avoid diplopia. If the face turn is marked, and in cases of incapacitating diplopia, mechanical occlusion of one eye will offer the most complete removal of symptoms.

The patient with paralytic esotropia due to sixth nerve paresis or palsy, either bilateral or unilateral, should be assessed in standard procedure at the first examination and in follow-up examinations thereafter. This would involve the assessment of visual acuity, measurement of the esotropia in primary position and in all positions of gaze at near and at distance, and assessment of the degree of lateral rectus dysfunction. For instance, grading of ductions could be estimated on a scale of 0 (normal) to –4 (complete palsy), with –5 indicating an inability of the affected eye to even reach the midline from adducted position, presumably due to medial rectus contracture (Figure 23.1). From a diag-

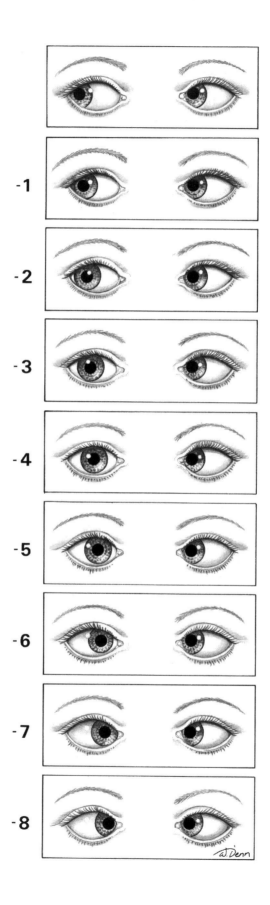

nostic point of view, and also for evaluation of the degree of secondary medial rectus contracture, the forced duction test is useful and can more readily be done on adults and cooperative teenagers than on children under 10 years of age.

The field of binocular single vision can be assessed by either the method of Fitzsimmons and White (1990) or that of Woodruff and colleagues (1987) using the binocular Goldmann visual field perimeter. More simply, the monocular single visual field might be assessed using the Worth four-dot test apparatus in distance fixation, and, beginning in any binocular visual field for distance, by moving the patient's head to one side or the other until fusional responses break down. The degree of movement of the patient's head to the right and left, during which a fusional response is maintained, will give an approximation of the binocular single visual field and can be noted on the patient's chart, but is certainly less standard than the perimetry method. A Lee screen or Hess screen can similarly be used to assess and follow abduction deficits.

The compensatory face turn can be estimated clinically, although this may be variable, and in my opinion is a less useful parameter than prismatic measurement of the paralytic esotropia present in primary fixation.

Any invasive procedures such as botulinum injection should be avoided until the neurologic evaluation is complete. The paralytic esotropia may be observed over time to assess its progress. Once stability and diagnosis have been achieved, then botulinum injection may be considered.

Occlusion

Theoretically, alternate occlusion of the eyes should help prevent secondary contracture of the medial rectus muscle in the paretic eye(s). Occlusion of the good eye, with fixation with the paretic eye, can sometimes lead to a sense of disorientation or vertigo in certain patients, and patching regimens should be tailored to each patient's needs and rate of acceptance. Some patients are content to simply fixate in an alternating fashion or monocularly, tending to ignore the diplopic image.

In children susceptible to the ambliogenic effect of occlusion and/or esotropia, occlusion *should* be alternated on the eyes to maintain the freely alternating mode of visual fixation or visual acuity in

◀ **FIGURE 23.1** *Eye movement deficits can be graded between 0 (normal) and –8 (eye is fixed in extreme adduction). A grade of –4 indicates that the eye moves to the midline, but no farther. This patient is gazing to the right.*

each eye. For instance, one might patch a 2-year-old child's eyes half the day (one-half day patching per eye) or alternate a full day on each eye if no amblyopia is present. If one eye is preferred for fixation with presumed amblyopia, however, one might patch the preferred eye 75% of the time and the nonpreferred eye 25% of the time, and modify this regimen according to the response of the child.

Prisms

The use of Fresnel press-on prisms may allow binocular single vision in the primary and downgaze positions, which are ultimately the most essential positions of visual use. The advantages of press-on prisms are their light weight and easy changeability as paralytic esotropia improves. Some patients, however, find unacceptable the slight decrease in acuity caused by the prism and the incomplete symptomatic relief with changes of gaze.

Botulinum Injection

Botulinum injection of the medial rectus muscle early in acute sixth nerve palsy can be used to prevent contracture of the ipsilateral medial rectus muscle during convalescence of the sixth nerve palsy. It is hoped that this would improve alignment of the eyes and also improve the secondary anomalous head position in some patients. The findings of Lee (1992), however, suggest that acute use of botulinum toxin on the medial rectus muscle does not appear to influence rate of recovery of the abduction paralysis. In those patients who seem to be improving only a little, but eventually will be unsuitable for surgical therapy because of systemic disease, repetitive injections of botulinum into the medial rectus muscle may similarly improve their diplopia or make it more amenable to prismatic treatment and improve head position.

Lee (1992) has reported a cure with botulinum toxin injected into the medial rectus muscle alone in 20 patients with chronic sixth nerve palsy, who showed no signs of spontaneous improvement at the time of injection. He attributed this cure to the relief of a reversible contracture and lengthening of the medial rectus muscle. Furthermore, Lee (1992) suggested a diagnostic use of botulinum injection into the medial rectus muscle in chronic sixth nerve palsy to alleviate medial rectus contracture, and thus allow more accurate determination of the ability of the eye to abduct in order to distinguish partial from complete palsies. The determinations would then also allow more appropriate amounts of horizontal rectus surgery to be performed eventually. A second diagnostic use would be in patients whose diplopia might be due to central disruption of fusion in cases of major head trauma or severe strokes, to produce temporary realignment of the eyes in prognostication for the possibility of binocular single vision in the future, if healing proceeds favorably.

Chronic Sixth Nerve Palsy Management

Patients with sixth nerve palsy should be observed on a regular basis to assess their evolution, resolution, or at least stabilization. In cases in which the etiology is unclear, one must continue to be vigilant about the possibility of progression of systemic disease such as brain tumor, despite the presence of negative neuroimaging studies in the past. Hence, if the strabismus increases or if other cranial nerve involvements or other neurologic symptoms and signs appear, the patient should be re-evaluated neurologically and symptomatic treatment of the diplopia and paralytic strabismus should be continued. Botulinum should be avoided in cases that are unclear from a diagnostic point of view or in cases in which there appears to be a progression of neurologic problems to suggest a changing diagnosis. Such an assessment should be made in consultation with a neurologist or neurosurgeon, so that there is a clear understanding as to which treatments are being used from an ophthalmic point of view. Despite the progression of certain neurologic diseases such as multiple sclerosis or brain tumor, it may still be necessary to use botulinum injection into the medial rectus muscle on a maintenance and palliative basis to treat the patient's symptoms.

In other well-defined cases of sixth nerve palsy, in which the degree of weakness of abduction has stabilized, one can contemplate further surgical intervention after a waiting period of approximately 6 months. The ultimate goal of extraocular surgery is to eliminate the strabismus, improve abduction, and enhance the binocular single visual field as much as possible, especially in primary position and in downgaze.

Partial Sixth Nerve Palsy Management

The partial nature of the sixth nerve weakness is seen clinically as some residual ability of the eye to abduct. The final result of surgical intervention in this type of case is generally satisfactory. Rosenbaum (1989) believes that saccadic velocity measurements and forced generation testing are necessary to determine the presence of clinically significant residual lateral rectus muscle function. In such a case, saccadic velocity measurement would be much greater than 175 degrees per second and the forced generation test would be present but reduced.

Lee (1992) suggested the use of botulinum paresis of the medial rectus muscle to fully assess the abducting ability of one or both eyes, and hence more appropriately assess whether two, three, or four horizontal recti muscles should be operated on to achieve surgical correction. A traction test at the time of surgery will corroborate the presence of any medial rectus contracture. Depending on the degree of strabismus and whether the case is bilateral or unilateral, the surgeon can then proceed with a recession of the contractured medial rectus muscle on an adjustable suture and resection of the paretic lateral rectus muscle. In bilateral cases, the fellow eye can also be treated similarly with the medial rectus muscle being recessed and the lateral rectus resected. Again, an adjustable suture can be placed on the second medial rectus muscle as well. In all cases, it is advisable to warn the patient with regard to residual diplopia postsurgically. Following a waiting period of approximately 4 months, or longer, reoperation may be planned to enhance the effect of the previous surgery.

Complete Abducens Palsy Management

If the sixth nerve palsy is judged to be complete, with no abduction whatsoever, saccadic velocity measurements less than 100 degrees per second, and no forced generation ability, then one should consider some type of transpositional procedure to enhance abduction, instead of a lateral rectus resection. Resection of the paretic lateral rectus muscle complex may produce a transient mechanical effect, but ultimately fails to enhance surgical correction of the problem. A transposition procedure may be necessary in complete palsies. The surgical results are less satisfactory in these more severe cases of sixth nerve weakness.

A variety of transposition procedures to improve abduction while at the same time maintaining an adequate blood supply to the anterior segment to prevent ischemic complication has been described (Helveston, 1971). In most cases the procedure is accompanied by simultaneous recession of the antagonist medial rectus muscle. Transposition alone without medial rectus weakening procedures results in further limitation of ocular movement and retraction of the globe on attempted abduction.

In the Jensen procedure, the superior, inferior, and lateral recti are split and adjacent halves of the vertical and lateral rectus muscle strips are joined with a nonabsorbable suture. A medial rectus recession is performed simultaneously. The Jensen procedure was popularized as a means of avoiding the complication of anterior segment ischemia, since the vertical rectus muscle insertions are not disturbed. The Hummelsheim procedure, whereby only half the vertical recti are transposed, also spares the circulation (Figure 23.2).

Full tendon transposition includes disinsertion of both the superior and inferior recti muscles, with replacement of these muscles above and below the lateral rectus muscle (Figure 23.3). Both transposition procedures can produce postoperative vertical deviations that may require secondary procedures. The medial rectus recession can be placed on an adjustable suture in older and more cooperative children. The use of an adjustable suture on the medial rectus muscle can help overcome the overcorrection sometimes

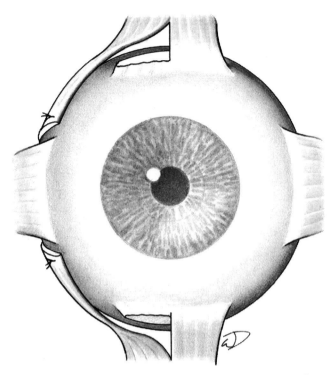

FIGURE 23.2   *In the Hummelsheim procedure, the superior and inferior rectus muscles are split. The lateral half of these muscles is joined to the superior or inferior half of the lateral rectus muscle.*

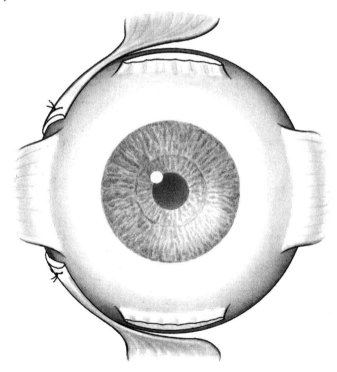

FIGURE 23.3   *In full tendon transposition, the entire muscle is transferred temporally above (superior rectus) and below (inferior rectus) the lateral rectus muscle.*

achieved with a muscle transposition. Reoperation on the transposition of Jensen is more difficult compared to that following a full muscle transposition procedure.

To eliminate or greatly reduce the chance of anterior segment ischemia when surgery is performed on more than two rectus muscles, some investigators have advocated the use of botulinum toxin to weaken the contracted medial rectus muscle before, during, or after transposition surgery to the vertical rectus muscles (Fitzsimmons et al., 1988). Because of the possibility that botulinum might induce a vertical deviation, Rosenbaum and colleagues (1989) prefer to inject botulinum postoperatively (following transposition surgery), to identify any vertical component induced by transposition surgery itself. If a vertical deviation is present secondary to the transposition maneuver, then the vertical deviation correction and the medial rectus muscle recession on an adjustable suture can be undertaken as a second procedure.

One must also keep in mind, in reaching a surgical strategy, that vertical deviations in cases of traumatic sixth nerve palsies may be due to an accompanying fourth nerve palsy (or skew deviation). Treatment plans may need to take this into consideration.

Combining Surgery with Botulinum Neurotoxin

In Lee's series (1992), the typical course in 8 of 51 patients who had ipsilateral medial rectus toxin injection 2–20 days preoperatively and who then underwent a full tendon transfer of the vertical rectus muscles (except for 1 patient who had a Jensen procedure) was one of an initial moderate reduction of the paralytic esotropia after botulinum and a transient overcorrection after transposition surgery, followed by an esotropic drift as the effect of the toxin dissipated.

Lee's results have made possible some useful observations regarding prognosis and outcome of the treatment of severe sixth nerve palsies. In patients with a unilateral complete sixth nerve palsy undergoing combined treatment with botulinum toxin injection in the medial rectus muscle and transposition procedures, he found that 33% require additional surgery for esotropia and that 84% achieve a centrally placed field of binocular single vision. In bilateral palsies with partial unilateral recovery, similar treatment will give a satisfactory result in 40% of patients, but 60% will require further surgery. In addition, 60% will also achieve a useful field of binocular single vision. He found that in bilateral palsies, 83% of patients will require further surgery for the esotropia—2.8 reoperations for the average patient. In this group, even fewer patients (50%) will achieve a field of binocular single vision.

Abducens Plus Other Cranial Neuropathy Management

Complex combined palsies of sixth nerve plus third and/or fourth nerve pose additional difficulties, but the principles of conservative treatment for diplopia are unchanged. Prisms are less often useful because of the multiplanar nature of the diplopia, although prisms may be more successful following strabismus surgery. Horizontal deviations should be corrected first. This will allow better assessment of the vertical component, which can then be attacked with another procedure aimed at both vertical and further horizontal correction.

In summary, noninvasive treatments are aimed at relieving symptoms secondary to paralytic esotropia in unilateral or bilateral cases. Once the diagnosis and etiology have been established and fully investigated and the deviations stabilized, surgical intervention is advised in most cases for significant residual esotropia. Botulinum toxin can be used early on to alleviate diplopia and for diagnostic reasons and as palliative care in selected cases. Partial sixth nerve palsies, unilateral or bilateral, can be treated by weakening the medial rectus muscle and resecting the lateral rectus muscle. Adjustable sutures in the medial rectus muscle are suggested whenever possible. In some cases, botulinum toxin injection of the medial rectus muscle alone can relieve contracture and achieve normal binocularity without any further treatment. In total unrecovered palsies, a transposition procedure is necessary, combined with medial rectus weakening or chemodenervation. Treatment with prisms postoperatively may be necessary, as well as reoperation to eliminate any residual horizontal or vertical deviation.

REFERENCES

Bajandas FJ. Neuro-Ophthalmology Board Review Manual. Thorofare, NJ: Charles B. Slack, 1980;71.

Fitzsimmons R, Lee JP, Elston J. Treatment of sixth nerve palsy in adults with combined botulinum toxin chemodenervation and surgery. Ophthalmology 1988;95:1535–1542.

Fitzsimmons R, White JS. Functional scoring of the field of binocular vision. Ophthalmology 1990;97:33–35.

Glaser J (ed). Neuro-Ophthalmology (2nd ed). Philadelphia: Lippincott, 1990;361–418.

Harley RD. Paralytic strabismus in children. Ophthalmology 1985;86:24.

Helveston EM. Muscle transposition procedures. Surv Ophthalmol 1971;16:92–97.

Knox DL, Clark DB, Schuster FF. Benign sixth nerve palsies in children. Pediatrics 1967;40:560.

Lee J. Modern management of sixth nerve palsy. Aust N Z J Ophthalmol 1992;20:41–46.

Robertson DM, Hines JD, Rucker CW. Acquired sixth nerve paresis in children. Arch Ophthalmol 1970;83:574.

Rosenbaum AL, Kushner BJ, Kirschner D. Vertical rectus muscle transposition and botulinum (Oculinum) to medial rectus for abducens palsy. Arch Ophthalmol 1989;107:820–823.

Woodruff G, O'Reilly C, Kraft SP. Functional scoring of the field of binocular vision in patients with diplopia. Ophthalmology 1987;94:1554–1561.

24

Third Nerve Palsy

J. Raymond Buncic

DIAGNOSIS

Of the three ocular motor nerve palsies, the clinical management of the third cranial nerve palsy remains the most difficult, incomplete, and least satisfying. In complete oculomotor palsy, the characteristic strabismus is a large exotropia due to unopposed action of the abducting lateral rectus (sixth cranial nerve), a small hypotropia due to the unopposed depressor action of the superior oblique muscle (fourth cranial nerve), and intorsion, again due to the unopposed action of the superior oblique muscle. Accommodation and pupillary function may or may not be involved. If the lid is at all open, the resultant diplopia is multiplanar and, thus, difficult to resolve with an anomalous head position or with simple prisms of any type. Similarly, with four of the six extraocular muscles paralyzed in a total palsy, the number of possible surgical solutions is limited.

ETIOLOGY

In the clinical assessment, investigation, and follow-up of these cases, knowledge of the neuroanatomy and function of the third cranial nerve will help to localize the lesion (Glaser, 1990; Bajandas, 1980). From the third nerve's nuclear complex located in the midbrain beneath the aqueductal gray matter and the superior colliculus, the fascicular fibers pass through the red nucleus and leave the midbrain ventrally on the medial aspect. In the interpeduncular space, the paired third nerves travel beneath the origin of the posterior cerebral artery in a position lateral to the posterior communicating artery, where aneurysms can easily impinge on the third nerve. The nerve bears a close relationship to the free edge of the tentorium as it passes forward to pierce the dura and enter into the cavernous sinus, eventually dividing into the superior and inferior divisions approximately 5 mm before the nerves enter the orbit through the superior orbital fissure. The superior branch supplies only two muscles: the superior rectus and the levator palpebra. The inferior branch, however, supplies the remaining muscles, the medial and inferior recti and inferior oblique, as well as the parasympathetic route for the ciliary ganglion, which eventually innervates the pupillary sphincter and ciliary muscle. In the analysis of bilateral ocular involvement, it is important to recall that the organization of the oculomotor nuclear complex is such that a single midline subnucleus innervates both lid levators, and the subnucleus of the superior rectus muscle innervates the contralateral superior rectus muscle. Two muscles, the superior rectus and the superior oblique (cranial nerve IV), are supplied by motor nuclei located contralateral to the involved eye.

In the midbrain, the medial longitudinal fasciculus (MLF) lies lateral to the third nuclear complex, but comes to lie medial to the abducens nucleus in the pons. Lesions of the MLF produce the complex of internuclear ophthalmoplegia, seen primarily as a failure of adduction of the ipsilateral eye to some degree during versions, usually accompanied by abducting nystagmus in the contralateral eye, and variably by skew deviation (vertical diplopia) and preservation of convergence. Paralytic exotropia can result from bilateral lesions of the MLF in the midbrain, or as part of the pontine exotropia in the one and one-half syndrome (Glaser, 1990). This latter syndrome consists of a gaze palsy to one side and contralateral adduction deficit.

NUCLEAR LESIONS

Nuclear lesions producing third nerve palsy are rare in clinical experience and may be minimal or extensive in involvement. Clear-cut cases would involve unilateral third nerve palsy, with contralateral involvement of the superior rectus muscle and bilateral ptosis, or bilateral third nerve palsy with sparing of levator action, with or without internal ophthalmoplegia. Daroff's clinical rules (Glaser, 1990) suggest that less clear-cut evidence of nuclear involvement would be bilateral total third nerve palsy, bilateral ptosis, bilateral internal ophthalmoplegia, bilateral medial rectus palsy, or single muscle involvement (with the exception of the levator and superior rectus muscle).

FASCICULAR LESIONS

Lesions involving the third nerve fasciculus also involve the surrounding brain stem structure and therefore produce accompanying signs of contralateral hemiplegia (Weber's syndrome) or contralateral intension tremor and ataxia (Benedikt's syndrome). Nuclear or fascicular third nerve palsies are most often caused by infarction, demyelination, or tumor involvement.

PERIPHERAL LESIONS

Peripheral third nerve involvements are more common and their causes are usually signaled by the history and surrounding nerve signs. In the interpeduncular course, the third nerves are subjected to compression by aneurysm, concussion by trauma, and inflammatory involvement by meningitis. Lesions of the third nerve within the cavernous sinus usually are accompanied by other involvements, namely those of the fourth, fifth, and sixth cranial nerves and the oculosympathetic plexus. The complete clinical cavernous sinus syndrome would be that of a closed eye, and underneath the lid, an eye frozen in primary position with a middilated pupil indicating involvement of both parasympathetic nerve supplies. Cavernous sinus syndromes can often be quite dramatic—the carotid cavernous fistula and the painful ophthalmoplegia of Tolosa-Hunt; or the more insidious intracavernous aneurysm seen in older individuals or with slowly growing tumors. Inflammatory lesions and rapidly growing malignancies produce a more acute course.

Ischemic oculomotor palsies are relatively common and often spare the pupillary function, producing the so-called pupil-sparing third nerve palsy (Asbury et al., 1970; Nadeau and Trobe, 1983). The ophthalmoplegia may present with acute pain in and around the involved eye and may be partial or complete. Recovery usually occurs in the first 3–4 months, usually without evidence of aberrant regeneration.

ORBITAL LESIONS

Orbital involvements include inflammatory pseudotumor as well as traumatic neuropathy and tumor involvement and, more often than not, produce other neuromyopathic soft-tissue or structural signs.

ABERRANT REGENERATION (MISDIRECTION) OF THE THIRD NERVE

Aberrant regeneration of the injured third nerve, usually unilateral and rarely bilateral, results in oculomotor synkinesis, which becomes evident approximately 2 months after acute ophthalmoplegia. This syndrome is seen frequently in congenital palsies, and occasionally it occurs in patients without any acute preceding palsy, usually caused by slowly growing mass lesions within the cavernous sinus (e.g., meningioma, aneurysm). This apparently spontaneous oculomotor synkinesis has been described as primary, as opposed to the more common or secondary type, which follows a clinically apparent third nerve palsy. Aberrant regeneration is most commonly recognized in association with trauma and aneurysm, very uncommonly with tumors, and virtually never with ischemic or demyelinative causes.

With aberrant regeneration of the third nerve, the exotropia in primary position may often be quite small and cosmetically acceptable. A variety of synkinetic movements can result: The upper lid may elevate on attempted adduction (inverse Duane's syndrome) (Figure 24.1) or depression (pseudo–von Graefe's sign); globe retraction (enophthalmos) or adduction may occur during attempted vertical movements; and an abnormal light-near pupillary dissociation, with the enlarged affected pupil constricting during adduction, may take place. Surgical correction of the ptosis in this situation requires special consideration (see discussion below).

INVESTIGATION

In general, acute onset of third nerve palsy, especially if non–pupil-sparing, should be investigated with prompt, appropriate neurologic studies. This is best done in conjunction with a neurologist or neurosurgeon, the urgency of consultation depending on the most likely cause.

Isolated third nerve palsy should bring to mind an aneurysm of the posterior communicating artery, especially when the pupil is involved and there is severe headache. If an aneurysm is suspected, urgent carotid angiography is essential. In other cases, neuroimaging of the pathways of the third cranial nerves should be carried out. In pupil-sparing cases, assessing fasting blood sugar is useful. In older individuals, a characteristic history and elevated sedimentation rate would suggest cranial arteritis with a need for temporal artery biopsy and quick institution of oral steroid therapy. A history of preceding viral illness suggests a viral mononeuropathy, and migraine-like headaches suggest a complicated migraine ophthalmoplegia. Third nerve palsies that are accompanied by other cranial nerve palsies should be investigated in conjunction with a neurologist for more complex disease. Any strabismus surgery should be deferred not only until the deviation has stabilized, but also until the neurologist feels that the underlying disease (and strabismus) is sufficiently controlled or unlikely to progress.

DIFFERENTIAL DIAGNOSIS

In cases of orbital trauma, the diagnosis is usually fairly evident. In certain cases, however, forced duction testing for muscle entrapment and

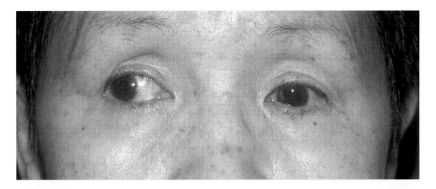

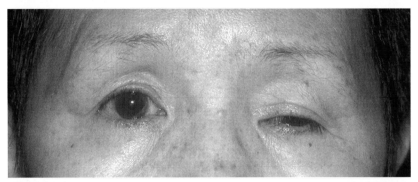

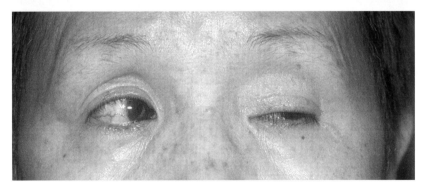

FIGURE 24.1 *In inverse Duane's syndrome, the upper eyelid elevates on attempted adduction. This occurs in aberrant regeneration and can be seen in this patient's left eye.*

computed tomographic scanning may be useful in securing the diagnosis. Similarly, pupil-sparing third nerve palsies of a probable ischemic nature should be watched in conjunction with a general physician.

MANAGEMENT

The management goals are short-term and long-term. Diplopia is difficult to treat with prisms because of its variable nature, and if the palsy is complete, the total ptosis provides a natural occlusive treatment.

Otherwise, occlusion with some mechanical means (e.g., a patch, opaque contact lens, blurred spectacle lens) is useful. Some patients will learn to tolerate some degree of diplopia, since the paretic eye frequently has a very blurred image. For children who are susceptible to amblyopia based on their age, appropriate spectacle correction and occlusion therapy are required to maintain visual acuity in the affected eye. Visual fixation patterns should be observed, because amblyopia occasionally occurs in the *uninvolved* eye (Miller, 1977). If the palsied eye is extremely exotropic and the refractive error is significant, corrective surgery should be considered all the earlier to promote efficient spectacle use.

The clinical course of the strabismus can be followed with prism cover tests to quantitate the deviation, and a Hess screen or Lees screen can document any change in muscle action. If any degree of binocular vision is present, its area can be measured using the Goldmann perimeter. Some standard form of estimation of limitation of muscle movements should be made on sequential visits.

The integrity of the fourth cranial nerve should be assessed. The mainly intorsional action of the superior oblique muscle is evident as the patient attempts to look downward. This torsion of the eye on attempted depression is the basis of examining the integrity of the fourth cranial nerve in the presence of a third nerve palsy.

Surgery

Surgical treatment of oculomotor palsy is imperfect and not totally satisfying for the majority of patients. The patient should be aware of this so that his or her expectations are realistic. Quite often, two or even more procedures are required to achieve an optimal result, i.e., produce or enlarge some degree of binocular single vision, if possible, and obtain the smallest deviation possible in primary position for cosmetic and psychosocial reasons (Jackson, 1952). Surgical correction of the ptosis should be left until the strabismus surgical management is complete and should be approached from a conservative point of view, since Bell's phenomenon of the affected eye may be significantly or even completely impaired. Surgical intervention should be reserved until spontaneous resolution of the third nerve palsy has had a chance to occur, that is, at least 6 months following the initial event, or until a partial recovery has stabilized—that is, the strabismus measurements and diplopia remain approximately the same on several sequential assessments. If there remains any function of the medial rectus muscle at all, then horizontal rectus muscle surgery by itself should be enough to correct the deviation. A large lateral rectus recession of the affected eye (14–16 mm) on an adjustable suture can be carried out, combined with a resection of the medial rectus muscle (approximately 4–6 mm) (Gottlob et al., 1991). Resection of a paretic muscle will have a variable effect; greater effect and predictability occur when there is greater medial rectus muscle recovery. The lateral conjunctiva should be recessed for further effects.

If the palsy is complete, with no medial rectus muscle action, resection of the medial rectus muscle will have only an immediate mechanical effect, but eventually this will be undone as the paretic muscle stretches. In this situation, a further adduction (maintenance) effect can be obtained by transposition of the insertion of the superior oblique tendon to a point 2 to 3 mm anterior to the medial side of the superior rectus muscle insertion (Scott, 1977; Saunders and Rogers, 1982), without trochleotomy (Scott procedure) (Scott, 1977). The tendon can be shortened sufficiently to produce some tonic elevation and adduction force to the globe in the primary position, although care must be taken to avoid overshortening the tendon and thus producing a leash effect with resultant hypertropia or paradoxic ocular movements. Combining trochleotomy with this transposition, as originally described, increases the technical difficulty intraoperatively, including the possibility of tendon severance within the trochlea, especially if the trochlea is calcified. The transposition procedure is meant to create a tonic adducting force to the globe to keep it in primary position rather than produce any true adductive force during horizontal gaze.

An alternative method for maintaining the operated globe in primary position would be to perform a large resection of the medial rectus muscle to act as a tethering mechanism, while adjustable traction sutures are used to maintain the eye in a slightly esotropic position for approximately 1 month to prevent any postoperative contracture of the recessed lateral rectus muscle.

If reasonable alignment in primary position is obtained with horizontal muscle surgery, but downgaze causes exotropia, tenotomy of the superior oblique may be helpful. The superior rectus and inferior rectus are usually involved to the same degree. Therefore, the vertical position is only slightly influenced by the depressor effect of the superior oblique in the abducted position.

Surgery is usually performed on the affected eye first. If the deviation is sufficiently large, however, horizontal muscle surgery may be necessary on the fellow eye. Assuming fixation with the unaffected eye, lateral rectus recession will enhance the adduction force of the paretic medial rectus muscle in the affected eye, thanks to Hering's law. This effect is especially useful when, in aberrant regeneration, enhanced adduction of the paretic eye is accompanied by elevation of the upper lid to help correct the ptosis.

In cases of palsy of the inferior division of the third nerve, resulting in hypertropia and exotropia, Knapp (1978) suggested transposition of the lateral rectus muscle to the site of insertion of the inferior rectus muscle and transposition of the superior rectus muscle to the medial rectus area, combined with tenotomy of the superior oblique muscle, to align the eyes in primary position.

If the operated eye remains hypertropic, the horizontal muscles may be moved downward. If the superior oblique tendon has already been transposed to the superior rectus muscle, the superior oblique tendon can be remobilized and inserted on the superior aspect of the medial rectus muscle (Peter-Jackson transposition) (Peter, 1934). Reinecke points out that a major advantage of the Scott transposition procedure (see discussion above) involving the superior oblique is that it can be undone in cases of hypertropia. Moreover, it can also be converted to the Peter-Jackson transposition if further adduction force is needed. In this case it is recommended that the superior oblique muscle be freed from the trochlea to promote a more horizontal alignment of the muscle.

Once the paralytic strabismus is treated maximally, the paralytic ptosis is treated with a frontalis type of procedure, taking care that the globe is not overly jeopardized because of the impaired or absent Bell's phenomenon. When aberrant regeneration of the third nerve is associated with synkinesis of adduction and lid elevation, recession of the lateral rectus muscle of the normal eye will produce elevation of the affected lid by inducing adduction in the paretic medial rectus muscle through Hering's law, as mentioned previously.

When the acquired third cranial nerve palsy is bilateral and one eye has been centered surgically as best as possible, the second eye may be left closed to avoid diplopia, or if the patient understands the imperfection of the surgical solution to his or her overall problem, then one could treat the second eye in the same fashion as the first.

Again, it should be pointed out to the patient or parents that several operations will most likely be necessary to straighten the eyes, and both patience and understanding are important throughout the course of treatment.

REFERENCES

Asbury AK, Aldredge H, Hershberg R, Fisher CM. Oculomotor palsy in diabetes mellitus: a clinico-pathological study. Brain 1970;93:555–566.

Bajandas FJ. Neuro-Ophthalmology Board Review Manual. Thorofare, NJ: Charles B. Slack, 1980;85–90.

Glaser JS. Neuro-Ophthalmology (2nd ed). Philadelphia: Lippincott, 1990;372–378.

Gottlob I, Catalano RA, Reinecke RD. Surgical management of oculomotor nerve palsy. Am J Ophthalmol 1991;111:71–76.

Jackson E. Surgery of the Eye (3rd ed). New York: Grune & Stratton, 1952;405.

Knapp P. Paretic Squints. Symposium on Strabismus. Transactions of the New Orleans Academy of Ophthalmology. St. Louis: Mosby, 1978;350.

Miller NR. Solitary oculomotor nerve palsy in childhood. Am J Ophthalmol 1977;83:106–111.

Nadeau SE, Trobe JD. Pupil-sparing in oculomotor palsy. A brief review. Ann Neurol 1983;13:143.

Peter LC. The use of the superior oblique as an internal rotation in the third nerve paralysis. Am J Ophthalmol 1934;17:294–300.

Saunders RA, Rogers GL. Superior oblique transposition for third nerve palsy. Ophthalmology 1982;89:310–316.

Scott AB. Transposition of the superior oblique. Am Orthop J 1977;27:11–14.

VIII

Strabismus and Neurologic Disease

25

Children, Neurologic Disease, and Strabismus

Luis C. F. deSa

Strabismus and other eye movement disorders are common in children with neurologic disease. Strabismus may be the first manifestation of brain damage (Buckley and Seaber, 1981), but most children with infantile strabismus do not have other neurologic problems other than a deficit in binocular vision and possible vision loss (amblyopia).

STATIC ENCEPHALOPATHY (CEREBRAL PALSY)

Cerebral palsy (CP), also called *static encephalopathy,* indicates nonprogressive brain damage with clinical findings of movement disorder, disordered posture, and other symptom complexes (Bax, 1964; Minear, 1956). Patients may show spasticity, athetosis, ataxia, or rigidity, or variations of all of these. Hemiplegia, diplegia, and tetraplegia can occur. Prenatal etiologies include infections, anoxia, or maternal metabolic causes. Perinatal causes include abnormalities of the birth process, metabolic disturbances, cardiorespiratory defects, and prematurity. Postnatal causes include infections, trauma, toxicoses, vascular abnormalities, genetic abnormalities, and neurologic developmental (structural) defects.

The most common visual problems in these children are optic atrophy and strabismus (Taylor, 1990). Less commonly, ocular anomalies of visual field defects, retinal dysplasias, congenital cataracts, choroiditis, colobomas of the macula, cornea and iris abnormalities, ptosis, spastic eyelids, abnormal head postures, and retinopathy of prematurity have been described (Breakey, 1955; Lossef, 1962).

The incidence of strabismus in children with CP has been reported to be 15% to 62% (Hiles et al., 1975). Esotropia is most frequent, occurring in 11–70% of patients. Exotropia may occur in 4–27% (Hiles et al., 1975). A few patients present a variety of hypertropias not related to horizontal strabismus.

Dyskinetic strabismus is a characteristic pattern of strabismus that may occur in patients with CP (Buckley and Seaber, 1981). The strabismus patterns fluctuate from esotropia to exotropia, but in children of dyskinetic strabismus age, exotropia predominates. Dyskinetic strabismus can be the first indication that a child suffers static encephalopathy and is more common in children with athetosis from basal ganglia disease. Surgical treatment is not indicated until a stable angle develops.

Amblyopia is also associated with strabismus in children with static encephalopathy. It is common and occurred in 37% of the patients described by Hiles and colleagues. Many of these children (33%) suffered strabismic amblyopia (Hiles et al., 1975). Treatment for amblyopia in children with static encephalopathy is usually successful.

HYDROCEPHALUS

Hydrocephalus is a frequent feature in children with neurologic impairment and can be congenital or acquired. Hydrocephalus can be caused by excess secretion of cerebrospinal fluid, obstruction within the ventricular system (noncommunicating hydrocephalus), and an absorptive block within the subarachnoid space (communicating hydrocephalus) (Menkes et al., 1990).

Ocular complications caused by hydrocephalus include sensory and motor (movement) abnormalities. Visual handicap may result from optic atrophy (long-standing papilledema or direct compression) or from cortical abnormalities due to increased intracranial pressure and cortical hypoxia (Moore, 1990; Huber, 1976).

The most common eye movement disorders are the "setting sun sign," nystagmus, and strabismus. The setting sun sign is a tonic downward deviation caused by a vertical gaze deficit. This sign occurs only in infants, usually premature babies who have suffered an intraventricular hemorrhage. It is attributed to pressure on the posterior commissure by the third ventricle, aqueduct, or suprapineal recess (Tamura and Hoyt, 1987; Leigh and Zee, 1991). Nystagmus may be secondary to decreased visual acuity (pendular nystagmus) or associated with specific damage to the central nervous system (e.g., horizontal jerk nystagmus in cases of gaze paretic nystagmus, or vertical nystagmus in Chiari malformation) (Moore, 1990). Opsoclonus, third nerve palsy, and fourth nerve

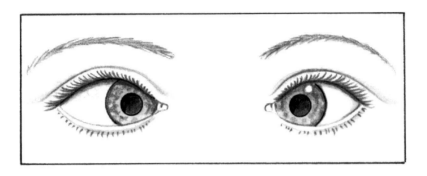

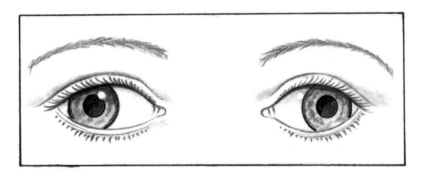

FIGURE 25.1 *In dyskinetic strabismus, the child's eyes vary from esotropic to exotropic. Dyskinetic strabismus may indicate neurologic damage.*

palsy caused by hydrocephalus have also been described (Shetty and Rosman, 1972; Clements and Kaushal, 1970; Rush and Younge, 1981).

Strabismus is the most common ocular complication, occurring in perhaps 50% of patients with hydrocephalus (France, 1975). It may appear in response to rising intracranial pressure (Rabinowicz, 1974). Strabismus may be divided into concomitant and incomitant types. Incomitant strabismus usually results from involvement of the third or sixth cranial nerve (Moore, 1990). Esotropia is more common and develops in hydrocephalus after unilateral or bilateral sixth nerve paresis (France, 1975; Moore, 1990; Wybar and Walker, 1980); lateral rectus weakness is often not demonstrable, although a convergent deviation greater for distance than for near suggests bilateral sixth nerve paresis.

A-pattern esotropia with bilateral superior oblique overaction is more common in children with neurologic disorders, including hydrocephalus and meningomyelocele (France, 1975; Rothstein et al., 1974) (Figure 25.1). It is not clear why the incidence of A pattern is so high, but disease at the cervicomedullary junction may have a role, or A patterns may be caused by a sort of alternating skew deviation on lateral gaze (Hamed et al., 1993a, b).

DOWN'S SYNDROME

A variety of ocular problems have been described in patients with Down's syndrome, including an increased incidence of mongoloid-type palpebral fissure, epicanthus, blepharoconjunctivitis, keratoconus, iridic changes (Brushfield spots), vascular changes at the optic disc, lens opacities, myopia, strabismus, and nystagmus (Hiles et al., 1974; Williams et al., 1973).

Strabismus has been reported in 33–50% of children diagnosed with Down's syndrome. Lowe (1949) showed a 20-fold increased risk of strabismus in these patients. Esotropia is much more common than exotropia; in some series, there have been no cases of exotropia (Hiles et al., 1974). Spontaneous resolution of strabismus is known to occur in later years, but most reports show a relatively constant rate throughout life (Hiles et al., 1974).

Hiles and associates (1974) treated a group of patients with standard therapy and obtained good results. Esotropia occurred in 81% of the patients with strabismus; 47% of these presented an accommodative esotropia and all but one responded to conventional treatment (including lenses or miotics). Nonaccommodative esotropia was treated with surgery in nine patients and eight (88.8%) achieved a postoperative alignment within 12 prism diopters of orthotropia. One patient was overcorrected. These results are encouraging. In our experience with neurologically impaired children, surgical results may worsen with time (deSa et al., 1992).

MANAGEMENT

In otherwise healthy children, successful management of esotropia may have a beneficial effect on overall development (Rogers et al., 1982). Whether this is true in neurologically impaired children is unknown.

Static Encephalopathy

Conservative treatment of strabismus in these children with lenses, prisms, or other occlusion has been used but without specific guidelines. Many authorities would delay surgery in the setting of static encephalopathy because the angle of strabismus may vary according to attention, emotion, fatigue, and illness (Figure 25.2). In some children the angle may spontaneously lessen to a cosmetically acceptable range (Guibor, 1953). Nevertheless, patients with static encephalopathy and strabismus, when treated using standard principles of strabismus therapy, may obtain good results (Hiles et al., 1975; Holman and Merritt, 1986). Most patients with static encephalopathy and esotropia present with nonaccommodative esotropia (72%), but 28% have accommodative esotropia. Accommodative esotropia can be treated with lenses (full

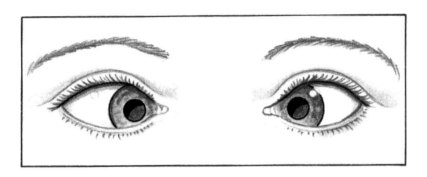

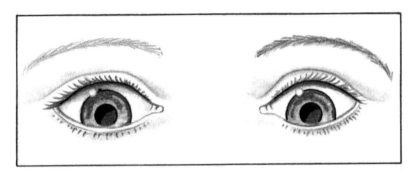

FIGURE 25.2 *A-pattern esotropia may indicate neurologic disease, particularly in white children. Note that the eyes are nearly aligned in downgaze.*

cycloplegic hypermetropic refractive error or bifocals, when necessary) or miotics; 90% of these patients achieve orthotropia or a small-angle tropia within 10 prism diopters of orthotropia. Patients with nonaccommodative esotropia treated with surgery ultimately have a satisfactory alignment in 77% of cases, with an average of 1.1 operations per patient. The treatment of exotropia was predominantly surgical in Hiles and colleagues' study: 57% of the patients were operated on, and 86% of patients treated with surgery achieved angles within 10 prism diopters of orthotropia. Only five patients (2%) reduced their angles spontaneously.

We also studied a group of neurologically impaired children (40% of the patients had static encephalopathy) with strabismus and treated them with standard strabismus therapy (deSa et al., 1992). Although 81% of the patients' eyes were aligned at 2 weeks postoperatively, only 53% remained aligned (compared to 70.5% in children without neurologic impairment).

Hydrocephalus

If strabismus is sudden in onset in hydrocephalus, a neurologic workup should be performed, especially in patients with central nervous system shunts, since strabismus can be associated with shunt failure (Moore, 1990). These patients should receive conservative treatment for 6 months to 1 year after intracranial pressure has been controlled, before considering strabismus surgery.

France (1975) advocates conservative treatment with patching for at least 6 months to prevent amblyopia and contraction of the antagonist muscle in cases of incomitant strabismus. For concomitant strabismus, patients can be patched, as necessary, to improve ductions and reduce amblyopia.

The surgical management of esotropia in hydrocephalus can be unsuccessful if **A** patterns are unrecognized (Wybar and Walker, 1980). These authors note that when the **A** pattern is associated with superior oblique overaction and downdrift or even a downshoot of each eye in adduction, these muscles must be weakened. When the **A** pattern is not associated with downdrift in adduction, then the pattern is not the result of sagittalization of the superior obliques, but related to a primary underaction of the lateral rectus muscles. In these cases, bilateral medial rectus recession should be combined with superior tendon transposition. In the unusual case of **V** esotropia with overaction of the inferior oblique muscles, Wybar and Walker (1990) recommend inferior oblique recession and even anteroposition; if there is no overaction of the inferior oblique muscles, recession and lowering the insertion of the medial rectus muscles are indicated.

REFERENCES

Bax MCO. Terminology and classification of cerebral palsy. Dev Med Child Neurol 1964;6:295–297.

Breakey AS. Ocular findings in cerebral palsy. Arch Ophthalmol 1955;53:852–856.

Buckley E, Seaber JH. Dyskinetic strabismus as a sign of cerebral palsy. Am J Ophthalmol 1981;91:652–657.

Clements DB, Kaushal K. A study of the ocular complications of hydrocephalus and meningomyelocele. Trans Ophthalmol Soc UK 1970;40:383–390.

deSa LCF, Good WV, Hoyt CS. Results of initial surgery for comitant strabismus in 25 neurologically impaired children. Binoc Vis 1992;7:165–172.

France TD. Strabismus in hydrocephalus. Am Orthopt J 1975;25:101–105.

Guibor GP. Some eye defects seen in cerebral palsy, with some statistics. Am J Phys Med 1953;32:342–347.

Hamed LM, Fang EN, Fanous MM et al. The prevalence of neurologic dysfunction in children who have superior oblique overaction. Ophthalmology 1993a;100:1483–1487.

Hamed LM, Maria BL, Quisling RG, Meckle JP. Alternating skew on lateral gaze: neuroanatomic pathway and relationship to superior oblique overaction. Ophthalmology 1993b;100:281–286.

Hiles DA, Hoyme SH, McFarlane F. Down's syndrome and strabismus. Am Orthopt J 1974;24:63–68.

Hiles D, Wallar PH, McFarlane F. Current concepts in the management of strabismus in children with cerebral palsy. Ann Ophthalmol 1975;7:789–798.

Holman RE, Merritt JC. Infantile esotropia: results in the neurologic impaired and "normal" child at NCMH (six years). J Pediatr Ophthalmol Strabismus 1986;23:41–45.

Huber A. In FC Blodi (ed), Eye Signs and Symptoms in Brain Tumors. St. Louis: Mosby, 1976;159–165.

Leigh RJ, Zee DS. The Neurology of Eye Movements. Philadelphia: FA Davis, 1991;439–447.

Lossef S. Ocular findings in cerebral palsy. Am J Ophthalmol 1962;54:1114–1118.

Lowe RF. The eyes in mongolism. Br J Ophthalmol 1949;33:131–174.

Menkes JH, Till K, Gabriel RS. Malformations of the Central Nervous System. In JH Menkes (ed), Textbook of Child Neurology (4th ed). Philadelphia: Lea & Febiger, 1990;252–272.

Minear WL. A classification of cerebral palsy. Pediatrics 1956;18:841–852.

Moore A. Hydrocephalus. In D Taylor (ed), Pediatric Ophthalmology. Cambridge, MA: Blackwell Scientific, 1990;498–504.

Rabinowicz IM. Visual function in children with hydrocephalus. Trans Ophthalmol Soc UK 1974;94:353–366.

Rogers GL, Chazan S, Fellows R, Tsou BH. Strabismus surgery and its effect upon infant development in congenital esotropia. Ophthalmology 1982;89:479–483.

Rothstein TB, Romano PE, Shoch D. Meningomyelocele. Am J Ophthalmol 1974;77:690–693.

Rush JA, Younge BR. Paralysis of cranial nerves III, IV, and VI. Course and prognosis in 1000 cases. Arch Ophthalmol 1981;99:76–79.

Shetty T, Rosman NP. Opsoclonus in hydrocephalus. Arch Ophthalmol 1972;88:585–589.

Tamura EE, Hoyt CS. Ocular motor consequences of intraventricular hemorrhages in premature infants. Arch Ophthalmol 1987;105:533–535.

Taylor D. The Visually Handicapped Baby and The Family. In D Taylor (ed), Pediatric Ophthalmology. Cambridge, MA: Blackwell Scientific, 1990;81–88.

Wheeler MB, Stonesifer K, Kenny M. Developmental evaluation in congenital esotropia. Ophthalmology 1979;86:2161–2164.

Williams EJ, McCormick AQ, Tischler B. Retinal vessels in Down's syndrome. Arch Ophthalmol 1973;89:269–271.

Wybar K, Walker J. Surgical management of strabismus in hydrocephalus. Trans Ophthalmol Soc UK 1980;100:475–478.

26

Myasthenia Gravis

Michael C. Brodsky

ETIOLOGY

Myasthenia gravis is an autoimmune disorder in which an antibody-mediated attack on the nicotinic acetylcholine receptors (AChRs) at the neuromuscular junction produces skeletal muscle weakness and fatigability (Maselli et al., 1991). The pathogenetic mechanisms by which circulating autoantibodies reduce the number of AChRs include accelerated degradation of AChRs, blockade of AChR-binding sites, and complement-mediated damage to the neuromuscular junction (Drachman et al., 1988). During repetitive activation of motor nerves, the amount of acetylcholine released at the nerve terminals normally declines to a plateau value that depends on firing frequency. In myasthenia, there is a decrease in the density of available AChRs, and this diminishes the probability that an end-plate potential will be generated, thus predisposing to failure of neuromuscular transmission (Leigh and Zee, 1991).

The natural history of myasthenia in adults consists of three general stages:

1. An active stage lasting 5–10 years in which there is progressive weakness with a labile course, maximal mortality, and best response to immunotherapy;
2. An inactive stage lasting 5–10 years in which there is less fluctuation and lability in symptoms, lower mortality, and less clinical benefit from immunotherapy;
3. A "burned-out stage" in which there is minimal fluctuation in symptoms and relatively static weakness (Finley and Pascuzzi, 1990; Verma and Oger, 1992a).

Three general categories of pediatric myasthenia have been described:

1. *Transient neonatal myasthenia:* This condition may develop in infants of mothers with myasthenia due to passive transfer of immunoglobulin G across the placenta to the fetus. Affected infants present with a feeble cry and difficulty sucking and swallowing at birth or within the first 48 hours after birth. Some of these children require mechanical ventilation. Ptosis and ophthalmoplegia may be present but are difficult to detect. The condition usually resolves in 1–6 weeks without sequelae (Verma and Oger, 1992a).

2. *Congenital myasthenia:* This is a rare condition resulting from structural abnormalities at the myoneural junction. It occurs in infants of nonmyasthenic mothers and may be familial (Engel et al., 1984). Unlike other forms of myasthenia gravis, it is not antibody- or immune-mediated. As such, it does not tend to remit. However, it is rarely life threatening and may even be benign. Typically, there is marked involvement of the ocular musculature. Some cases of congenital myasthenia respond to pyridostigmine bromide (Prostigmin).

3. *Juvenile myasthenia:* This is a condition similar to adult myasthenia, but it is more frequently familial, more likely to cause severe ophthalmoplegia, and more likely to have slower progression and a higher proportion of spontaneous remissions. Therapy is similar to that in adult myasthenia gravis.

DIAGNOSIS

No single physical finding, laboratory test, or provocative test is diagnostic of myasthenia gravis. To diagnose myasthenia gravis, clinicians must rely on constellations of findings, variability in the findings, and an understanding of the differential diagnosis. Even the Tensilon test can be misleading, since patients with other neuromuscular disorders (e.g., Guillain-Barré syndrome, botulism, poliomyelitis) occasionally respond with improvement (Rowland, 1955; Schwab and Perlo, 1966). Myasthenia gravis is notorious for mimicking other ocular motor abnormalities.

Systemic Findings

Myasthenia gravis is characterized by weakness of skeletal and cranial nerve-innervated muscles. Patients experience fatigability that typically increases as the day progresses and becomes worse with exertion. Systemic symptoms of myasthenia may involve bulbar-innervated musculature and include difficulty and fatigability with breathing, swallowing, or chewing. Acute respiratory failure and death may occur in severe cases (Phillips and Melnick, 1990). With proximal limb muscle weakness, patients experience difficulty climbing stairs or getting out of a chair.

Eye Findings

Approximately 50% of patients with myasthenia gravis present with ocular symptoms, and close to 90% develop ocular symptoms at some point in the disease process (Grob et al., 1987). Most patients with ocular myasthenia gravis who develop systemic weakness do so within 2 years of onset.

Ocular motor abnormalities in myasthenia gravis reflect impaired neuromuscular transmission and central nervous system adaptive mechanisms that attempt to compensate for extraocular muscle weakness (Feldon et al., 1982). Extraocular muscles differ from other skeletal muscles in that they have higher discharge rates, fewer AChRs in nontwitch fibers, and chemical differences in the nature of the receptors. All these differences may predispose to extraocular muscle involvement in myasthenia gravis (Leigh and Zee, 1991). Myasthenia gravis may mimic a single muscle palsy, a cranial nerve palsy, or a supranuclear or internuclear ophthalmoplegia (Burde et al., 1985). It is the mimicry found in myasthenia gravis that makes it one of the most challenging of diagnoses.

Ptosis, limitation of ductions, and strabismus are the most common ocular abnormalities associated with myasthenia gravis (Figures 26.1 and 26.2). Ptosis typically is improved after sleep and is worse at the end of the day. Strabismus is usually incomitant and accompanied by diplopia. Ocular motility measurements may change from one examination to the next. If pupillary abnormalities or pain accompany incomitant strabismus, the diagnosis of myasthenia is effectively excluded (Miller, 1985).

Specific Neuro-Ophthalmic Signs

Levator Fatigability

With sustained upgaze, myasthenic ptosis gradually worsens (see Figure 26.2). (Levator fatigability is a sensitive and specific sign of myasthenia gravis.) Levator fatigability results from decreasing recruitment of muscle fibers during repetitive stimulation, as seen on electromyographic tracings from myasthenic patients.

Cogan's Lid Twitch

The patient with myasthenic ptosis is asked to sustain downgaze and then to look quickly into primary gaze. The upper eyelids will momentarily overshoot, then descend to their final position, producing the appearance of a twitch (Cogan, 1965). This phenomenon is caused by

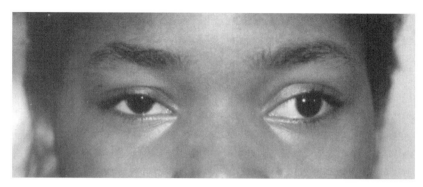

FIGURE 26.1 *A 17-year-old girl with myasthenia gravis, demonstrating upper right eyelid ptosis and exotropia in primary gaze.*

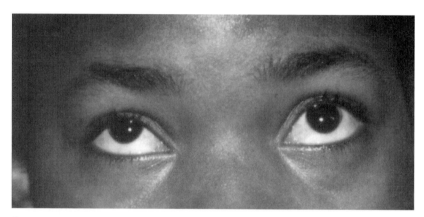

A

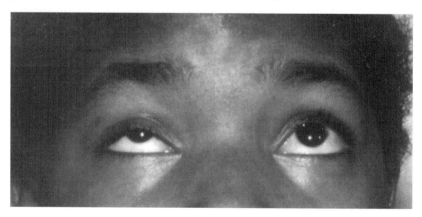

B

FIGURE 26.2 *A. Same patient as in Figure 26.1, demonstrating levator fatigability. Minimal upper right eyelid ptosis on upgaze. B. Marked upper right eyelid ptosis 45 seconds later.*

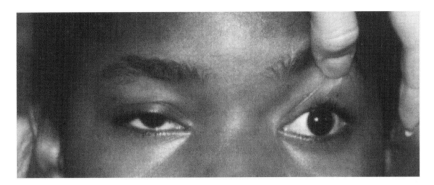

FIGURE 26.3 *Same patient as is Figures 26.1 and 26.2, demonstrating a marked increase in upper right eyelid ptosis with manual elevation of the contralateral lid.*

rapid recovery (the overshoot) and easy fatigability (eyelid descent) of the levator muscle in myasthenia gravis.

Quiver Movements

In myasthenia, a tiny backward drift of the eyes may occur immediately after a saccade (Cogan et al., 1976). Global (predominantly fast-twitch) fibers, which are relatively inactive during fixation, produce a normal pulse of activity during a saccadic eye movement. On the other hand, orbital (primarily tonic) fibers are fatigued and are unable to sustain the innervation, allowing the eyes to drift backward (Leigh and Zee, 1991).

Increased Ptosis with Contralateral Lid Elevation

In patients with ptosis of any etiology, elevation of the contralateral eyelid by the examiner produces an ipsilateral increase in ptosis (Figure 26.3). The effect is markedly accentuated in myasthenia gravis. Hering's law applies to levator muscle innervation. When the amount of innervation to one levator muscle is decreased (by the examiner lifting the lid), the innervation to the other levator automatically diminishes, and ptosis worsens.

Unilateral Eyelid Retraction

Unilateral eyelid retraction may be a physiologic correlate to increased ptosis with contralateral lid elevation, as noted above. Some patients with myasthenia gravis show unilateral eyelid retraction but no visible ptosis in the contralateral eye. This paradoxical finding presumably represents bilaterally increased levator innervation producing a compensated ptosis (Kansu and Subutay, 1987). That is, the ptotic eye is innervated so that it opens. Hering's law mandates that the fellow eye receive equal innervation, thus eyelid retraction occurs.

Saccadic Abnormalities

Saccades may be slow in myasthenia gravis, as in any disease involving the peripheral nerve, muscle, or neuromuscular junction (Yee et al., 1987). Large saccades may exhibit intrasaccadic fatigue and appear to "slow down in midflight." "Stutter-like" and "stair-step" saccades resulting from intermittent block of peripheral conduction suggest myasthenia gravis, but are also seen in Guillain-Barré syndrome and botulism poisoning (Feldon et al., 1982; Hedges et al., 1983).

Orbicularis Oculi Weakness

Most patients with myasthenia gravis can close their eyelids, but the examiner can easily pry them open. Rarely, an inability to close the lids leads to exposure keratopathy (Walsh, 1985). The combination of ptosis, ophthalmoplegia, and orbicularis oculi weakness is virtually diagnostic of myasthenia gravis.

Mimicry of Oculomotor Disorders

Myasthenia gravis mimics other neuro-ophthalmologic disorders. It can cause a pseudointernuclear ophthalmoplegia (Glaser, 1966) (Figure 26.4), isolated inferior rectus palsy (Figures 26.5 and 26.6), and virtually any other disorder of eye movements. We have seen myasthenia gravis simulate accommodative esotropia and fourth nerve palsy in the same patient at different times. Variability in the examination, from one date to the next, is most helpful in diagnosing myasthenia gravis when it mimics other disorders.

DIAGNOSTIC TESTS

Tensilon Test

The Tensilon (edrophonium chloride) test is the primary diagnostic test in the patient with suspected myasthenia gravis. Tensilon is an anticholinesterase agent that acts rapidly and hydrolyzes quickly. Tensilon competes with acetylcholine for the enzyme anticholinesterase, and thus causes a reduction in the activity of this enzyme at the neuromuscular junction (Miller, 1985).

Tensilon (10 mg in a 1-ml tuberculin syringe) is first administered intravenously as a small 0.2-ml bolus. The patient is observed for 1–2 minutes. If no significant side effects occur, the remaining 0.8 ml can be injected in 1–3 more bolus injections (Burde et al., 1985). Atropine (0.4 mg in a 1-ml syringe) should be on hand in the unlikely event that cholinergic side effects occur (e.g., bradycardia, tearing, salivation, gastrointestinal distress, flushing, sweating).

In performing the Tensilon test, it is crucial to have a measurable quantitative response to evaluate. While the Tensilon test is both

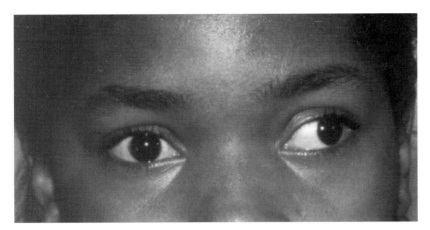

FIGURE 26.4   *The same patient as in Figures 26.1, 26.2, and 26.3, demonstrating a marked adduction deficit in the right eye. This mimics internuclear ophthalmoplegia.*

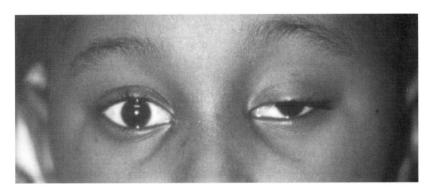

A

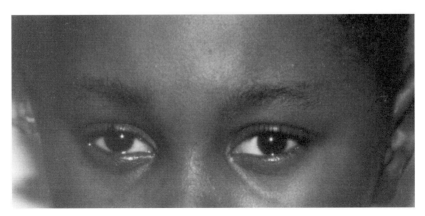

B

FIGURE 26.5   *An 8-year-old girl with myasthenia gravis. A. Marked upper left eyelid ptosis on initial presentation. B. Resolution of ptosis immediately after 30 minutes of sleep.*

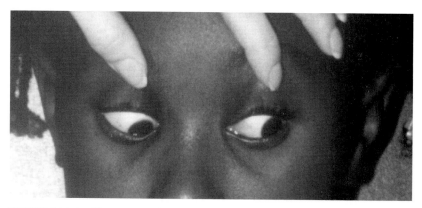

FIGURE 26.6   *The same patient as in Figure 26.5, showing weakness of the left inferior rectus muscle.*

sensitive and specific for the diagnosis of myasthenia gravis, false-positive and false-negative results are seen occasionally. A negative Tensilon test in a patient with a history and physical findings of myasthenia gravis should be repeated. Conversely, a positive Tensilon test will rarely occur in patients with ophthalmoplegia caused by cranial nerve compression from aneurysms or tumors (Moorthy et al., 1989). False-positive tests also occur in botulism, Guillain-Barré syndrome, transverse myelitis, poliomyelitis, Eaton-Lambert syndrome, and amyotrophic lateral sclerosis (Odel et al., 1991). A "paradoxical" Tensilon test in which ocular motor abnormalities worsen or reverse is inconclusive.

In children, pyridostigmine bromide (neostigmine) can be administered intramuscularly according to the formula: weight in kg × 1.5 = dose in milligrams. This produces a more prolonged beneficial response in patients with myasthenia gravis. The patient is examined 30–45 minutes after injection.

Odel and colleagues (1990) have advocated the "sleep test" to establish the diagnosis of myasthenia gravis. The patient is re-examined after 30 minutes of sleep (or closed eyelids). In myasthenia gravis, marked clinical improvement in upper eyelid ptosis and ophthalmoplegia occurs. A positive sleep test obviates the need for a Tensilon test.

Acetylcholine Receptor Antibody Test

The AChR antibody test (from the patient's serum) is positive in 85–90% of patients with generalized myasthenia gravis, and in 50–70% of patients with ocular myasthenia (Verma and Oger, 1992a). Patients with seronegative myasthenia gravis have a lower incidence of thymoma (Verma and Oger, 1992b). False-positive AChR antibody tests are rare (Miller, 1985).

Electromyography

Electromyographic abnormalities occur in 76% of patients with systemic myasthenia gravis and in 34% of patients with ocular myasthenia (Phillips and Melnick, 1990). The primary electrophysiologic technique used in the diagnosis of myasthenia gravis consists of eliciting a decremental response to repetitive supramaximal motor nerve stimulation (Miller, 1985). Single-fiber electromyography is more sensitive in establishing the diagnosis of myasthenia gravis but currently has limited availability (Phillips and Melnick, 1990).

DIFFERENTIAL DIAGNOSIS

Having emphasized that myasthenia gravis mimics other ocular motor disturbances, we must also note that certain conditions may mimic myasthenia. Ocular pseudomyasthenia was described by Moorthy and associates (1989) as a myasthenia-like syndrome occurring in patients with serious intracranial disease (tumor, aneurysm). Occasionally, patients with intracranial disease show variable ocular motor abnormalities and may even improve with Tensilon. Myasthenia gravis can also coexist with other central nervous system disease.

Thyroid myopathy can emulate myasthenia gravis. Early in the course of thyroid myopathy, patients may experience intermittent diplopia and fatigability, with symptoms worse at the end of the day. Among patients with Graves' disease, 5% also have myasthenia gravis. Orbital computed tomographic scanning will usually demonstrate enlarged extraocular muscles, indicating thyroid myopathy, but an evaluation for coexisting myasthenia gravis still may be necessary.

Other conditions that can mimic myasthenia gravis are progressive external ophthalmoplegia, botulism (early in the disease course), brain stem hypoxic-ischemic encephalopathy in neonates, and the various causes of variable strabismus.

MANAGEMENT

Systemic Evaluation

Verma and Oger (1992a) suggest a comprehensive evaluation of the patient with myasthenia gravis because of the potentially serious complications of myasthenia and its treatment:

1. Anti-AChR antibodies and electromyographic testing to confirm the diagnosis of myasthenia gravis (if not already done)
2. A computed tomographic scan of the chest to rule out thymoma

3. Careful assessment of baseline motor weakness by a neurologist
4. Evaluation by an internist for pathogenetically related diseases such as systemic lupus erythematosus, rheumatoid arthritis, and thyroid disease
5. Evaluation for systemic conditions such as asthma, diabetes, ulcer disease, or tuberculosis, which may make the patient prone to respiratory failure or which may contraindicate treatment with oral steroids
6. Evaluation of respiratory function
7. Referral to local self-help groups

Medical Management

Treatment of myasthenia is aimed at enhancing neuromuscular transmission and/or suppressing the immune system (Drachman et al., 1988; Maselli et al., 1991; Tokya et al., 1988; Verma and Oger, 1992a).

Pyridostigmine bromide is the initial treatment for both ocular and systemic myasthenia gravis. Pyridostigmine is an anticholinergic agent that enhances neuromuscular transmission by inhibiting the activity of cholinesterases, leading to prolongation of the action of acetylcholine on the motor end-plate. Pyridostigmine produces improvement in myasthenic symptoms but is rarely sufficient to eliminate symptoms. Pyridostigmine is usually used in conjunction with oral steroids. Myasthenic ocular motor paresis responds poorly to pyridostigmine.

Oral prednisone is usually the second treatment in myasthenia gravis. The complex immunosuppressive effects of oral prednisone are sufficient to produce complete remission in 40–80% of myasthenic patients, and partial remission in 20–40% (Verma and Oger, 1992a), but the full therapeutic effect of prednisone does not become clinically evident for several months.

Myasthenic patients are often hospitalized when systemic thyroid therapy is commenced, since steroid therapy can cause an acute exacerbation of myasthenic symptoms, leading to extreme weakness and possible respiratory failure. Acute worsening of symptoms is less frequent and less severe when low doses of steroids are started and gradually increased. However, high-dose initial treatment yields a more rapid therapeutic response and a greater overall remission rate (Finley and Pascuzzi, 1990). Steroids are often avoided in the treatment of ocular myasthenia gravis, because long-term steroid treatment can be life-threatening, whereas ocular myasthenia is not (Verma and Oger, 1992a). In children, steroids stunt growth and should be used with great caution. Oral steroids should be viewed as a life-long commitment, since most patients cannot discontinue them without relapse (Finley and Pascuzzi, 1990). Patients taking long-term prednisone should be placed on a low-salt, low-calorie, high-protein diet and take supplemental potassium, calcium, and, if appropriate, estrogens. Early thymectomy may reduce the overall need for steroids in myasthenia gravis.

Thymectomy is the safest and most effective therapeutic modality aimed at curing myasthenia gravis. The incidence of thymoma in generalized myasthenia is 10–25%. In generalized myasthenia, thymectomy hastens the onset and increases the frequencies of remissions. Complete remission occurs in 10–15% of patients, partial remission in nearly 50%, and some degree of improvement in 30% (Verma and Oger, 1992a). The peak effect of thymectomy is noted after 3 years.

Which patients should have thymectomy? Thymoma remains an absolute indication for thymectomy. In nonthymomatous myasthenia gravis, early thymectomy is currently being recommended for patients with generalized myasthenia and for moderate to severe bulbar myasthenia. Early thymectomy may eventually be recommended for mild generalized myasthenia and for purely ocular myasthenia, since the surgical risks of thymectomy are almost negligible.

Thymoma is diagnosed by computed tomographic scanning. Thymectomy in children often is avoided for fear of compromising the developing immune system, but reports of thymectomy in children have shown favorable results without immune compromise (Finley and Pascuzzi, 1990). Scanning may also show enlargement of the thymus due to thymic hyperplasia. The presence of antistriated antibodies in myasthenic patients correlates highly with the presence of thymoma (Rivener and Swift, 1990).

Nonsteroidal immunosuppressive agents may be helpful in some cases. The pharmacologic mechanism by which azathioprine improves neuromuscular transmission in myasthenia gravis is unknown. In one study, the best response occurred in older males with a brief duration of disease, high AChR antibody titer, and thymoma (Finley and Pascuzzi, 1990). Azothioprine should be considered in patients whose symptoms are disabling but not life threatening, or in whom there are major concerns about complications of steroid treatment (Finley and Pascuzzi, 1990). The therapeutic effects of azothioprine do not become clinically apparent for several months (Rivener and Swift, 1990). The major toxic effects of azothioprine include bone marrow suppression, elevated hepatic enzymes, and infection.

Plasmapheresis provides transient improvement in myasthenic symptoms lasting weeks to months, although patients do not generally improve to the point of clinical remission. Finley and Pascuzzi (1990) outlined the indications for plasmapheresis in the treatment of myasthenia gravis as:

1. Acute, severe, or rapidly progressive myasthenia with rapidly impending myasthenic crises when prolonged mechanical ventilation is judged to be hazardous;
2. Preoperative stabilization of myasthenia prior to thymectomy or other elective surgery in patients with marginal therapeutic control; and
3. Disabling myasthenia refractory to other therapeutic modalities.

Myasthenia gravis may develop during treatment with penicillamine, which is frequently used in patients with severe rheumatoid arthritis (Kuncl et al., 1986). Aminoglycoside antibiotics, anticholinergics, corticosteroids, anticonvulsants, cardiac medications, and quinine derivatives may impede neuromuscular transmission and aggravate the symptoms of myasthenia gravis (Verma and Oger, 1992a).

Surgical Management

Before considering strabismus surgery or botulinum toxin injection for strabismus in myasthenia gravis, every attempt should be made to maximize anticholinesterase therapy. Systemic steroids generally are avoided in ocular myasthenia, since ocular symptoms are not life threatening.

Various authors have cautioned against strabismus surgery in active myasthenia gravis (Kushner et al., 1989). Diplopia is often variable and spontaneous exacerbations and remissions are the rule. Hoyt and Good (1989) suggested that patients with chronic stable myasthenia gravis may be poor surgical candidates, since AChR loss at the neuromuscular junction results in tenuous motor fusion, even if ocular alignment is restored surgically.

A role for botulinum toxin in establishing ocular alignment in myasthenia gravis has not been explored. Because botulinum toxin provides a neuromuscular blockade similar to that produced by myasthenia gravis, it stands to reason that a lower dose of botulinum toxin would be necessary to paralyze extraocular muscles in myasthenia.

Strabismus surgery can be considered in patients with chronic myasthenia whose ocular misalignment has remained stable on long-term follow-up (at least 1 year) and in whom high-dose pyridostigmine and prednisone have failed to restore ocular alignment (Acheson et al., 1991). In cases where one or more muscles underact, the secondarily overacting muscle should be weakened. For example, an underacting medial rectus muscle causing exotropia could be managed with an ipsilateral lateral rectus recession. The addition of a resection of the involved muscle may also be helpful (e.g., medial rectus resection in this hypothetical case).

Matching the eye movement abnormality by weakening the yoke muscle may also be helpful (Acheson et al., 1991). Using the example of a weak medial rectus muscle causing exotropia, the lateral rectus muscle in the fellow eye could be weakened (via very large recession or a Faden suture) to match the ipsilateral adduction defect. Due to the highly unpredictable nature of surgery in myasthenia gravis, adjustable sutures are advised (Rosenbaum et al., 1977; Fells, 1981).

REFERENCES

Acheson JF, Elston JS, Lee JP, Fells P. Extraocular muscle surgery in myasthenia gravis. Br J Ophthalmol 1991;75:232–235.

Burde RM, Savino PJ, Trobe JD. Clinical Decisions in Neuro-Ophthalmology. St. Louis: Mosby, 1985;175–178, 251–255.

Cogan DG. Myasthenia gravis: a review of the disease and a description of the lid twitch as a characteristic sign. Arch Ophthalmol 1965;74:217–221.

Cogan DG, Yee RD, Gittinger J. Rapid eye movements in myasthenia gravis: clinical observations. Arch Ophthalmol 1976;94:1083–1085.

Drachman DB, McIntosh KR, DeSilva S et al. Strategies for the treatment of myasthenia gravis. Ann NY Acad Sci 1988;540:176–186.

Engel AG. Myasthenia gravis and myasthenic syndromes. Ann Neurol 1984;16:519–534.

Feldon SE, Stark L, Lehman SL, Hoyt WF. Oculomotor effects of intermittent conduction block in myasthenia gravis and Guillain-Barré syndrome. Arch Neurol 1982;39:497–503.

Fells P. The use of adjustable sutures. Trans Ophthalmol Soc UK 1981;101:279–283.

Finley JC, Pascuzzi RM. Rational therapy of myasthenia gravis. Semin Neurol 1990;10:70–82.

Glaser JS. Myasthenic pseudo-internuclear ophthalmoplegia. Arch Ophthalmol 1966;75:363–366.

Grob D, Arsura EL, Brunner NG, Namba T. The course of myasthenia gravis and therapies affecting outcome. Ann NY Acad Sci 1987;505:472–499.

Hedges TR 3rd, Jones A, Stark L, Hoyt WF. Botulin ophthalmoplegia: clinical and oculographic observations. Arch Ophthalmol 1983;101:211–213.

Hoyt CS, Good WV. Management of ocular motility problems in myasthenia gravis. Binoc Vis Q 1989;4:187–192.

Kansu T, Subutay N. Lid retraction in myasthenia gravis. J Clin Neuro-Ophthalmol 1987;7:145–150.

Kuncl RW, Pestronk A, Drachman DB, Rechthand E. The pathophysiology of penicillamine-induced myasthenia gravis. Ann Neurol 1986;20:740–744.

Kushner BJ, Buckley EG, Hoyt CS et al. A case of myasthenia gravis with extraocular muscle pareses, complicated by prior glaucoma filtration surgery. Binoc Vis Q 1989;4:187–192.

Leigh JR, Zee DS. The Neurology of Eye Movements (2nd ed). Philadelphia: FA Davis, 1991;338–344.

Maselli RA, Richman DP, Wollman RL. Inflammation at the neuromuscular junction in myasthenia gravis. Neurology 1991;41:1497–1504.

Miller NR. Walsh and Hoyt's Clinical Neuro-Ophthalmology (4th ed). Vol 2. Baltimore: Williams & Wilkins, 1985;840–862.

Moorthy G, Behrens MM, Drachman DB et al. Ocular pseudomyasthenia or ocular myasthenia "plus": a warning to clinicians. Neurology 1989;39:1150–1154.

Nossal GJ. Possible strategies for the treatment of myasthenia gravis and other autoimmune diseases. Ann NY Acad Sci 1987;505:610–618.

Odel JG, Winterkorn JM, Behrens MM. The sleep test for myasthenia gravis: a safe alternative to Tensilon. J Clin Neuro-Ophthalmol 1991;11:288–292.

Phillips LH 2nd, Melnick PA. Diagnosis of myasthenia gravis in the 1990s. Semin Neurol 1990;10:62–69.

Rivener MH, Swift TR. Thymoma: diagnosis and management. Semin Neurol 1990;10:83–88.

Rosenbaum AL, Metz AS, Carlson M, Jampolsky AJ. Adjustable rectus muscle recession surgery. A follow-up study. Arch Ophthalmol 1977;95:817–820.

Rowland LP. Prostigmine-responsiveness and the diagnosis of myasthenia gravis. Neurology 1955;5:612–624.

Schwab RS, Perlo VP. Syndromes simulating myasthenia gravis. Ann NY Acad Sci 1966;135:350–366.

Tokya KV, Hohlfeld R, Heininger K. Myasthenia gravis. New therapeutic strategies. Monogr Allergy 1988; 25:108–115.

Verma P, Oger J. Treatment of acquired autoimmune myasthenia gravis: a topic review. Can J Neurol Sci 1992a;19:360–375.

Verma PK, Oger JJ. Seronegative generalized myasthenia gravis: low frequency of thymic pathology. Neurology 1992b;42:586–589.

Walsh TJ. Neuro-Ophthalmology: Clinical Signs and Symptoms (2nd ed). Philadelphia: Lea & Febiger, 1985.

Yee RD, Whitcup SM, Williams IM et al. Saccadic eye movements in myasthenia gravis. Ophthalmology 1987;94:219–225.

27

Management of Nystagmus

ETIOLOGY

Nystagmus is of great interest to strabismus specialists because it may lead to unusual and potentially harmful adaptations. Some patients with congenital nystagmus find a null point—a position where the nystagmus is dampened. This null zone is often eccentric—that is, it is not in primary gaze position. To optimize vision, patients with an eccentric null zone turn their heads so that they point their "null position" toward the object of visual interest (Figure 27.1). Head turning can be slight or pronounced and can lead to an unattractive appearance and problems with daily activity. A constantly turned head may lead to neck pain and even cervical spine abnormalities. Arguably, nystagmus also diminishes visual acuity (Dickinson and Abadi, 1985; Abadi and Worfolk, 1989). In cases of congenital motor nystagmus (CMN), where there is no known ocular defect, nystagmus may diminish foveation time and thereby reduce acuity. It is understandable, then, that over the years a variety of efforts have been made to try to help diminish patients' nystagmus. This chapter examines null zone management and nystagmus management.

DIAGNOSIS

Congenital sensory nystagmus (CSN) appears early in infancy, usually in the first 6–12 weeks of life, or after the onset of a vision abnormality. It is caused by bilateral anterior visual pathway disease (i.e., diseases of the eyes or optic nerves) and persists throughout life. A careful oph-

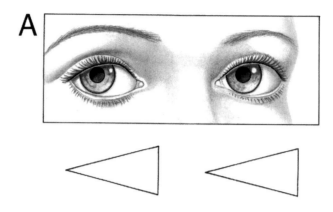

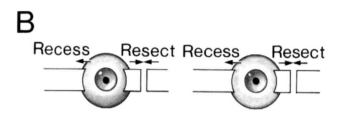

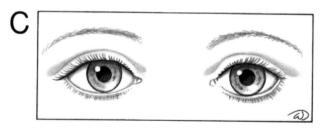

FIGURE 27.1 *Prism glasses to manage nystagmus should be oriented with the apex pointing toward the null zone. Surgical management for the same patient ideally would move the null point to a primary position.*

thalmologic examination may reveal such causes as optic nerve hypoplasia, optic atrophy, bilateral retinal disease, or even untreated bilateral congenital cataract. In the absence of any physical findings, retinal disease should be suspected. In many cases, an electroretinogram will reveal that a patient suffers hereditary or congenital retinal dystrophy. If the electroretinogram examination is normal, then CMN may be diagnosed, as long as there are no signs of neurologic disease.

In CSN and CMN, nystagmus may have any waveform. Horizontal waveforms predominate, but vertical nystagmus has also been noted (Good et al., 1991). There are some characteristics of nystagmus that suggest possible specific causes. Monocular nystagmus or asymmetric nystagmus may be caused by optic glioma. In this situation, a neuroimaging study is probably indicated (Reinecke et al., 1990). A very fast frequency, small amplitude nystagmus may indicate congenital achromatopsia (Yee, 1981). This can be diagnosed by electroretinography. Nystagmus that presents after 3 months of life may also be caused by neurologic disease, and in this clinical scenario, a neuroimaging study is also advisable.

Congenital nystagmus, either CSN or CMN, has other clinical characteristics. It may be dampened by convergence, thereby leaving children with better near vision than distance vision (Good, 1990). Congenital nystagmus is often increased by attempts at visual fixation. Strabismus commonly accompanies nystagmus.

MANAGEMENT

Prisms

Prior to 1953, the only treatment for head turns associated with nystagmus consisted of prisms. Prisms were oriented in such a way as to shift the visual axis either to the left or to the right. Occasionally, prisms were used in a base-out fashion to induce convergence, thereby dampening nystagmus.

Certainly, for small angles of head turn, the use of prisms may be beneficial. In the usual case where the patient complains about a head turn, though, the amount of prism necessary to change the null point is so large and cosmetically unacceptable that it is not even worth trying, except perhaps as a trial to determine if the head turn can be alleviated.

The orientation of prisms would be as follows: If the patient had a left head turn with eyes deviated to the right to dampen nystagmus, the prisms would be oriented with the base in, in front of the right eye, and the base out, in front of the left eye (see Figure 27.1). The reverse would apply if the eyes had to be moved to the left (head turn to the right) to dampen nystagmus. Note: the prism should be positioned so that the apex points to the null zone.

Surgical Management of Horizontal Eye Turns Associated with Nystagmus

Most authors would agree that surgery is indicated for significant torticollis, usually amounts greater than 20–30 degrees, but the evaluation of nystagmus in a patient prior to surgery should include a number of other important features. (Obviously, it is paramount to demonstrate that visual acuity improvement occurs in the null position.) A shifting null zone can occur in periodic alternating nystagmus (PAN) and can be diagnosed by observing the patient for approximately 4 minutes. Multiple head positions can occur in the absence of PAN (Abadi and Whittle, 1991) and, again, should be searched for in a careful examination. Some patients search out a neutral zone rather than a null zone for gaze preference (Abadi and Whittle, 1991). The neutral zone represents the position at which the nystagmus fast phase changes direction when the patient changes gaze from left to right or right to left (Daroff et al., 1978). It does not necessarily coincide with the null zone. Recognition of neutral zone and alternating fixation patterns could lead to variations in surgical intervention, or no intervention at all.

The measurement of the head turn in degrees or prism diopters can be performed, although some authors simply estimate the amount of deviation to the nearest 15 degrees—that is, 15 degrees, 30 degrees, or 45 degrees. Another classification scheme for head turn would be mild, moderate, or marked. Kestenbaum (1954) measured the distance between the position of the limbus in primary position and the optimal eye position and used this number to determine the number of millimeters that the rectus muscle should be moved. It is also possible to determine the strength of the prism necessary to eliminate the head turn and to use this number of prism diopters as a guide to how much surgery to perform.

There are also special devices for measurement of head turn. A headlight that projects onto a scale on the wall adjacent to an eye chart can be used (Schatz and Urist, 1971), or eye movement recordings can be used to determine the position of the null zone (Dell'Osso and Flynn, 1979).

Kestenbaum (1954) and Anderson (1953) independently proposed similar approaches to congenital nystagmus with torticollis. Kestenbaum proposed surgically moving both eyes the same amount and in the same direction as the head turn. In other words, a right head turn would be treated with a right medial rectus recession and left lateral rectus recession, combined with resections of the right lateral and left medial rectus muscles.

Several modern approaches to quantitation of surgery have been taken. Parks (1973) recommended the same amount of surgery for all patients with moderate to marked head turns. This approach eliminates the necessity of taking prism diopter or degrees of turn measurements. Parks, for example, recommended a 5-mm medial rectus muscle recession, 6-mm medial rectus resection, an 8-mm lateral rectus recession, and 7-mm lateral rectus resection. He acknowledged that this amount of surgery will not fully correct a large head turn, but at least it does not restrict ductions postoperatively. Fells and Dulley (1976) followed the guidelines proposed by Parks. On the other hand, Ohmi and colleagues (1978) recommended a 7- to 8-mm recession of the yoke muscles responsible for the slow phase of nystagmus in both eyes, no matter what the amount of the head turn, and several investigators have advocated so-called augmented Kestenbaum procedures to attempt to eliminate the postoperative return of torticollis (Nelson et al., 1984; Calhoun and Harley, 1973; Biglan et al., 1989). Augmentation might include increasing the amount of surgery performed at each muscle by 60% (over conventional surgery amounts).

As a second approach, Schlossman (1962, 1972) simply recommends the use of recessions bilaterally for moderate head turns, but adding resection (thereby performing bilateral recession/resection procedures) for marked head turns.

Yet another approach would involve tailoring the amount of surgery to the individual patient (Kestenbaum, 1954). Kommerell (1974) recommends equal amounts of recessions and resections on both eyes in the manner proposed by Kestenbaum, but other authors do unequal amounts of recession and resection on the medial and lateral rectus muscles in order to take into account the differences in effects of surgery on these different muscles.

A Faden suture can also be combined with rectus muscle surgery (Berard, 1978; Muhlendyck, 1978). Another wrinkle to surgery for null point includes deliberately giving the patient a postoperative divergence, which then must be compensated for by convergence. Convergence often dampens nystagmus and may further improve visual acuity (Priglinger and Priglinger, 1981; Roggenkamper, 1982; Economopoulos, 1985). Patients should be given a trial of base-out prisms (which induce exotropia and force the patient to converge). A successful trial with base-out prisms will indicate that the patient can tolerate iatrogenic divergence.

In general, the best results from nystagmus surgery are noted in the first few months after surgery. Generally, after 1 year, the amount of residual head turn is stable (Dell'Osso and Flynn, 1979). The surgery certainly should result in a decrease in the torticollis and may also result in better-than-expected visual acuity, based on preoperative null zone acuity measurements. The null zone may be broadened and the amount of nystagmus may be less intense surrounding the null zone (Dell'Osso and Flynn, 1979). Eye movement recordings also show that there is a decrease in the velocity of both the quick and the slow phase following Kestenbaum-Anderson surgery, yet another reason for improved visual acuity (Ohmi et al., 1978).

Management of Strabismus Associated with Congenital Nystagmus

One of two approaches can be taken to manage strabismus associated with nystagmus. The first is to attempt to correct the strabismus at the same time as the null point problems (Schlossman, 1972). The surgeon can write down the amount of surgery necessary to correct the null point. Then he or she can add to this the amount of surgery that would be required to correct the strabismus abnormality.

The other approach, and one that appears to be more widely accepted, involves two separate operations: surgery for torticollis, followed by a second operation for residual strabismus.

Management of Nystagmus in the Chin-Up or Chin-Down Position

In the case of vertical head tilt to dampen nystagmus, various authors recommend vertical recess/resect procedures or recession alone (Pierse, 1959; Sternberg-Rabb, 1963; Schlossman, 1972; Parks, 1973; Muhlendyck, 1978). For example, a chin-up position (with eyes rotated down) could be managed with bilateral inferior rectus recessions or with inferior rectus recessions combined with superior rectus resections.

Management of Nystagmus and Head Tilt

Head tilting to reduce nystagmus is less common but still can be corrected with surgery on the eye's cyclotorsional muscles (Schlossman, 1972; de Decker, 1980; Conrad and de Decker, 1982) (Figure 27.2). Surgery to induce incyclotorsion could consist of an inferior oblique recess, ipsilateral superior oblique tuck, or even transposition of the insertion of the superior oblique muscle anteriorly to get more torsional effect and, it is hoped, avoid shifting the eye vertically (Conrad and de Decker, 1984). Surgery to induce excyclotorsion might include a superior oblique tenotomy or recession. A patient with nystagmus and a right head tilt, for example, dampens nystagmus with right eye incyclotorsion and left eye excyclotorsion. Treatment could consist of creating right eye excyclotorsion (e.g., superior oblique tenotomy) and left eye incyclotorsion (e.g., superior oblique tuck, inferior oblique recession). In other words, the surgery should tort the eyes in the direction of the shoulder toward which the patient tilts his or her head.

Management of Nystagmus

Given the fact that nystagmus itself can probably reduce visual acuity (Dickinson and Abadi, 1985; Abadi and Worfolk, 1989), it is understandable that many authorities have attempted to effect a cure for nystagmus per se, whether or not a null zone is present. Attempts at treating nystag-

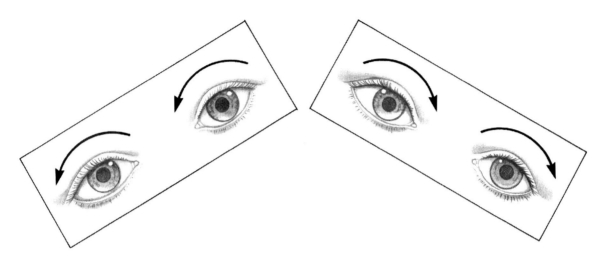

FIGURE 27.2 *Cyclotorsional surgery for nystagmus dampened by a head tilt should rotate the eyes toward the side of the tilt.*

mus have fallen into three arenas: the use of contact lenses, the use of botulinum neurotoxin injections, and large rectus muscle recessions (Bietti, 1956; Bietti and Bagolini, 1960; von Noorden and Sprunger, 1991).

Contact Lens Use
Several authorities have commented on the value of contact lenses in dampening nystagmus (Abadi, 1979; Dell'Osso et al., 1988.) The weight of the contact lens may in some manner reduce nystagmus. More likely, some sort of sensory feedback may occur when the edge of the lens bumps the inside of the eyelids. The feedback reduces nystagmus (Dell'Osso et al., 1988). In one case, eye movement recordings documented a rebound nystagmus following cessation of contact lens use (Safran and Gambazzi, 1992). Our experience with contact lenses has been less gratifying, although we do occasionally see patients who feel satisfied with some improvement with the use of contacts.

Medication
A variety of medications have been used in an attempt to manage acquired nystagmus, but usually to no avail. The exception to this statement is baclofen, which appears to help in acquired periodic alternating nystagmus (PAN) (Larmande, 1982; Halmagyi et al., 1980). Baclofen is a gamma-aminobutyric acid drug. In other kinds of acquired nystagmus, however, there is insufficient evidence to allow enthusiasm for the use of medication.

Botulinum Neurotoxin Injection
Helveston and Pogrebniak (1988) used botulinum neurotoxin injections in retrobulbar fashion in a successful effort to control nystagmus

associated with brain stem stroke. Two patients responded favorably and without complication to repeated injections of 25 U of botulinum toxin given in only one eye. Leigh and associates (1992) also reported on the effectiveness of botulinum toxin injected into the rectus muscles in acquired nystagmus. Leigh and associates' patients showed slightly improved vision, but at the expense of increased nystagmus in the noninjected eye and of gaze-holding eye trajectory abnormalities in the injected eye.

Surgery for Nystagmus

von Noorden and Sprunger (1991) reported improvement in visual acuity in patients undergoing large horizontal rectus muscle recessions. Patients with horizontal nystagmus had both medial and lateral rectus muscles recessed behind the equator and reported improvement in visual acuity, both objectively and subjectively. Others have advocated a cautious approach to surgery for nystagmus until further studies are performed (Flynn et al., 1991). Future studies may confirm or refute the value of a surgical approach to nystagmus.

COMPLICATIONS. Because surgery for nystagmus is performed infrequently, the surgeon should be very careful to record and carefully consider the desired surgery preoperatively. The patient's records and surgical plan probably should be brought to the operating room, where they can serve as a backup in case the surgeon needs it. In principle, the eyes should be moved toward the direction of the head turn and away from the position of the null zone.

Vedel-Jensen (1962) noted a patient who had surgery that resulted in moving the eyes in the wrong direction. For the first 2 weeks postoperatively, the nystagmus and vision improved in primary position, but after 2 weeks the nystagmus returned at a larger amplitude than previously in the primary position. When she underwent a second operation about 6 months later to correct this error, she did well, with decreased nystagmus and better visual acuity.

REFERENCES

Abadi RV. Visual performances with contact lenses and congenital idiopathic nystagmus. Br J Physiol Optics 1979;33:32–37.

Abadi RV, Whittle J. The nature of head postures in congenital nystagmus. Arch Ophthalmol 1991;109:216–220.

Abadi RV, Worfolk R. Retinal slip velocities in congenital nystagmus. Vision Res 1989;29:195–205.

Anderson JR. Causes and treatment of congenital eccentric nystagmus. Br J Ophthalmol 1953;37:267–281.

Berard PV, Mouillac N, Reydy R, Spielmann A. Surgical Treatment of Congenital Nystagmus with Horizontal Torticollis. In RD Reinecke (ed), Strabismus. Orlando, FL: Grune & Stratton, 1978;169–176.

Bietti GB. Note di tecnica chirurgica oftalmologica. Boll d'oculist 1956;35:642–656.

Bietti GB, Bagolini B. Traitement medicochirurgical du nystagmus. L'Anne Ther Clin Ophtalmol 1960;11:268–293.

Biglan AW, Hiles DA, Ying-Fen Z et al. Results after surgery for null point nystagmus with abnormal head position. Am Orthop J 1989;39:134–142.

Calhoun JH, Harley RD. Surgery for abnormal head position in congenital nystagmus. Trans Am Ophthalmol Soc 1973;71:70–87.

Conrad HG, de Decker W. Torsional Kestenbaum Procedure: Evolution of a Surgical Concept. In Reinecke RD, ed, Strabismus II. Orlando, FL: Grune & Statton, 1982;301–314.

Daroff RB, Troost BT, Dell'Osso LF. Nystagmus and Related Oscillations. In JS Glaser (ed), Neuro-Ophthalmology. New York: Harper & Row, 1978;221–243.

de Decker W. Kestenbaum transposition operation for treatment of the Duane I retraction syndrome. Trans Ophthalmol Soc UK 1980;100:479–482.

Dell'Osso LF, Flynn JT, Daroff RB. Hereditary congenital nystagmus: an intrafamilial study. Arch Ophthalmol 1974;92:366–374.

Dell'Osso LF, Traccis S, Abel LA, Erzurum SI. Contact lenses and congenital nystagmus. Clin Vision Sci 1988;3:229–232.

Dell'Osso LF, Flynn JT. Congenital nystagmus surgery. A quantitative evaluation of the effects. Arch Ophthalmol 1979;97:462–469.

Dickinson CM, Abadi RV. The influence of nystagmoid oscillation on contrast sensitivity in normal observers. Vision Res 1985;25:1089–1096.

Economopoulos NK, Damanakis AG. Modification of the Kestenbaum operation for correction of nystagmic torticollis and improvement of visual acuity with the use of convergence. Ophthalmic Surg 1985;16:309–314.

Fells P, Dulley B. Surgical management of compensatory head posture. Trans Ophthalmol Soc UK 1976;96:90–95.

Flynn JT, Scott WE, Kushner BJ et al. Large rectus muscle recessions for the treatment of congenital nystagmus [letter]. Arch Ophthalmol 1991;109:1636–1638.

Good WV. Behaviors of visually impaired children. Semin Ophthalmol 1991;6:158–160.

Good WV, Brodsky MC, Hoyt CS, Ahn JC. Upbeating nystagmus in infants: a sign of anterior visual pathway disease. Binoc Vis Q 1990;5:158–163.

Gottlob I, Zubcov A, Catalano RA et al. Signs distinguishing spasmus nutans (with and without central nervous system lesions) from infantile nystagmus. Ophthalmology 1990;97:1166–1175.

Halmagyi GM, Rudge P, Gresty MA et al. Treatment of periodic alternating nystagmus. Ann Neurol 1980;8:609–611.

Helveston EM, Pogrebniak AE. Treatment of acquired nystagmus with botulinum A toxin. Am J Ophthalmol 1988;106:584–586.

Kestenbaum A. A nystagmus operation. Proceedings of the XVII International Congress on Ophthalmology, 1954;2:1071.

Kommerell G. Surgical management of altered head posture in patients with congenital nystagmus. [Nystagmusoperationnen zur korrectur verschiedener kopszwangshaltungen]. Klin Monatsbl Augenheilkd 1974;164:172–191.

Larmande P. Baclofen as a treatment for nystagmus. Ann Neurol 1982;11:213–217.

Leigh RJ, Tomsak RL, Grant MP et al. Effectiveness of botulinum toxin administered to abolish acquired nystagmus. Ann Neurol 1992;32:633–642.

Muhlendyck H. The Faden operation in the treatment of congenital nystagmus. In RD Reinecke (ed), Strabismus. Orlando, FL: Grune & Stratton, 1978;235.

Nelson LB, Ervin-Mulvey LD, Calhoun JH et al. Surgical management for abnormal head position in nystagmus: the augmented modified Kestenbaum procedure. Br J Ophthalmol 1984;68:796–800.

Ohmi E, Fujita J, Tuboi T. Electrophysiological analysis of congenital nystagmus before and after Anderson's surgery. In RD Reineke (ed), Strabismus. Orlando, FL: Grune & Stratton, 1978;159.

Parks MM. Congenital nystagmus surgery. Am Orthopt J 1973;23:35–39.

Pierse D. Operation on the vertical muscles in cases of nystagmus. Br J Ophthalmol 1959;43:230–233.

Priglinger S, Priglinger S. Numerische ueberlegungen zu wechselnder kopfzwangshaltung bei nystagmus undbinokularen funktionen. Klin Monatsbl Augenheilkd 1981;178:10–19.

Roggenkamper P. Combination of artificial divergence with Kestenbaum operation in cases of torticollis caused by nystagmus. In RD Reinecke (ed), Strabismus II. Orlando, FL: Grune & Stratton, 1982;329–333.

Safran AB, Gambazzi Y. Congenital nystagmus: rebound phenomenon following removal of contact lenses. Br J Ophthalmol 1992;76:497–498.

Schatz H, Urist M. An instrument for measuring ocular torticollis (head turn, tilt, and bend). Trans Am Acad Ophthalmol Otolaryngol 1971;75:650–653.

Schlossman A. Nystagmus with strabismus: surgical management. Trans Am Acad Ophthalmol Otolaryngol 1972;76:1479–1486.

Schlossman A. The surgical treatment of nystagmus. Eye Ear Nose Throat Monthly 1962;41:549.

Sternberg-Raab A. Anderson-Kestenbaum operation for asymmetrical gaze nystagmus. Br J Ophthalmol 1963;47:339–345.

Vedel-Jensen N. Operative treatment of congenital nystagmus. Acta Ophthalmol 1962;40:629–635.

von Noorden GK, Sprunger DT. Large rectus muscle recessions for the treatment of congenital nystagmus. Arch Ophthalmol 1991;109:221–224.

Yee RD, Baloh RW, Honrubia V. Eye movement abnormalities in rod monochromacy. *Ophthalmology* 1981;88:1010–1018.

28

Superior Oblique Myokymia

Luis C. F. deSa

ETIOLOGY

Superior oblique myokymia (SOM) is an uncommon eye movement disorder characterized by a unilateral, vertical, and torsional, high-frequency microtremor of one eye. It was first noted by Duane in 1906, but Hoyt and Keane (1970) defined and named this distinct entity. The use of the term *superior oblique myokymia* has been questioned (Breen et al., 1983). Variations of the usual movements found in SOM may occur, prompting the use of other terms, such as macrorotatory deviation (Rosenberg and Glaser, 1983). Nevertheless, superior oblique myokymia is the term used by most authorities.

The etiology of SOM is unknown. Disturbance of the trochlear nucleus, causing neuron membrane threshold alterations, might be responsible. This is the case in facial muscle myokymia, where facial nucleus involvement is etiologic (Hoyt and Keane, 1970). Superior oblique myokymia may occur after superior oblique palsy, suggesting a postdenervation phenomenon. In postdenervation phenomenon, repetitive firing of a nerve causes symptomatic contraction of the muscles it innervates. This occurs in disorders such as aberrant regeneration of the oculomotor nerve, cyclic oculomotor spasm, cyclic esotropia, spring pupil, and facial myokymia (Lee, 1984). In an electromyographic study, the cause of SOM was attributed to regeneration of trochlear motor neurons and defective supranuclear control (Kommerell and Schaubele, 1980). Some authors have speculated that a virus or vascular or inflammatory abnormality could cause damage to only a few of the motor (trochlear) neurons (Kommerell and Schaubele, 1980; Keltner, 1983), but enough to cause SOM.

DIAGNOSIS

Superior oblique myokymia is a rare, chronic disease with a variable course (Hoyt and Keane, 1970). It affects adults. To date, it has not been described in children. Some patients experience spontaneous improvement or remission (Roper-Hall and Burde, 1978), but most seek medical treatment. The diagnosis can be missed by the primary physician, or SOM can erroneously be considered a functional disorder (von Noorden, 1991).

Visual symptoms of SOM consist of shimmering oscillopsia and/or torsional diplopia. These symptoms occur during the episode of myokymia. Most patients have bursts of microtremor that last from seconds to several minutes. Careful observation, including magnification with slit-lamp microscopy or an ophthalmoscopic view of the fundus, may be necessary to diagnose SOM. Patients usually have many episodes of myokymia during the day; the frequency of these episodes often increases with time. In some patients, symptoms become constant (Susac et al., 1973). An attack may be precipitated when the patient's eye returns to the primary position after looking in the field of action of the superior oblique muscle (Leigh and Zee, 1991). Looking directly into the field of action of the superior oblique muscle, reading, driving, and watching television also may worsen symptoms (Susac et al., 1973).

The superior oblique muscle may underact in the resting phase of SOM, causing a hypertropia of the affected side. It may overact with hypotropia in the active phase (Roper-Hall and Burde, 1978). Intermittent Brown's syndrome with limitation of elevation on adduction has been described (Rosenberg and Glaser, 1983). The disorder usually does not signify serious central nervous system disease, although it has been reported to be associated with intracranial tumor (Morrow et al., 1990) and adrenoleukodystrophy (Neetens and Martin, 1983).

MANAGEMENT

Treatment of SOM should begin with reassurance that symptoms are real, commonly self-limiting, and usually not associated with significant central nervous system disease. Although SOM can resolve within months or years, its symptoms may pose a significant and troubling visual handicap severe enough to require medical therapy.

Medical Management

Successful medical management has been reported with anticonvulsants, muscle relaxants, hypnotic/sedatives, and beta blockers. Carbamazepine (Susac et al., 1973), propranolol (Tyler and Ruiz,

TABLE 28.1 Surgical outcome in superior oblique myokymia

Series	Surgical Cases	Surgeries per Patient	Outcome
Hoyt and Keane, 1970	1	1	Improved
Susac et al., 1973	1	1	Improved
Kommerell and Schaubel, 1980	1	More than 1	Improved
Miller, 1983	1	1	Improved
Gittinger, 1984	1	1	Temporary improvement
Palmer and Schultz, 1984	3	2, 1, and 1	Overall improvement
Staudenmaier, 1986	1	2	Improved
Ruttum and Harris, 1988	1	3	Improved
deSa et al., 1992	4	2, 1, 1, and 1	Improved

1990), benzodiazepines (Rosenberg and Glaser, 1983; Keltner, 1983), and phenytoin (Rosenberg and Glaser, 1983; Roper-Hall and Burde, 1978) are used most often. Carbamazepine was one of the first drugs used for SOM (Susac et al., 1973), and it remains the most popular drug, despite potential side effects of aplastic anemia and cardiovascular collapse (Rall and Schleifer, 1985).

Surgical Management
When symptoms persist with medication or when side effects develop, surgery may be indicated. Only 14 patients have been treated and reported with this modality at the time of this writing (deSa et al., 1992) (Table 28.1).

Superior oblique tenotomy/tenectomy combined with myectomy of the ipsilateral inferior oblique muscle has been used most often, but superior oblique tenotomy/tenectomy alone, and even superior oblique myectomy with trochlectomy, have been used to treat SOM (Ruttum and Harris, 1988). Palmer and Shults (1984) were the first to report a series of surgical cases. They observed that all three of their patients improved. Only one patient was completely satisfied and has required two surgeries.

After weakening the superior oblique muscle, diplopia may occur in extreme positions of gaze, especially in the gaze to the side opposite the involved eye or in downgaze. Many authorities have attempted to overcome this complication of superior oblique weakening surgery by combining the superior oblique tenotomy with an ipsilateral inferior oblique myectomy. This treatment has been advocated for Brown's syndrome (Parks and Eustis, 1987), in which superior oblique weakening is also advised.

Superior oblique myokymia occasionally recurs after surgery. Recurrence may be due to reattachment of the tendon to the globe (Ruttum and Harris, 1988) or to the inability of the tendon to retract due to fibrillar attachments between the tendon, its sheath, and the globe (Berke, 1947). Tenectomy may be more effective than tenotomy for treating oscillopsia and preventing recurrence, but may induce a greater amount of postoperative vertical inconcomitance, with diplopia in downgaze (Staudenmaier, 1986).

Diplopia in downgaze following superior oblique tenotomy might best be managed with a weakening procedure on the inferior rectus muscle of the fellow eye (e.g., a Faden suture) (Kushner, personal communication, 1993). Whether this should be performed simultaneously with the superior oblique tenotomy depends on the surgeon's own experience with surgical outcome for this procedure. In our experience, we noted diplopia in downgaze in one of four patients undergoing superior oblique tenotomy, but the patient has been managed effectively without further surgery (deSa et al., 1992).

REFERENCES

Berke R. Tenotomy of superior oblique muscle for hypertropia. Arch Ophthalmol 1947;38:605–644.

Breen LA, Gutmann L, Riggs JE. Superior oblique myokymia. A misnomer. J Clin Neuro-Ophthalmol 1983;3:131–132.

deSa LC, Good WV, Hoyt CS. Surgical management of myokymia of the superior oblique muscle. Am J Ophthalmol 1992;114:693–696.

Duane A. Unilateral rotary nystagmus. Trans Am Ophthalmol Soc 1906;11:63–67.

Gittinger JW Jr. Homonymous hemianopia and disc pallor after severe head injury. Surv Ophthalmol 1984;28:333–338. Clinical conference.

Hoyt WF, Keane JR. Superior oblique myokymia. Arch Ophthalmol 1970;84:461–466.

Keltner JL. The monocular shimmers—your patient isn't deluded! Surv Ophthalmol 1983;27:313–316.

Kommerell G, Schaubel G. Superior oblique myokymia. An electromyographical analysis. Trans Ophthalmol Soc UK 1980;100:504–506.

Lee JP. Superior oblique myokymia. A possible etiologic factor. Arch Ophthalmol 1984;102:1178–1179.

Leigh RJ, Zee DS. The Neurology of Eye Movements. Philadelphia: FA Davis, 1991;329.

Morrow MJ, Sharpe JA, Ranalli PJ. Superior oblique myokymia associated with a posterior fossa tumor: oculographic correlation with an idiopathic case. Neurology 1990;40:367–370.

Neetens A, Martin JJ. Superior oblique myokymia in a case of adrenoleukodystrophy and in a case of lead intoxication. Neuro-Ophthalmol 1983; 3:103–108.

Palmer EA, Shults WT. Superior oblique myokymia: preliminary results of surgical treatment. J Pediatr Ophthalmol Strabismus 1984;21:96–101.

Parks MM, Eustis HS. Simultaneous superior oblique tenotomy and inferior oblique recession in Brown's syndrome. Ophthalmology 1987; 94:1043–1048.

Rall TW, Schleifer LS. Drugs Effective in the Therapy of Epilepsies. In AG Gilman, LS Goodman (eds), Goodman and Gilman's The Pharmacological Basis of Therapeutics (7th ed). New York: MacMillan, 1985;457–459.

Roper–Hall G, Burde RM. Superior oblique myokymia. Am Orthopt J 1978;28:58–63.

Rosenberg ML, Glaser JS. Superior oblique myokymia. Ann Neurol 1983;13:667–669.

Ruttum MS, Harris GJ. Superior oblique myectomy and trochlectomy in recurrent superior oblique myokymia. Graefes Arch Clin Exp Ophthalmol 1988;226:145–147.

Staudenmaier C. Superior oblique myokymia: when treatment is necessary. Can J Ophthalmol 1986;21:236–241.

Susac JO, Smith JL, Schatz NJ. Superior oblique myokymia. Arch Neurol 1973;29:432–434.

Tyler TD, Ruiz RS. Propranolol in the treatment of superior oblique myokymia [letter]. Arch Ophthalmol 1990;108:175–176.

von Noorden GK. Binocular Vision and Ocular Motility: Theory and Management of Strabismus (4th ed). St. Louis: Mosby, 1990;509–512.

IX

Management Techniques

29

Botulinum Neurotoxin

The application of botulinum neurotoxin for strabismus management was introduced by Alan Scott (Scott et al., 1973; Scott, 1980, 1981). Since its introduction, botulinum neurotoxin has been used for many different strabismus conditions, with variable results. Botulinum neurotoxin has been used in the management of sixth nerve palsy (Fitzsimons et al., 1988), for surgical overcorrections (Biglan et al., 1989), in the management of consecutive exotropia (Lee et al., 1988), for infantile strabismus (Magoon, 1984; Magoon and Scott, 1987), for strabismus following retinal detachment surgery (Scott, 1991), for thyroid myopathy (Scott, 1984; Dunn et al., 1986), and to dampen the oscillations in nystagmus (Helveston and Pogrebniak, 1988). In this chapter we discuss the pharmacology of botulinum neurotoxin, methods of administration of the toxin into extraocular muscles, and specific indications.

Botulinum neurotoxin is produced by *Clostridium botulinum*. Type A toxin is used in the management of strabismus. The toxin causes an irreversible blockade of cholinergic junctions at the motor endplate. The toxin's effect is to block the release of acetylcholine, thereby effectively denervating the muscle.

The onset of action after injection is 1–7 days (Magoon, 1985; Scott, 1981), and the duration of the effect is 6–9 months (Scott et al., 1973; Gammon, 1984). After the paralytic effects of botulinum toxin have worn off, permanent changes in ocular alignment may occur (Scott et al., 1973; Scott, 1981).

Most authorities choose to inject botulinum toxin directly into an extraocular muscle under electromyographic control (Figure 29.1). Using this technique, the surgeon receives an audible signal, which indicates that the needle has entered the extraocular muscle. Once this

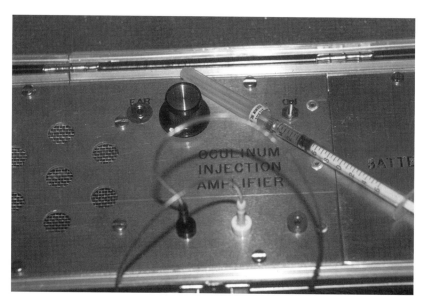

FIGURE 29.1   *An electromyographic machine like the one shown here is used for needle guidance. When the needle is in the muscle, a signal increases in intensity.*

signal has been achieved, the muscle can be injected with a predetermined number of units of botulinum neurotoxin.

The actual technique for inserting the needle into the muscle involves penetrating the conjunctiva and Tenon's fascia and passing the needle posteriorly into the belly of the extraocular muscle. In some cases, it may be useful to have the patient attempt to use the muscle, because this will increase the rate of firing and make it apparent when the needle is actually in the muscle.

The number of units chosen to inject may vary from 2 to as many as 15. Typically, a solution of sterile, nonpreserved saline is made so that the number of units desired is available in 0.1 ml of solution. In this manner, the surgeon can avoid having to inject a large bolus of fluid, which might extravasate into the surrounding tissue and paralyze other muscles.

A topical anesthetic agent is employed prior to inserting the needle. We have not found it necessary to administer subconjunctival anesthesia, and we have had very few problems with patients experiencing pain.

INDICATIONS

Sixth Nerve Palsy

Botulinum neurotoxin is widely used and, arguably, most successful in the management of sixth nerve palsy. In patients with acute sixth nerve palsy who are awaiting the possibility of actual recovery of the nerve, some binocular vision can be restored by injecting botulinum neurotoxin into the antagonistic muscle, the medial rectus muscle (Scott and Kraft, 1985; Scott, 1985; Wagner and Frohman, 1989). The injection may also help to prevent contracture of the medial rectus muscle, a problem that requires surgical treatment even when the lateral rectus muscle recovers.

The long-term effects on sixth nerve palsy are debated (Metz and Mazow, 1988; Lee et al., 1988). Certainly, patients receive short-term benefit if botulinum toxin is effective. On the other hand, the effects of the neurotoxin wear off after a number of months, and subsequent injections may be necessary if the sixth nerve palsy does not resolve. Evaluating sixth nerve palsy in patients is very important neurologically, and should not be delayed on account of botulinum neurotoxin treatment.

Esotropia

Infantile esotropia can also be managed with botulinum neurotoxin. Scott (1989) showed that approximately 37% of children can be satisfactorily aligned with botulinum neurotoxin alone after one injection. After a second injection, 63% of patients have good ocular alignment. The duration of satisfactory alignment (once it is achieved) is at least 2 years in 85% of this study group (Magoon, 1989). Unfortunately, the use of botulinum neurotoxin requires extremely good restraint, low-dose ketamine, or anesthetic inhalant. If a child has to have an anesthetic agent, botulinum therapy loses some of its advantage over surgery.

Graves' Myopathy

Botulinum neurotoxin has been proposed for use in Graves' myopathy, particularly in its early stages, and prior to the fibrotic stage. Lyons and colleagues (1990) showed that toxin can reduce the angle of deviation by an average of 75% when used early in the disease. However, the toxin's duration of action is typically about 2 months, at which point either the medicine has to be reinjected or the patient has to be subjected to an operation. Five of six patients in the study by Lyons and colleagues eventually needed surgery. Nevertheless, these authors accurately make the point that in the active stage of the disease, patients suffer very troublesome double vision and are not good candidates for surgery due to disease activity. The angle of misalignment can be reduced with botulinum toxin. Patients may have some restitution of binocular fields with the use of small amounts of Fresnel or other types of prisms.

Scott (1984) and Dunn and associates (1986) also studied the use of botulinum neurotoxin for thyroid myopathy. However, these authors found no trend toward improvement with the use of this medicine.

Surgical Undercorrections and Overcorrections

In some cases, patients undergoing surgery are inadvertently under- or overcorrected, even as much as 20–30 prism diopters. The best results in using botulinum toxin for this problem probably are achieved in adults who have small or medium amounts of horizontal misalignment. McNeer (1990) showed that consecutive esodeviations respond to botulinum better than consecutive exodeviations, presumably because patients with exodeviations are more likely to have had multiple previous operations on their lateral rectus muscles (Osako and Keltner, 1991). Patients who present either with primary large angles of strabismus or with the unusual circumstance of having a very large overcorrection typically will not respond very well or completely with botulinum neurotoxin. This is particularly true when the patient lacks fusion (Carruthers et al., 1990).

Strabismus After Retinal Detachment Surgery

Botulinum neurotoxin has been studied in patients with strabismus following retinal detachment surgery (Petitto and Buckley, 1991; Scott, 1990). Scott (1990) was successful in re-achieving fusion in primary gaze in 60% of patients. Toxin injection for this problem has been more disappointing in our hands, but we still prefer it as an alternative to surgery, because retinal redetachment (via removal of exoplant) is a risk during strabismus surgery.

Nystagmus

The use of botulinum neurotoxin for the treatment of nystagmus is discussed in Chapter 28.

COMPLICATIONS OF TREATMENT

Even when large doses of botulinum neurotoxin are injected into extraocular muscles, systemic side effects have not been reported. However, local side effects occur with some regularity. Ptosis may occur in 15–20% (Scott, 1989) of patients. Extravasation of the fluid containing the botulinum neurotoxin can lead to partial paralysis of other extraocular muscles and worsening of diplopia. The oblique muscles are most difficult to treat with botulinum. Injection of the superior rectus muscle is most likely to cause ptosis (Metz, 1984; Magoon, 1987). Therefore, injection of the inferior rectus muscle is advised for management of vertical strabismus (Osako and Keltner, 1991).

We have noted dry eyes, decreased lacrimation, and foreign body sensation in some of our patients. Pupillary dilatation can occur, as can diminished accommodation (Scott, 1989).

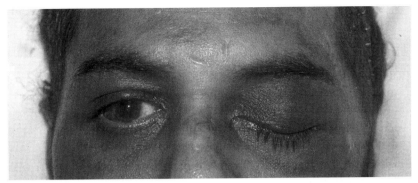

A

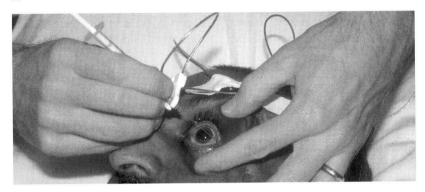

B

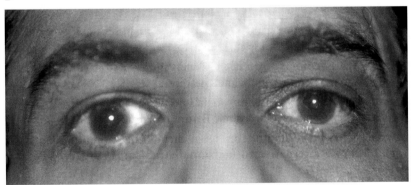

C

FIGURE 29.2 *A. This 40-year-old man suffered a traumatic left oculomotor nerve palsy. B. One month later his left lateral rectus muscle was injected in an attempt to prevent contracture of the muscle. C. One week after the injection his palsy resolved. He attributed this to the injection. This case highlights difficulties in evaluating the use of botulinum neurotoxin for paralytic strabismus. Some cases resolve spontaneously.*

Inadvertent injection of the medicine into the eye can occur (Scott, 1989), but probably does not have any neurotoxic effects on the retina (Wienkers et al., 1984). However, the hole in the retina could lead to subsequent retinal detachment (Figure 29.2).

REFERENCES

Biglan AW, Burnstine RA, Rogers GL, Saunders RA. Management of strabismus with botulinum A toxin. Ophthalmology 1989;96:935–943.

Carruthers JD, Kennedy RA, Bagaric D. Botulinum vs. adjustable suture surgery in the treatment of horizontal misalignment in adult patients lacking fusion. Arch Ophthalmol 1990;108:1432–1435.

Dunn WJ, Arnold AC, O'Connor PS. Botulinum toxin for the treatment of dysthyroid ocular myopathy. Ophthalmology 1986;93:470–475.

Fitzsimons R, Lee JP, Elston J. Treatment of sixth nerve palsy in adults with combined botulism toxin chemodenervation and surgery. Ophthalmology 1988;95:1535–1542.

Gammon JA, Gemmill M, Tigges J, Lerman S. Botulinum chemodenervation treatment of strabismus. J Pediatr Ophthalmol Strabismus 1985; 22:221–226.

Helveston EM, Pogrebniak AE. Treatment of acquired nystagmus with botulinum A toxin. Am J Ophthalmol 1988;106:584–586.

Lee J, Elston J, Vickers S et al. Botulinum toxin therapy for squint. Eye 1988;2:24–28.

Lyons CJ, Vickers SF, Lee JP. Botulinum toxin therapy in dysthyroid strabismus. Eye 1990;4:538–542.

Magoon EH. Chemodenervation of strabismic children. A 2- to 5-year follow-up study compared with shorter follow-up. Ophthalmology 1989;96:931–934.

Magoon EH. Botulinum chemodenervation for strabismus and other disorders. Int Ophthalmol Clin 1985;25:149–159.

Magoon EH. Botulinum toxin chemodenervation for strabismus in infants and children. J Pediatr Ophthalmol Strabismus 1984;21:110–113.

Magoon EH. The use of botulinum toxin injection as an alternative to strabismus surgery. Contemp Ophthalmic Forum 1987;5:222–229.

Magoon EH, Scott AB. Botulinum toxin chemodenervation in infants and children. An alternative to incisional strabismus surgery. J Pediatr 1987;110:719–722.

McNeer KW. An investigation of the clinical use of botulinum toxin A as a postoperative adjustment procedure in the therapy of strabismus. J Pediatr Ophthalmol Strabismus 1990;27:3–9.

Metz HS. Botulinum injections for strabismus. J Pediatr Ophthalmol Strabismus 1984;21:199–201.

Metz HS, Mazow M. Botulinum toxin treatment of acute sixth and third nerve palsy. Graefe's Arch Clin Exp Ophthalmol 1988;226:141–144.

Osako M, Keltner JL. Botulinum A toxin (Oculinum) in ophthalmology. Surv Ophthalmol 1991;36:28–46.

Petitto VB, Buckley EG. The use of botulinum toxin in strabismus surgery after retinal detachment surgery. Ophthalmology 1991;98:509–513.

Scott AB. Botulinum toxin injection into extraocular muscles as an alternative to strabismus surgery. Ophthalmology 1980;87:1044–1049.

Scott AB. Botulinum toxin injection of eye muscles to correct strabismus. Trans Am Ophthalmol Soc 1981;79:734–770.

Scott AB. Injection treatment of endocrine orbital myopathy. Doc Ophthalmol 1984;48:141–145.

Scott AB. Botulinum toxin treatment of strabismus. Am Orthopt J 1985;35:28–29.

Scott AB. Botulinum Toxin Treatment of Strabismus. Focal Points 1989: Clinical Modules for Ophthalmologists. San Francisco: American Academy of Ophthalmology, 1989;7:1–11.

Scott AB. Botulinum treatment of strabismus following retinal detachment surgery. Arch Ophthalmol 1990;108:509–510.

Scott AB. When considering oculinum (botulinum toxin type A) injection for the treatment of strabismus, can the surgeon anticipate different results in patients who have had previous strabismus surgery? Arch Ophthalmol 1991;109:1510.

Scott AB, Kraft SP. Botulinum toxin injection in the management of lateral rectus paresis. Ophthalmology 1985;92:676–683.

Scott AB, Magoon EH, McNeer KW, Stager DR. Botulinum treatment of strabismus in children. Trans Am Ophthalmol Soc 1989;87:174–184.

Scott AB, Rosenbaum A, Collins CC. Pharmacologic weakening of extraocular muscles. Invest Ophthalmol Vis Sci 1973;12:924–927.

Wagner RS, Frohman LP. Long-term results: botulinum for sixth nerve palsy. J Pediatr Ophthalmol Strabismus 1989;26:106–108.

Wienkers K, Helveston EM, Ellis FD, Cadera W. Botulinum toxin injection into rabbit vitreous. Ophthalmic Surg 1984;15:310–314.

30

Complications of Strabismus Surgery

Complications of strabismus surgery are uncommon, but their recognition is important. In this chapter we discuss the main side effects of strabismus surgery, many of which can be prevented through forethought and appropriate surgical technique. Other side effects result from surgical manipulation, including long-term ocular effects of anterior ischemia and potentially life-threatening cardiac vagal response to stimulation by manipulation of rectus muscles. The key is to prevent or manage expected complications and to be as prepared as possible for the unexpected.

MANAGEMENT OF THE LOST MUSCLE

Etiology
MacEwen and colleagues (1992) have grouped lost or detached rectus muscles into four categories, according to etiology. In the first group, muscles may be inadvertently cut during strabismus surgery. In the second group, a muscle can be accidentally snapped as the result of excess traction with a muscle hook. The third group involves a slipped muscle early in the postoperative period. This etiology has also been discussed in detail by Plager and Parks (1988, 1990). The fourth group involves patients in whom the muscle is damaged as the result of actual fascial or orbital trauma.

Unfortunately, patients in whom the muscle is inadvertently cut often experience this complication when most or all fascial attachments to the muscle have been deliberately surgically excised. The loss of these attachments may make it very difficult to retrieve the muscle. Plager and Parks (1990) noted that the medial rectus muscle was most difficult to retrieve due to its lack of attachments to oblique muscles. The medial rectus muscle also does not arc around the globe as much as the other rectus muscles, and tends to retract directly posteriorly into the orbit. This adds to the difficulty in finding it when it is lost.

Diagnosis

When an inferior rectus muscle is lost, the eye will rotate inferiorly only to approximately the horizontal position (Figure 30.1). Presumably, this is due to the ability of the superior oblique muscle to bring the eye down to this position, beyond which the inferior rectus must provide force on the globe. Similarly, a lost superior rectus results in an inability to elevate the eye at about the midposition (Figure 30.2). Again, the inferior oblique muscle presumably can elevate the eye to the midposition, but beyond this, the superior rectus must provide the elevating force. A lost lateral rectus will cause esotropia in primary gaze and a marked abduction deficit (Figure 30.3). Conversely, a lost medial rectus muscle causes a large-angle exotropia in primary gaze with great difficulty adducting the eye.

On the other hand, a *slipped* muscle will result in a mild to moderate deficit of eye movement in the field of gaze of the slipped muscle. Plager and Parks (1988) have commented on a useful finding that occurs with a slipped medical rectus muscle: The interpalpebral fissure may widen on attempted adduction.

Management

Perhaps the best form of management of lost extraocular muscles involves taking steps to prevent the complication. Plager and Parks (1988, 1990) advocate a full-thickness suture placed through the rectus muscle. In this way, the surgeon avoids inadvertently placing a superficial suture through the muscle capsule, which can then allow the muscle to slip and retract in the capsule after recession.

Wright (1990) recommended preserving posterior intermuscle septum ligaments, so that if the muscle is lost, it can be retrieved more easily. We would add to these recommendations that the surgeon place a suture through a suspected rectus muscle at the time of surgery, particularly in cases where previous operations have distorted the anatomy and made it difficult to successfully identify the extraocular muscle initially. If the muscle is inadvertently detached from the globe, the suture can be used to help pull it back into the operative field.

An excellent review of management issues in lost and slipped muscles is provided by MacEwen and associates (1992). The first issue

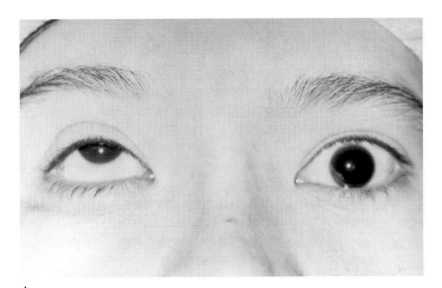

A

B

FIGURE 30.1 *A. This man underwent surgery in a country other than the United States, at which time his right inferior rectus muscle slipped off a hook and was lost. B. It was found in a subsequent operation and readvanced, resulting in a satisfactory outcome. Note that the eye rotates down to the midline, but not farther.*

involves the timing of searching for the lost muscle. Almost all authorities advocate looking for the lost muscle (if its loss is recognized at the time) during the same surgical setting. The fascial planes are more predictable and identifiable prior to the scarring response brought on by surgery. The likelihood of finding the muscle is greater if it is searched for as soon as feasible after it is lost.

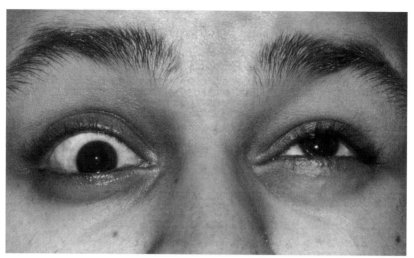

A

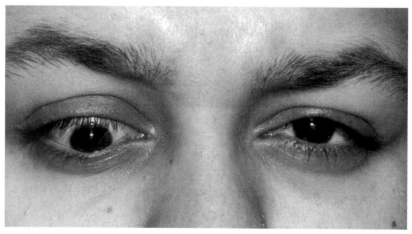

B

FIGURE 30.2 *With a lost superior rectus muscle, the eye rotates up to midposition, but not higher. A. Upgaze. B. Primary gaze. The right superior rectus muscle had been lost.*

The quest for the lost muscle involves indirect and direct examinations for muscle fibers. The surgeon may occasionally be able to take advantage of the oculovagal response induced by traction on a rectus muscle, using the slowing of the heart rate to confirm that the lost muscle has been located by pulling on it (Apt and Isenberg, 1980). We also occasionally find it helpful to note a bradycardic response when muscle fibers are placed on traction. For that reason, the anesthesiologist should be advised to terminate the use of anticholinergic agents or to avoid them at the outset of surgery.

A skilled assistant is invaluable. Skilled hands help prevent the mismanagement and resulting obscuring of fascial planes. The operat-

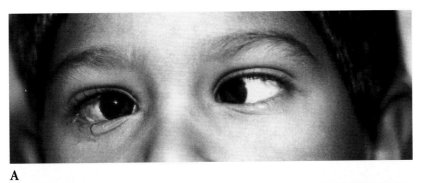

A

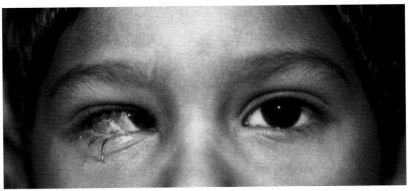

B

C

FIGURE 30.3 *When the lateral rectus muscle is lost, a large-angle esotropia occurs with abduction deficit. The right lateral rectus muscle was lost. In gaze right (A), the right eye only goes to midline. In primary and left gaze (B and C), the medial rectus rotates the right eye.*

ing microscope is occasionally helpful in identifying and retrieving lost muscles.

Surgeons should note, as pointed out earlier, that the medial rectus muscle tends to follow a course directly posteriorly and does not arc back along the course of the globe. Failure to take note of this fact could result in inadvertent damage to the optic nerve on the medial aspect of the retracted globe.

Ideally, the muscle can be found and reattached at the desired location. If the muscle cannot be found, then fascia adjacent to the muscle can be brought anteriorly and sutured to the globe in a manner and location based on forced duction and spring-back examinations. The surgeon may choose to recess the antagonist muscle. We agree with MacEwen and colleagues (1992) that additional transposition of extraocular muscles at the initial exploration for a lost muscle is probably ill advised. Any decision to modify the strabismus further can be based on postoperative motility examinations.

SCLERAL PERFORATION DURING EYE MUSCLE SURGERY

Etiology

Due to the thinness of the sclera and the fact that extraocular muscles must be reattached to it after recession or resection, scleral perforations caused by the suture needle can occur. Past studies of scleral perforations have placed the incidence at 9% to 12% (Gottlieb and Castro, 1970; Rojas et al., 1979; Kaluzny et al., 1977). Faden sutures may be prone to result in scleral perforations and, due to their more posterior location, more likely to lead to retinal detachment (Alio and Faci, 1984). Recently, a survey of members of the American Association for Pediatric Ophthalmology and Strabismus indicated that *recognized* scleral perforations occurred in 0.13% of cases of eye muscle surgery performed by the reporting surgeons. Patients for which residents or fellows were the primary surgeon were more likely to suffer this complication than when attending surgeons performed the procedures (Simon et al., 1992). Scleral perforation was most likely to occur during placement of the scleral suture; however, scleral perforation also occurred during disinsertion of the operated muscle, dissection of the operated muscle, passage of a traction suture (for example, underneath the lateral rectus muscle), and during preplacement of a muscle suture.

Of patients in this study, 99% suffered no vision loss. However, 14 patients out of a total of 728 (0.02%) cases of scleral perforation had a retinal detachment, and eight of these resolved without complications.

Endophthalmitis after strabismus surgery is presumably related to suture placement. Estimates of the incidence of endophthalmitis range from 1 in 3,500 (Knobloch and Lorenz, 1962) to 1 in 8,000 (Weinstein et al., 1979). In the national survey (Simon et al., 1992), the incidence of endophthalmitis was only 1 in every 185,000 operated cases.

Other complications associated with scleral perforation include lens dislocation (Hittner, 1979), phthisis bulbi (Apple et al., 1985), and vitreous hemorrhage (Greenberg et al., 1988). We have also noted a small hyphema associated with a limbal scleral traction suture.

Management

Perhaps the best form of management is prevention. The use of a "hang-back" technique for passage of scleral sutures may be advisable, particularly in the setting of surgery performed by residents or fellows. The inexperienced surgeon is less likely to create a retinal hole in an area where a retinal detachment could result. Exposure and visualization are of obvious importance, and again may be especially important when residents and fellows are operating (Simon et al., 1992).

In the setting of a recognized scleral perforation, pupillary dilatation is advisable. The role of retinal cryopexy has been debated (Mittelman and Bakos, 1984). We would prefer to leave retinal perforations in the area of the vitreous base alone. However, a more posterior perforation might be more likely to cause a retinal detachment. In this scenario, consultation with a retinal surgeon is advisable.

CONJUNCTIVAL REACTION TO STRABISMUS SURGERY

Conjunctival reactions to strabismus surgery can take one of three forms: irritation indicated by hyperemia, conjunctival granuloma, and inclusion cyst (Figure 30.4). The first two types of reactions probably represent inflammatory responses to suture material and surgery. The last reaction, epithelial inclusion cyst, may occur in the setting of conjunctival surgery of any variety, and therefore is not necessarily related to the suture per se.

Inflammation caused by suture material is relatively common. In fact, in order for Vicryl suture to be absorbed and degraded, it must attract blood vessels and accompanying inflammatory cells. Therefore, some degree of local irritation is to be expected.

On the other hand, granulomas are uncommon with modern strabismus surgery, perhaps due to the fact that Vicryl suture material is coated with polyglactin, a substance that is relatively inert. Suture granulomas have the appearance of a bump, usually at the anterior edge of the Vicryl suture material. The bump can be elevated and can cause considerable discomfort.

Cysts are presumably caused by inclusion of epithelial lining cells underneath the surface during closure of the conjunctiva. A cyst can be virtually any size, but large ones may be fluid filled, unsightly, and

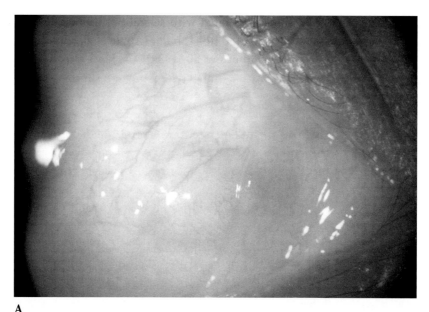

A

B

FIGURE 30.4   *A. This patient developed a conjunctival cyst over the right medial rectus after recession with a Vicryl suture. B. This patient has a granuloma in the region of the right lateral rectus, also after Vicryl suture. Note the granuloma's more solid and inflamed appearance.*

uncomfortable. In contrast to inflammatory conjunctival reactions, epithelial cysts do not appear inflamed.

Management

The management of local irritation or conjunctival granulomas is usually nonsurgical. Most cases of conjunctival reaction are self-limited and resolve with time. Occasionally, the use of topical steroids, in either ointment or drops, may be indicated and helpful. A slow tapering of steroids once the granuloma has resolved is indicated.

Dellen Management

Rarely will local conjunctival swelling, a cyst, or a granuloma lead to dellen formation in the area of sclera or cornea most proximal to the swelling. The dellen has all of the characteristics of dellen seen in other settings. Its management consists of vigorous lubrication. Prophylaxis against infection may be indicated in some cases and can be provided in the form of antibiotic ointment. Efforts at reducing the conjunctival swelling responsible for the dellen are also advisable.

FAT ADHERENCE

Etiology

Syndromes of fat adherence are discussed in Chapter 22. An inadvertent incision through the extraocular muscle cone, posterior to the equator of the globe, can lead to fat exposure. In most cases, fat exposure goes unnoticed and is considered when restrictive strabismus develops. In some cases, fat exposure can be pronounced and cosmetically unsatisfactory. This occurs particularly with incisions in the inferior temporal quadrant of the eye during inferior oblique weakening surgery and in the superonasal quadrant of the eye during superior oblique surgery.

Management

Once again, the best form of management for this type of complication is to avoid it in the first place. So-called stripping of the extraocular muscles with cotton-tipped applicators probably increases the risk of fat adherence syndrome. An understanding of the anatomy of the eye and its fat compartments is also important. Posterior incisions are likely to result in extrusion of fat, and so should be avoided.

When fat exposure has occurred, it can be dissected free of its conjunctival attachments, but with great care. The fat can be removed and the conjunctiva sutured back approximately in its original position.

BLEEDING

The amount of bleeding that occurs in strabismus surgery is usually trivial. Even in patients who are anticoagulated, bleeding can be easily controlled with cauterization. Rarely will patients with hemophilia require strabismus surgery, and in this scenario it is best to admit the patient, provide the patient with factor replacement, and monitor the patient in the hospital postoperatively for several days. At least in the setting of hemophilia, we have encountered unexpected and prolonged bleeding with the simple procedure of nasolacrimal duct probing.

On the other hand, severance of one of the vortex veins can lead to a large amount of bleeding and potentially result in fibrofatty (scarring) proliferation (adherence syndrome). The vortex veins vary from individual to individual. As a rule, there are vortex veins in the superonasal, superotemporal, inferonasal, and inferotemporal quadrants. These vortex veins are located between 6 and 8 mm posterior to the equator of the globe. The superior vortex veins are located more posteriorly than the inferior vortex veins.

Inferior oblique surgery runs the potential risk of damaging the inferotemporal vortex vein. Similarly, superior oblique surgery runs the risk of damaging the superonasal vortex vein.

Management

If the vein is inadvertently cut, hemostasis can usually be achieved simply by applying pressure. Every effort should be made to achieve hemostasis promptly, because prolonged and excessive bleeding can lead to a scarring response, which in turn can aggravate the very strabismus for which the patient is undergoing surgery.

SUTURE ABSCESS

Fortunately, suture abscesses rarely occur. When they do occur, they are noted in the first few days or week after strabismus surgery. The danger of the suture abscess is that it can lead to erosion of the underlying sclera and potential endophthalmitis.

Diagnosis

Suture abscess should be distinguished from suture granuloma and epithelial cysts. The suture abscess is more liquid, occurs in the immediate postoperative period, and, on close inspection, resembles a collection of exudate. On the other hand, granulomas usually occur several weeks after surgery, are solid appearing, and usually are not liquified at all.

Management

Suture abscesses should be managed with cultures to identify the causative organism and with intensive antibiotic coverage. The patient should be examined on a daily basis until the abscess starts to regress. A careful fundus examination is indicated to ensure that the infection is not penetrating the globe itself. In some cases, the suture should be removed to eliminate the nidus of infection.

CELLULITIS

Cellulitis is more common than endophthalmitis, although estimates of the incidence of cellulitis are hard to come by. Presumably, infections are introduced into the operative field at the time of surgery. Occasionally, an occult or unrecognized nasolacrimal duct obstruction can contribute. All children with planned ocular surgery should be examined for the possibility of nasolacrimal duct obstruction (Good et al., 1990).

Diagnosis

Infection may be difficult to distinguish from postoperative edema (caused by surgical trauma) or even allergy. Infectious disease is suggested by upper and lower eyelid edema, diffuse chemosis, pain, an elevated white blood cell count, and exudate.

Management

The suspicion of infectious disease should be an indication for prompt management. Cultures of a conjunctival smear should be obtained. A white blood cell count should be determined. The patient should be aggressively treated with systemic antibiotics. In some cases where the infection has been caught early, oral antibiotics may suffice. In many cases, an intravenous course of antibiotics is indicated. The choice of antibiotics should be dictated by the suspected pathogen. In our experience, gram-positive organisms are likely to be the cause.

ANTERIOR SEGMENT ISCHEMIA

Etiology

Anterior segment ischemia is a rare complication of surgery and may develop in 1 of 13,000 patients who undergo strabismus surgery (France and Simon, 1986). The anterior ciliary arteries that supply the anterior segment of the eye course through the rectus muscles. Although there is some individual variation, most humans have two

TABLE 30.1   Risk factors for anterior segment ischemia

Three or more rectus muscles operated simultaneously
Older age
Contiguous rectus muscle surgery
Transposition procedure
Previous buckle for retinal detachment
Abnormal extraocular muscles
Previous local radiation therapy
Graves' myopathy

ciliary arteries in each rectus muscle, with the exception of the lateral rectus, which usually has one ciliary artery running in it. An episcleral blood supply, not necessarily linked to anterior ciliary arteries, exists in primates (Morrison and VanBuskirk, 1983), but its existence in humans is debated (Saunders and Phillips, 1988). The potential for its existence has led Guyton to propose that fornix conjunctival incisions may be less compromising than limbal incisions (Guyton, personal communication, cited in Saunders and Phillips, 1988).

It is not possible to predict the development of anterior segment ischemia entirely, but certain risk factors are apparent (Table 30.1).

With increasing numbers of muscles operated on, the risk for ischemia also increases (Saunders and Phillips, 1988; France and Simon, 1986; Simon et al., 1984). The vertical rectus muscles are particularly important in bringing blood to the anterior segment (Olver and Lee, 1992). Anterior ischemia is probably more likely when three rectus muscles are operated on at the same time, especially if two are vertical muscles. Nevertheless, anterior segment ischemia has been reported after recession of two muscles, and even one (Fells and Marsh, 1978; Saunders and Sandall, 1982). Operating on contiguous muscles (e.g., medial and inferior rectus muscles) may also increase the chances of ischemia (Wilcox et al., 1981). Transposition procedures may also cause anterior segment ischemia (von Noorden, 1976). Combining vertical rectus transposition with a medial rectus recession can cause ischemia. Even injection of the medial rectus muscle with botulinum neurotoxin does not necessarily avert ischemia when combined with a vertical rectus muscle transposition (Keech et al., 1991).

Older patients are probably more vulnerable to postoperative ischemia, but younger patients may also be affected (France and Simon, 1986). Other risk factors for ischemia include absent (agenesis) rectus muscles (Wong and Jampolsky, 1974) and a previous buckling procedure for retinal detachment (Robertson, 1975). Thyroid myopathy could predispose to necrotizing scleritis, which may be similar to anterior ischemia in pathogenesis (Kaufman et al., 1989).

Diagnosis

Anterior segment ischemia begins shortly after surgery and occurs along a continuum from mild to severe. Corneal edema, uveitis, corectopia, cataract, and atonic pupil can occur (Forbes, 1959; Girard and Beltranena, 1960; Helveston, 1971). The clinical course may be prolonged, but the survey reported by France and Simon (1986) shows that most patients recover without significant vision loss.

Management

Surgical planning should take into consideration the risk factors for ischemia (see Table 30.1). Operating on two muscles is safe, except in unusual cases of congenital fibrosis syndrome (Wong and Jampolsky, 1974). After two-muscle surgery in one eye, waiting to operate on a third muscle is advisable. Even so, iris-filling defects may last 6 months or longer after disruption of anterior ciliary blood supply (Hayreh and Scott, 1978). Therefore, staged surgery is no guarantee that ischemia will be avoided. Tendon-splitting procedures may spare part of the ciliary blood supply, but ischemia still can occur (von Noorden, 1976).

Treatment for ischemia can include topical steroids. Hyperbaric oxygen may prove useful (De Smet et al., 1987) but requires further investigation. In many cases, patiently waiting for symptoms to subside is the mainstay of treatment.

ANESTHETIC COMPLICATIONS

Although anesthetic complications are usually outside the purview of the ophthalmologist, a working relationship with the anesthesiologist is paramount, because anesthetic interventions may affect the strabismus operation in important ways.

Laryngeal masks are preferred over endotracheal intubation in some centers. Laryngeal masks are usually well tolerated but occasionally dislodge (Bogetz et al., 1995). The surgeon is closest to the patient's airway and may be the first to notice mask dislocation.

Traction on extraocular muscles can cause a vagal response. In our center, most patients are not atropinized in advance, but if profound bradycardia or a hypotensive effect is noted with strabismus surgery, the patient should receive an anticholinergic agent. The surgeon should notify the anesthesiologist before pulling on a rectus muscle.

Nausea and vomiting occur commonly after strabismus surgery. To some extent, this complication can be prevented with perioperative management with antiemetic agents (e.g., droperidol). Nevertheless, some patients will have problems with emesis when they awaken from anesthetic. Ideally, this can be recognized in the recovery room before the patient is discharged home.

REFERENCES

Alio JL, Faci A. Fundus changes following Faden operation. Arch Ophthalmol 1984;102:211–213.

Apple DJ, Jones GR, Reidy JJ, Loftfield K. Ocular perforation and phthisis bulbi secondary to strabismus surgery. J Pediatr Ophthalmol Strabismus 1985;22:184–187.

Apt L, Isenberg SJ. The oculocardiac reflex as a surgical aid in identifying a slipped or "lost" extraocular muscle. Br J Ophthalmol 1980;64:362–365.

Bogetz M, Good WV, Hoyt CS, Way LR. Laryngeal mask for pediatric ophthalmology outpatient procedures. Presented at the American Association of Pediatric Ophthalmology and Strabismus, Orlando, FL, 1995.

De Smet MD, Carruthers J, Lepawsky M. Anterior segment ischemia treated with hyperbaric oxygen. Can J Ophthalmol 1987;22:381–383.

Fells P, Marsh RJ. Anterior Segment Ischemia Following Surgery on Two Rectus Muscles. In RD Reinecke (ed), Strabismus: Proceedings of the Third Meeting of the International Strabismological Association, May 10–12, 1978, Kyoto, Japan. New York: Grune & Stratton, 1978;375–380.

Forbes SB. Muscle transplantation for external rectus paralysis: report of case with unusual complications. Am J Ophthalmol 1959;48:248–251.

France TD, Simon JW. Anterior segment ischemia syndrome following muscle surgery: the AAPO&S experience. J Pediatr Ophthalmol Strabismus 1986;23:87–91.

Girard LJ, Beltranena F. Early and late complications of extensive muscle surgery. Arch Ophthalmol 1960;64:576–584.

Good WV, Taylor DSI, Hoyt CS et al. Postoperative endophthalmitis in children. J Pediatr Ophthalmol Strabismus 1990;27:383–385.

Gottlieb F, Castro JL. Perforation of the globe during strabismus surgery. Arch Ophthalmol 1970;84:151–157.

Greenberg DR, Ellenhorn NL, Chapman LI et al. Posterior chamber hemorrhage during strabismus surgery. Am J Ophthalmol 1988;106:534–535.

Hayreh SS, Scott WE. Fluorescein iris angiography. I. Normal pattern. Arch Ophthalmol 1978;96:1383–1389.

Helveston EM. Muscle transposition procedures. Surv Ophthalmol 1971;16:92–97.

Hittner HM. Lens dislocation after strabismus surgery. Ann Ophthalmol 1979;11:1115–1119.

Kaluzny J, Ralcewicz H, Perlikiewicz-Kikielowa A. Eye fundus periphery after operation for squint. Klin Oczna 1977;47:557–558.

Kaufman LM, Folk ER, Miller MT, Tessler HH. Necrotizing scleritis following strabismus surgery for thyroid ophthalmopathy. J Pediatr Ophthalmol Strabismus1989;26:236–238.

Keech RV. Superior oblique adjustable suture surgery. A rabbit model. Arch Ophthalmol 1991;109:1152–1154.

Knobloch R, Lorenz A. Uber ernste komplikationen nach schielopraetionen. Klin Monatsbl Augenheilkd 1962;141:344–353.

MacEwen CJ, Lee JP, Fells P. Aetiology and management of the "detached" rectus muscle. Br J Ophthalmol 1992;76:131–136.

Mittelman D, Bakos IM. The role of retinal cryopexy in the management of experimental perforation of the eye during strabismus surgery. J Pediatr Ophthalmol Strabismus 1984;21:186–189.

Morrison JC, VanBuskirk EM. Anterior collateral circulation in the primate eye. Ophthalmology 1983;90:707–715.

Olver JM, Lee JP. Recovery of anterior segment circulation after strabismus surgery in adult patients. Ophthalmology 1992;99:305–315.

Plager DA, Parks MM. Recognition and repair of the "lost" rectus muscle. A report of 25 cases. Ophthalmology 1990;97:131–137.

Plager DA, Parks MM. Recognition and repair of the "slipped" rectus muscle. J Ped Ophthalmol Strabismus 1988;25:270–274.

Robertson DM. Anterior segment ischemia after segmental episcleral buckling and cryopexy. Am J Ophthalmol 1975;78:871–874.

Rojas B, Vargas A, Riveros M. Retinal periphery after strabismus surgery. Arch Chil Oftalmol 1979;36:119–121.

Saunders RA, Phillips MS. Anterior segment ischemia after three rectus muscle surgery. Ophthalmology 1988;95:533–537.

Saunders RA, Sandall GS. Anterior segment ischemia syndrome following rectus muscle transposition. Am J Ophthalmol 1982;93:34–38.

Simon JW, Lininger LL, Scherage JL. Recognized scleral perforation during eye muscle surgery: incidence and sequelae. J Pediatr Ophthalmol Strabismus 1992;29:273–275.

Simon JW, Price EC, Krohel GB et al. Anterior segment ischemia following strabismus surgery. J Pediatr Ophthalmol Strabismus 1984;21:179–185.

von Noorden GK. Anterior segment ischemia following the Jensen procedure. Arch Ophthalmol 1976;94:845–847.

Weinstein GS, Mondino BJ, Weinberg RJ, Biglan AW. Endophthalmitis in a pediatric population. Ann Ophthalmol 1979;11:935–943.

Wilcox LM Jr, Gittinger JW Jr, Breinin GM. Congenital adduction palsy and synergistic divergences. Am J Ophthalmol 1981;91:1–7.

Wong GY, Jampolsky A. Agenesis of three horizontal rectus muscles. Ann Ophthalmol 1974;6:909–915.

Wright KW. Discussion on recognition and repair of the lost rectus muscle. Ophthalmology 1990;97:136–137.

Index

In this index, the letter "(t)" after a page number represents a table and "(f)" represents a figure.